369 0051829

DATE DUE

D1613354

Atlas of Procedures in GYNECOLOGIC ONCOLOGY

Douglas A Levine
Gynecology Service, Department of Surgery
Memorial Sloan-Kettering Cancer Center
New York, New York

Richard R Barakat
Chief
Gynecology Service, Department of Surgery
Memorial Sloan-Kettering Cancer Center
New York, New York

William J Hoskins
Director
Curtis and Elizabeth Anderson Cancer Institute
Memorial Health University Medical Center
Savannah, Georgia

MEMORIAL SLOAN-KETTERING CANCER CENTER

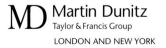
Martin Dunitz
Taylor & Francis Group
LONDON AND NEW YORK

First published in the United Kingdom in 2003
by Martin Dunitz, Taylor & Francis Group plc, 11 New Fetter Lane,
London EC4P 4EE

Tel.: 44 (0) 20 7583 9855
Fax.: +44 (0) 20 7842 2298
E-mail: info.dunitz@tandf.co.uk
Website: http://www.dunitz.co.uk

Although every effort has been made to ensure that drug doses and
other information are presented accurately in this publication, the
ultimate responsibility rests with the prescribing physician. Neither
the publishers nor the authors can be held responsible for errors or
for any consequences arising from the use of information contained
herein. For detailed prescribing information or instructions on the use
of any product or procedure discussed herein, please consult the
prescribing information or instructional material issued by the
manufacturer.

A CIP record for this book is available from the British Library.

ISBN (DVD: NTSC version) 1 84184 196 X
       (DVD: PAL version) 1 84184 372 5

Distributed in the USA by
Fulfilment Center
Taylor & Francis
10650 Tobben Drive
Independence, KY 41051, USA
Toll Free Tel.: +1 800 634 7064
E-mail: taylorandfrancis@thomsonlearning.cmo

Distributed in Canada by
Taylor & Francis
74 Rolark Drive
Scarborough, Ontario M1R 4G2, Canada
Toll Free Tel.: +1 877 226 2237
E-mail: tal_fran@istar.ca

Distributed in the rest of the world by
Thomson Publishing Services Limited
Cheriton House
North Way
Andover, Hampshire SP10 5BE, UK
Tel.: +44 (0)1264 332424
E-mail: salesorder.tandf@thomsonpublishingservices.co.uk

Composition by Scribe Design, Gillingham, Kent
Printed and bound in Spain by Grafos SA

Contents

For Yasemin, Cathy and Iffath

Contributors

Nadeem R Abu-Rustum
Gynecology Service, Department of Surgery
Memorial Sloan-Kettering Cancer Center
New York, New York

Kaled M Alektiar
Department of Radiation Oncology
Memorial Sloan-Kettering Cancer Center
New York, New York

Christopher S Awtrey
Gynecology Service, Department of Surgery
Memorial Sloan-Kettering Cancer Center
New York, New York

Richard R Barakat
Gynecology Service, Department of Surgery
Memorial Sloan-Kettering Cancer Center
New York, New York

Bernard H Bochner
Department of Urology
Memorial Sloan-Kettering Cancer Center
New York, New York

Carol L Brown
Gynecology Service, Department of Surgery
Memorial Sloan-Kettering Cancer Center
New York, New York

Dennis S Chi
Gynecology Service, Department of Surgery
Memorial Sloan-Kettering Cancer Center
New York, New York

Anne M Covey
Department of Radiology
Memorial Sloan-Kettering Cancer Center
New York, New York

Mary L Gemignani
Breast and Gynecology Services, Department of
Surgery
Memorial Sloan-Kettering Cancer Center
New York, New York

George I Getrajdman
Department of Radiology
Memorial Sloan-Kettering Cancer Center
New York, New York

William J Hoskins
Curtis and Elizabeth Anderson Cancer Institute
Memorial Health University Medical Center
Savannah, Georgia

Robert J Korst
Cardiothoracic Surgery and Genetic Medicine
Weill Medical College of Cornell University
New York

Eric Leblanc
Departement de Oncologie Gynécologique
Centre Oscar Lambret
Lille, France

Mario M Leitao Jr
Gynecology Service, Department of Surgery
Memorial Sloan-Kettering Cancer Center
New York, New York

Douglas A Levine
Gynecology Service, Department of Surgery
Memorial Sloan-Kettering Cancer Center
New York, New York

Michelle Montemarano
Gynecology Service, Department of Surgery
Memorial Sloan-Kettering Cancer Center
New York, New York

Marie Plante
Gynéco-Oncologie
Center Hospitalier Universitaire de Québec (CHUQ)
L'Hôtel-Dieu de Québec
Laval University
Québec City, Québec, Canada

Bhavana Pothuri
Gynecology Service, Department of Surgery
Memorial Sloan-Kettering Cancer Center
New York, New York

Elizabeth A Poynor
Gynecology Service, Department of Surgery
Memorial Sloan-Kettering Cancer Center
New York, New York

Denis Querleu
Department of Surgery
Institut Claudius Regand
Toulouse, France

Marie-Claude Renaud
Gynéco-Oncologie
Center Hospitalier Universitaire de Québec (CHUQ)
L'Hôtel-Dieu de Québec
Laval University
Québec City, Québec, Canada

Michel Roy
Gynéco-Oncologie
Center Hospitalier Universitaire de Québec (CHUQ)
L'Hôtel-Dieu de Québec
Laval University
Québec City, Québec, Canada

Mark A Schattner
Gastroenterology and Nutrition Service
Department of Medicine
Memorial Sloan-Kettering Cancer Center
New York, New York

Moshe Shike
Gastroenterology and Nutrition Service
Department of Medicine
Memorial Sloan-Kettering Cancer Center
New York, New York

Sang E Sim
Department of Radiation Oncology
Englewood Hospital and Medical Center
Englewood, New Jersey

Yukio Sonoda
Gynecology Service, Department of Surgery
Memorial Sloan-Kettering Cancer Center
New York, New York

Preface

This atlas has been designed for the purpose of providing a detailed overview of the major procedures performed by gynecologic oncologists, using full color photographs, and is accompanied by a DVD of live surgical footage with spoken commentary. Creating the basis of this text exclusively from color images of actual surgical procedures offers the reader a vantage point similar to that seen by the operating surgeon. Owing to the sophisticated computer technology that is currently on hand, all the photographs were captured on digital film and digital videotape. We have made great effort, except where absolutely necessary, to preclude the use of sketches or black-and-white photographs throughout *Atlas of Procedures in Gynecologic Oncology*.

This book should be valuable for those beginning their surgical training, as well as for senior practitioners. For the medical student and house officer, it will provide an introduction to basic gynecologic oncology procedures such as surgical staging, vulvar surgery, radical hysterectomy, and others. There are also sections on paracentesis, chest tube placement and central venous access. For the fellow in training, procedures, such as laparoscopic lymph node dissection, intraoperative radiation therapy, inguino-femoral lymphadenectomy, and others, will be indispensable when acting as the first assistant. For the senior surgeon, the text will introduce new technologies and advanced minimally invasive procedures that are not part of the usual surgical armamentarium. Procedures such as laparoscopic radical hysterectomy, sentinel lymph node biopsy, radical vaginal trachelectomy, and others are not typically taught during normal subspecialty training. All these procedures are illustrated in such detail that any surgeon can appreciate the adaptation of currently practiced surgical procedures to the minimally invasive approach, which may be readily learned from selected specialists in the field.

The chapters in *Atlas of Procedures in Gynecologic Oncology* are purposely presented in great detail, giving the reader a complete working knowledge of each procedure. While we would be amiss in believing that one could actually perform a new procedure simply by reviewing this text, with proper instruction the procedure should be readily grasped. Expertise in a particular procedure can be acquired more quickly on account of having a detailed knowledge of the procedure prior to performing it or observing it for the very first time. When one studies procedures in gynecologic oncology without the benefit of detailed operative color photographs, it can be quite surprising to see how different a real surgical procedure is from that depicted in sketches and diagrams; through the use of actual color photographs, the representations within this *Atlas* should approximate what is actually seen in the operating room.

Over one hour of actual surgical footage is included on an accompanying DVD with spoken commentary. The reader is able to review a procedure with full color photographs and then view selected procedures on video. The combination of photographs, written text, surgical footage, and spoken commentary is one of the most realistic approaches to understanding a complex surgical procedure without actually scrubbing into the case. Indeed, in some respects the material contained within may serve better to illustrate the procedures than actually being in the operating room as an observer: here, the reader will see the major portions of procedures without the surgical staff or the surgical drapes obstructing the view.

We have attempted to present all major procedures in our specialty. Some of the less frequently performed procedures are not illustrated owing to the lack of material or space within the text. Subsequent editions of this *Atlas* will replace some operations with new procedures and will expand as our specialty expands. Hopefully, we will have the opinions of our readers to allow each edition to be a better reference work than the preceding one. In addition to the commonly performed major procedures, we have also illustrated many advanced procedures currently performed only at specialized centers throughout the world. These procedures are likely to be practiced on a more widespread basis as physicians become sufficiently trained in minimally invasive surgery. We have tried to highlight important technical points for each step of the procedures in order to steer the reader away from potential complications.

The text here is limited to procedural descriptions and succinct introductory paragraphs explaining general indications without a comprehensive review of the literature. A discourse on the management of gynecologic malignancies is certainly readily available in many other well-written texts. This text is strictly focused on procedures, as will become apparent to the reader. We have attempted to design a high-quality, comprehensive *Atlas* and hope that the reader appreciates its distinctiveness and merit.

Douglas A Levine
Richard R Barakat
William J Hoskins

Acknowledgments

The editors are grateful to Martin Dunitz, Robert Peden, Abigail Griffin, David Hearn and Alison Campbell at Martin Dunitz Publishers in London for their help and patience throughout the development of this book. We would also like to thank the editorial staff at Memorial Sloan-Kettering Cancer Center, including George Monemvasitis, who served as lead copy-editor, and his colleagues Denise Buckley and Alexandra McDonald for their dedication and organizational skills. Our medical photographers, Richard DeWitt and Ethan Kavet, were invaluable to this project as was our technical consultant, Juan Rodriguez. The video department was very effective in obtaining operating room footage of open procedures, and includes Sam Palmucci and Richard Gontarek. We are grateful to our contributors who have provided not only their surgical expertise but also their patients and operating time to allow us to photograph ongoing procedures without sacrificing the highest level of performance during the diagnosis and treatment of cancer and allied diseases.

1 Laparotomy staging procedures

Bhavana Pothuri and Elizabeth A Poynor

Thorough surgical staging is the hallmark of treatment for early-stage endometrial and ovarian cancers. Comprehensive staging determines surgical stage and is important in guiding adjuvant chemotherapy or radiation therapy for patients with endometrial or ovarian cancer. In 1988, surgical staging replaced clinical staging for endometrial cancer due to significant under-reporting of disseminated tumor that was inherent in the former staging system. The current surgical staging system allows more accurate reporting of tumor distribution and better guidelines for additional therapy. Likewise, comprehensive staging is critical in early-stage ovarian cancer, since certain patients may not require further therapy following surgery. For patients with advanced ovarian cancer, surgical cytoreduction with tumor debulking is the standard of care and is discussed in detail elsewhere within this text. Surgical staging is usually not applicable due to the advanced nature of the disease; however, some gynecologic oncologists perform a complete lymph node dissection to ensure resection of all bulky tumor.

The standard procedure for surgical staging in early-stage ovarian carcinoma includes an adequate midline vertical incision, peritoneal washings, thorough exploration of the abdominal and pelvic cavities, biopsy of any suspicious lesions, random peritoneal biopsies, bilateral diaphragm sampling, total abdominal hysterectomy, bilateral salpingo-oophorectomy, bilateral pelvic and paraaortic lymph node dissection, and infracolic omentectomy. When performing the aortic lymph node dissection, it is important to remember that the lymphatic drainage pattern of the ovary follows that of the ovarian vein, which empties into the vena cava on the right and the renal vein on the left. Thus, these high aortic nodes should be removed in order to determine the extent of disease accurately and often a generous incision is required. If a tumor of mucinous histology is suspected or noted on frozen section, an appendectomy should also be performed. Many mucinous ovarian tumors may be metastases from the appendix or other gastrointestinal organs.

In endometrial carcinoma, surgical staging is nearly identical to the ovarian cancer staging procedure and for this reason they are presented together in this chapter. It includes a midline vertical incision, peritoneal washings, a thorough exploration of the abdomen and pelvis, a total abdominal hysterectomy, bilateral salpingo-oophorectomy, and pelvic and paraaortic lymph node dissection. Certain practitioners may elect to eliminate the nodal dissection for patients with minimally invasive tumors of favorable histologic grade and subtype due to the relatively low incidence of metastases. In general, this should be avoided due to the inaccuracies of frozen-section evaluation of depth of invasion and sampling errors of endometrial biopsies that may misrepresent final histologic grade or subtype. The risk of lymph node metastases in minimally invasive, low-grade endometrial tumors is approximately 3%, and the benefits of detecting metastases in these patients would outweigh the risks of the procedure. In certain individuals, such as those with significant medical co-morbidities, eliminating the lymph node dissection may be warranted. Ultimately, the risks of lymph node sampling for an individual patient must be balanced against the risks of spread based upon depth of invasion and tumor aggressiveness. If the endometrial tumor is predominantly serous or carcinosarcomatous, the aggressive nature of these tumors warrants additional staging procedures, including random peritoneal biopsies, subtotal omentectomy and lymph node dissection, regardless of the depth of invasion.

Abdominal exploration and specimen removal

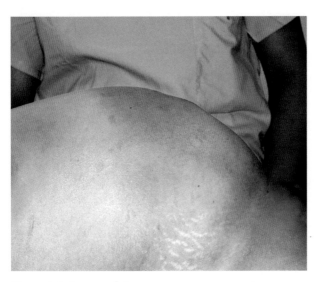

Figure 1.1. Large pelvic mass.
Ovarian tumors have a variety of presenting signs and symptoms. Shown here is a presentation of a large pelvic mass often seen in ovarian cancer. Note the protuberant, distended abdomen due to a large adnexal mass.

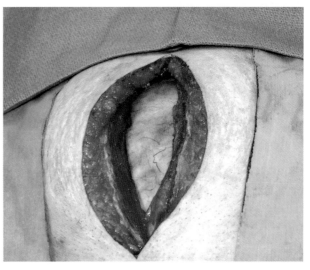

Figure 1.2. Abdominal entry.
A midline vertical incision is made in the skin using a scalpel. The subcutaneous fat and fascia are incised using either a scalpel or electrocautery. The linea alba between the two rectus abdominus muscles is identified, the underlying peritoneum is grasped with hemostats or forceps and is incised using Metzenbaum scissors or a scalpel. Shown is a large adnexal mass found upon entry into the abdomen.

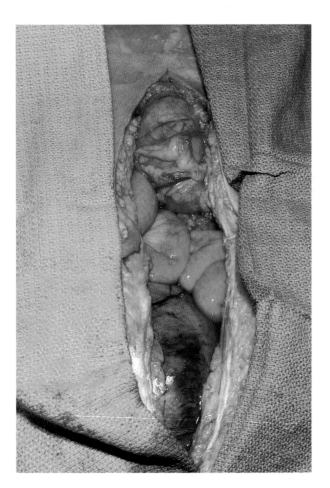

Figure 1.3. Extending the incision.
While a limited incision is appropriate to determine the malignant potential of a suspicious adnexal mass, the incision will usually need to be extended beyond the umbilicus. This is necessary to gain adequate exposure of the upper abdomen and to perform a full aortic node dissection.

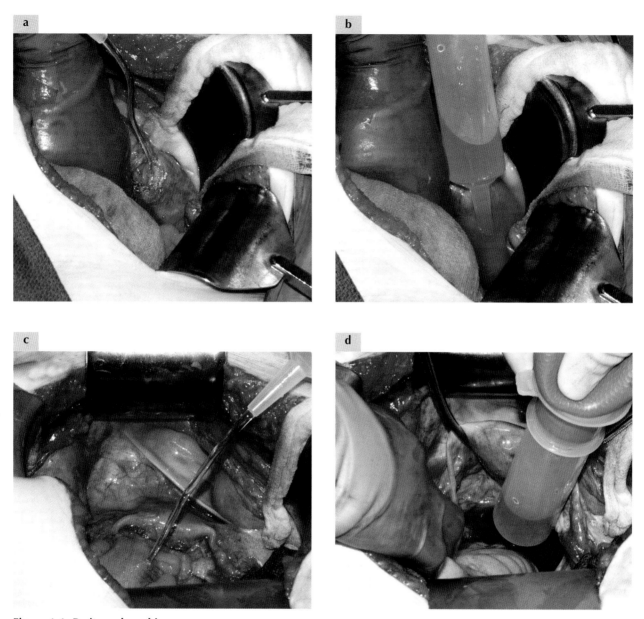

Figure 1.4. Peritoneal washings.
Immediately after entry into the abdomen, peritoneal washes are taken using warm saline and sent for cytology. Usually, washings are obtained from each diaphragm surface, each paracolic gutter, and from the pelvis. These may be combined prior to submitting them for cytologic evaluation. Shown in these figures are right paracolic gutter washings (**a** and **b**) and pelvic washings (**c** and **d**). The washings should be aspirated from the most dependent portion of the pelvis.

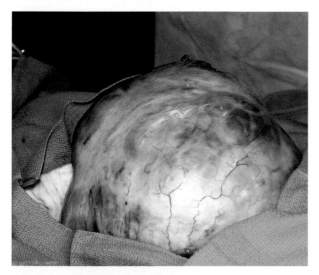

Figure 1.5. Delivery of the mass.
The mass is delivered through the incision in order to gain adequate mobility to perform the procedure.

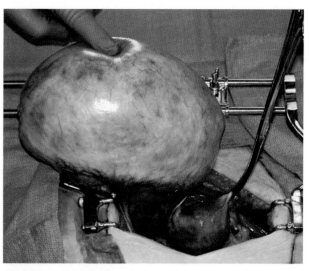

Figure 1.6. Placement of the retractor.
A self-retaining retractor is placed into the abdomen. In a relatively thin patient, a Balfour retractor with extension may be adequate to perform the procedure. In obese patients, the Bookwalter retractor is preferred.

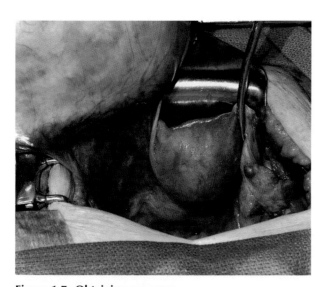

Figure 1.7. Obtaining exposure.
A large Kelly clamp is placed at the cornu of the uterus to provide traction. The uterus and mass are elevated. The lower blade of the Balfour retractor is inserted to protect the bladder and to provide additional traction.

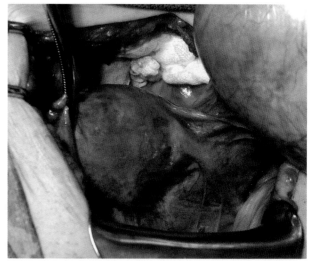

Figure 1.8. Specimen removal.
The small bowel is packed out of the operative field with large, moist lap sponges. This provides adequate exposure to identify the critical pelvic structures prior to removing the specimen. The steps of the technique are described in detail below.

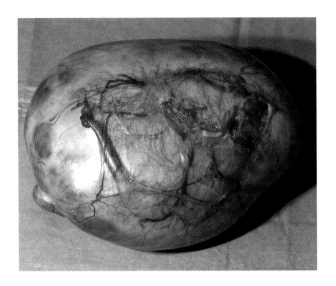

Figure 1.9. Detached mass.
Once the specimen is removed, it can be sent for intraoperative frozen section to determine the malignant potential. If a comprehensive staging procedure is required, the incision is extended as needed and the remainder of the procedure is performed. Described below is the standard staging procedure. Individualization is appropriate for those young patients who desire to retain the potential for future fertility. The risks of performing a conservative procedure must be weighed carefully against the potential for recurrence or residual disease in the remaining organs. The patient, after being appropriately counseled, must be an integral part of the decision-making process.

Hysterectomy and contralateral salpingo-oophorectomy

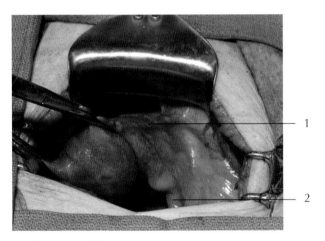

1 – Right round ligament
2 – Right infundibulopelvic ligament

Figure 1.10. Contralateral pelvic sidewall.
Attention is turned to the contralateral adnexa. The round ligament and infundibulopelvic ligament are identified.

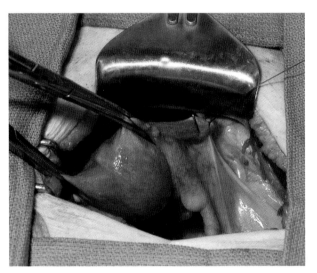

Figure 1.11. Ligation of the round ligament.
A suture is securely placed around the distal portion of the round ligament. It is passed beneath and then through the round ligament to ensure that the round ligament vessels are completely occluded. A small branch of the uterine artery, Samson's artery, provides blood supply to the round ligament. A large clip may be placed on the specimen side.

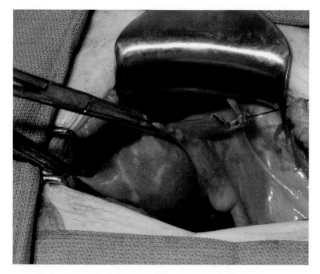

Figure 1.12. Transection of the round ligament.
The round ligament is then transected using
electrocautery or scissors. The round ligament suture is
held for traction, which is useful when opening the
pelvic sidewall.

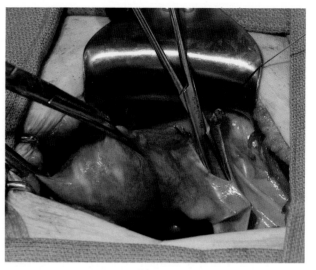

Figure 1.13. Opening the pelvic peritoneum.
The peritoneum is then dissected free from the
underlying areolar tissue with a right-angled clamp or
similar. The peritoneum is incised using electrocautery to
skeletonize the infundibulopelvic ligament.

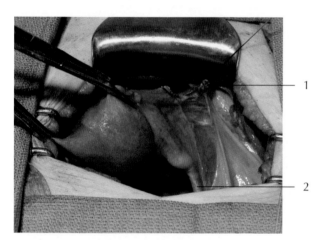

1 – Transected right round ligament
2 – Right infundibulopelvic ligament

**Figure 1.14. Skeletonizing the infundibulopelvic
ligament.**
The peritoneum has been opened further. The parallel
orientation of the peritoneal incision in relation to the
infundibulopelvic ligament is clearly seen.

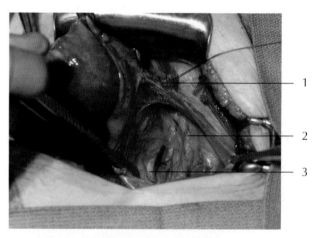

1 – Transected right round ligament
2 – Right external iliac vessels
3 – Right ureter

Figure 1.15. Identifying the ureter.
The back of a forceps can be used to dissect gently from
lateral to medial toward the sacrum in order to locate
the ureter. It is important not to dissect laterally as the
iliac vessels may be inadvertently injured. At this level in
the pelvis, the ureter can be identified on the medial leaf
of the broad ligament medial to the external and internal
iliac vessels.

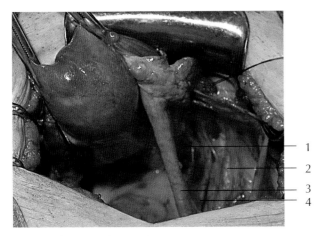

1 – Window in pelvic peritoneum
2 – Right external iliac vessels
3 – Right infundibulopelvic ligament
4 – Right ureter

Figure 1.16. Isolating the infundibulopelvic ligament.
A window is created in the peritoneum beneath the infundibulopelvic ligament, which contains the ovarian artery and vein, and above the ureter, which has been previously identified.

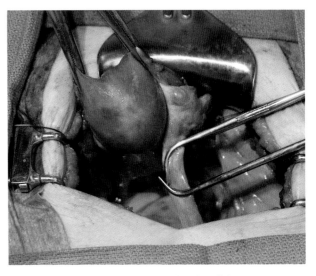

Figure 1.17. Clamping the infundibulopelvic (IP) ligament.
Two right-angled clamps or similar are placed across the IP ligament to occlude the ovarian vessels completely. Care is taken to ensure that no portion of the ovary is included in the clamp, since this will lead to an ovarian remnant where disease could recur or develop in the future.

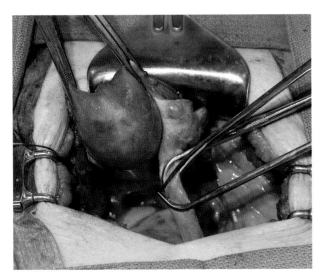

Figure 1.18. Transection of the infundibulopelvic ligament.
The IP ligament is transected using a Metzenbaum scissors, scalpel, or cautery.

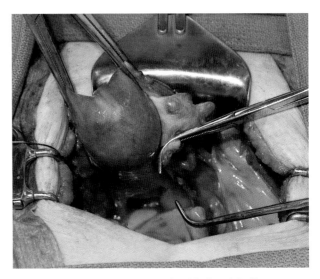

Figure 1.19. Ligation of the infundibulopelvic ligament.
The two ends of the IP ligament are now clearly separated. The distal side is ligated with a simple free tie, as it will be removed with the specimen. The proximal side of the IP ligament is first ligated with a free tie of delayed absorbable material and then a suture ligature on a CT-1 needle or smaller is placed above this free tie. It is important not to place the second suture below the first as this could result in the development of a retroperitoneal hematoma that may dissect along the ovarian vessels.

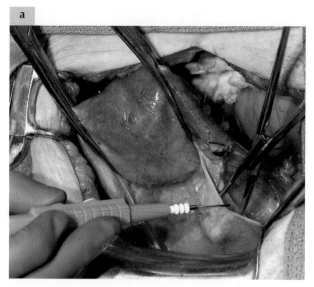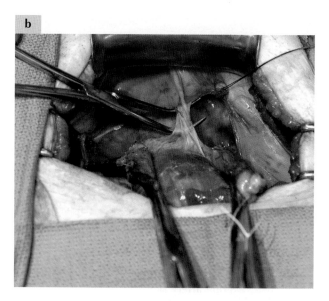

Figure 1.20. Creation of the bladder flap.
(**a**) Anteriorly, the bladder flap is created by using a right-angled clamp or similar to define the correct plane in the vesicouterine peritoneum just superior to the bladder reflection. The lower uterine segment is separated from the bladder, and electrocautery is used to incise the vesicouterine peritoneum. Blunt dissection with fingers or sponge sticks should not be used, as this can lead to inadvertent cystotomy, especially in those patients who have had previous pelvic surgery. (**b**) The vesicouterine peritoneum is completely transected to allow adequate caudad mobilization of the bladder.

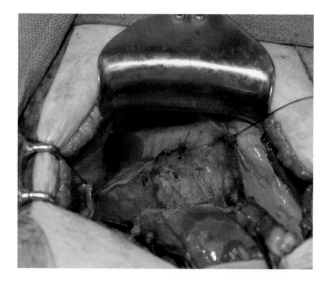

Figure 1.21. Completed bladder flap.
The bladder is now fully mobilized and away from the uterus and cervix to allow ligation of the uterine arteries.

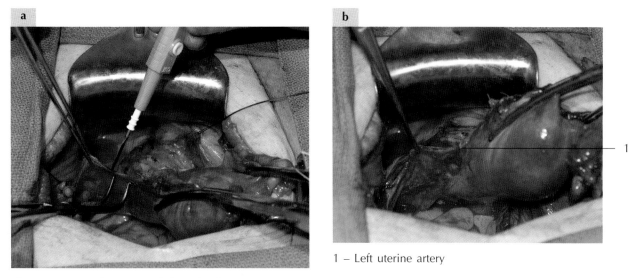

1 – Left uterine artery

Figure 1.22. Uterine artery skeletonization.
The uterine arteries are skeletonized by grasping the tissue laterally with a forceps in order to separate the tissue planes. (**a**) The tissues of the cardinal ligaments can be transected using electrocautery. (**b**) Once fully isolated, the uterine artery can be identified. If the uterine artery is not adequately skeletonized, excessive tissue may become incorporated when placing the clamp.

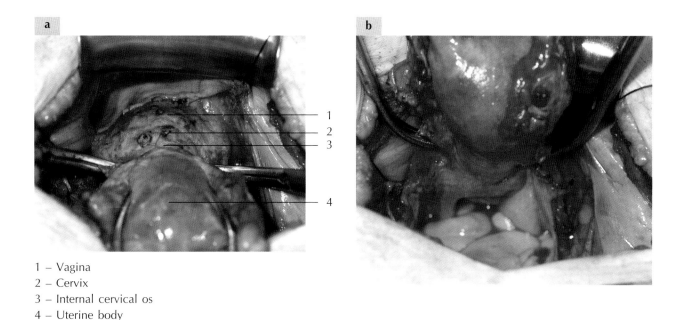

1 – Vagina
2 – Cervix
3 – Internal cervical os
4 – Uterine body

Figure 1.23. Transecting the uterine arteries.
The uterine arteries are clamped bilaterally with curved Zeppelin, Heaney, Gusberg, or similar clamps at the level of the internal cervical os or the uterine isthmus. Both uterine arteries are clamped prior to transecting either of them to diminish the backbleeding that will occur due to the collateral uterine circulation. The pedicle is transected using scissors or scalpel and then suture ligated with a delayed absorbable suture, such as polyglactin or polydioxanone. (**a**) Anterior and (**b**) posterior views are shown.

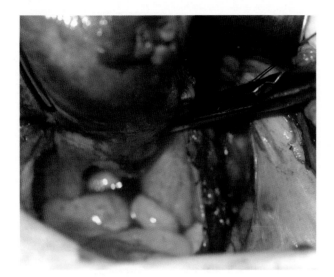

Figure 1.24. Clamping the cardinal ligament.
Once the uterine arteries have been ligated, the cardinal ligament is clamped with a straight clamp, transected and suture ligated. Each successive clamp should be placed medial to the previous one to allow transected tissues to fall away laterally. This minimizes the risk of injury to the ureter or to other adjacent structures. When completely dissected in patients or cadavers, the uterine artery passes several millimeters medially to the ureter at the level of the internal cervical os. Care should be taken always to place clamps as close to the uterine body as possible when performing a simple extrafascial hysterectomy.

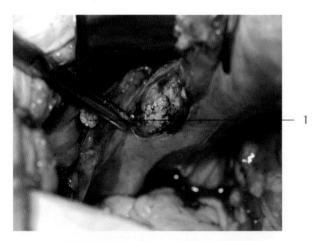

1 – Ligated left uterine artery

Figure 1.25. Transecting the cardinal ligament.
The cardinal ligaments are transected and suture ligated bilaterally. Shown here is the cut end of the left cardinal ligament, which will be suture ligated with the same material used on the uterine arteries. This clamp can be seen medial to and within the previous pedicle, which is the ligated uterine artery. A scalpel may be used to transect the tissues right along side the clamp as Heaney and Zeppelin clamps are designed to hold tissues without slippage.

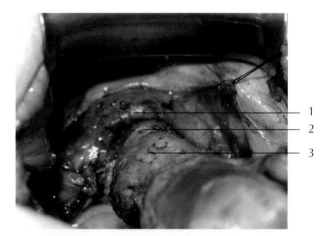

1 – Bladder
2 – Vagina
3 – Cervix

Figure 1.26. Preparation for removal.
Successive clamps are placed on the cardinal and uterosacral ligaments until the cervico–vaginal junction is reached. The pelvic structures are then reassessed to ensure that the bladder is sufficiently mobilized to allow clamps to be placed below the cervix during the transection of the vagina.

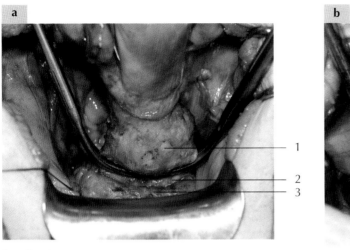

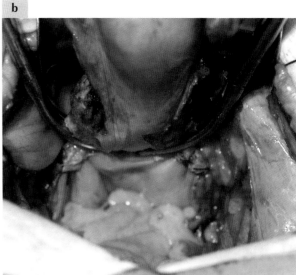

1 – Cervix
2 – Vagina
3 – Bladder

Figure 1.27. Clamping the vagina.
Curved Zeppelin clamps or similar are placed on the vagina at the cervico–vaginal junction bilaterally. The clamps do not need to reach entirely across the vaginal apex, although often will in patients with a normal sized uterus and cervix. Shown are (**a**) anterior and (**b**) posterior views of the vaginal clamps.

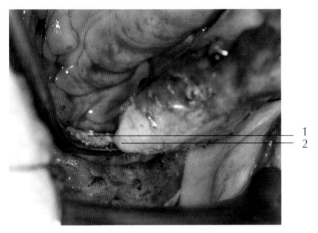

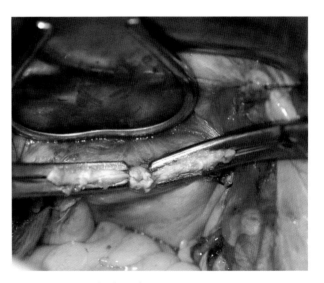

1 – Transected right vaginal angle
2 – Resected cervix

Figure 1.28. Transecting the vagina.
Heavy curved Mayo, Jorgenson, or Zeppelin scissors are used to transect the vagina and remove the specimen. Traction on the uterus facilitates this portion of the procedure.

Figure 1.29. Vaginal angles.
The specimen has been removed and the clamps remain on the vaginal angles. Each angle is suture ligated with delayed absorbable suture material. Transfixion or Heaney sutures are placed to secure the vaginal angles. These sutures are not cut but held for traction throughout the remainder of the hysterectomy. The remaining vaginal apex can be oversewn with a continuous running locked suture or interrupted figure-of-eight sutures. A sweetheart retractor is used to exclude the bladder during closure.

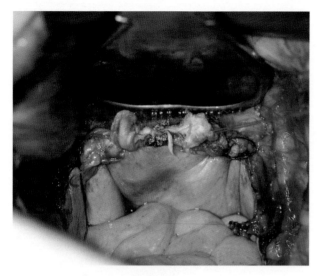

Figure 1.30. Closed vaginal cuff.
The vaginal cuff has now been closed and the pelvis is carefully inspected to search for uncontrolled vascular pedicles or bleeding from the posterior aspect of the bladder.

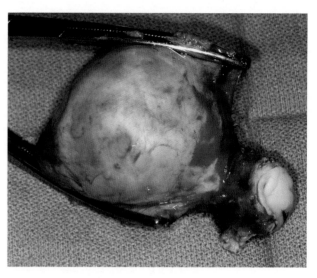

Figure 1.31. Specimen.
This particular specimen has had the adnexal structures previously removed. The specimen is either opened in the operating room or sent for intraoperative frozen section to determine depth of invasion for an endometrial carcinoma.

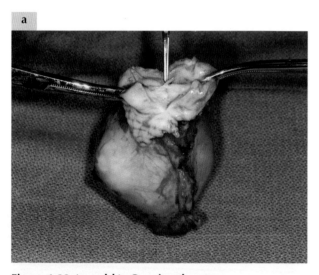

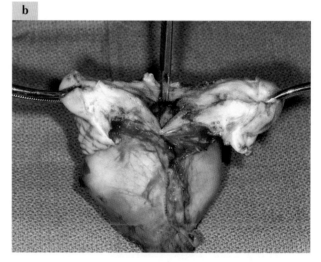

Figure 1.32 (a and b). Opening the uterus.
In the operating room, the specimen can be opened to assess depth of invasion for endometrial cancer. The uterus is bivalved from cervix to fundus along the lateral aspects in order to maintain orientation.

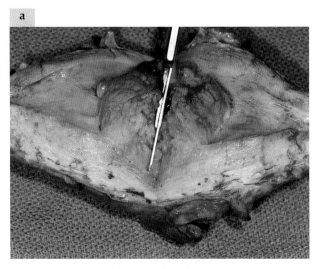 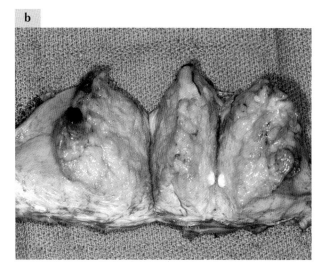

Figure 1.33 (a and b). Assessing the endometrium.
Once the uterus is bivalved, the endometrium should be bread-loafed to assess depth of invasion; thus, multiple sections can be visually inspected to find the location of greatest tumor burden. Opening the specimen in this manner does not interfere with a subsequent complete pathologic evaluation.

Pelvic lymph node dissection

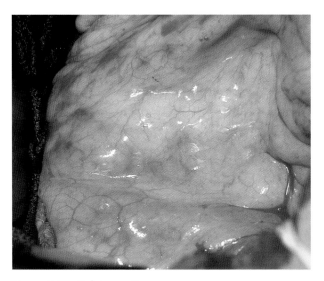

Figure 1.34. Pelvic peritoneum.
Prior to the start of the pelvic lymph node dissection, the pelvic peritoneum covers the pelvic sidewall and iliac vessels.

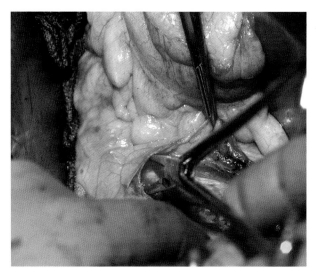

Figure 1.35. Opening the pelvic peritoneum.
The pelvic peritoneum is opened over the external iliac artery with electrocautery or Metzenbaum scissors. The incision in the peritoneum is extended toward the paracolic gutter to allow for adequate exposure to perform the lymph node dissection.

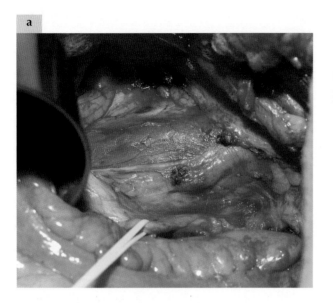

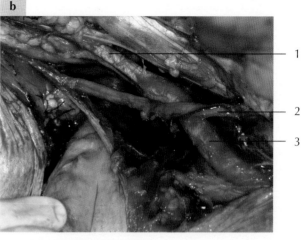

1 – Right external iliac artery
2 – Right ureter
3 – Right common iliac artery

Figure 1.36. Identifying the ureter.
The ureter normally crosses over the iliac vessels at the level where the common iliac artery bifurcates into the internal and external iliac arteries. Alternatively, it can be found on the medial leaf of the broad ligament lower in the pelvis. It should be clearly identified and a vessel loop can be placed for clear identification throughout the procedure. (**a**) The ureter after it has been dissected free from the pelvic peritoneum. (**b**) The ureter crossing over the iliac vessels at the bifurcation of the common iliac artery.

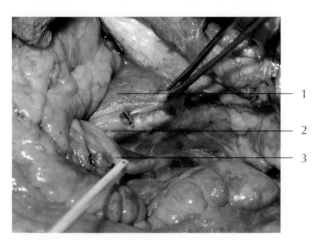

1 – Psoas muscle
2 – Left external iliac artery
3 – Left ureter

Figure 1.37. External iliac lymph node dissection.
The pelvic node dissection is started by grasping the lymphatic tissue overlying the external iliac artery. Singley forceps or similar is used to provide traction on the nodal tissue. The ureter is seen again in the foreground.

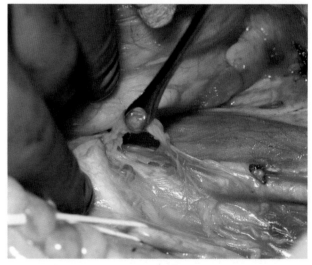

Figure 1.38. Creation of pedicles.
Pedicles are created with blunt or sharp dissection in order to delineate the nodal tissue to be removed.

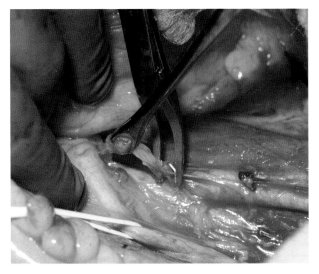

Figure 1.39. Clipping the pedicle.
Small perforating vessels and lymphatic channels can be occluded with hemostatic clips as shown here.

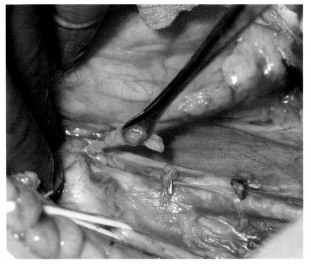

Figure 1.40. Excision of lymph node.
The pedicle has now been transected with Metzenbaum scissors. This process of creating pedicles, clipping, and excising is used throughout the nodal dissection.

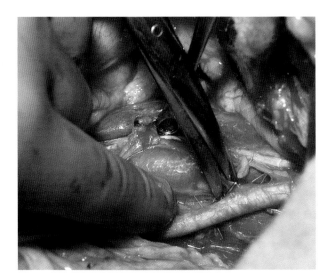

Figure 1.41. Further dissection.
Small perforators and lymphatics are clipped and cut in order to skeletonize the external iliac vessels and facilitate the dissection.

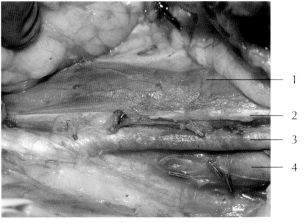

1 – Psoas muscle
2 – Left genitofemoral nerve
3 – Left external iliac artery
4 – Left external iliac vein

Figure 1.42. Genitofemoral nerve.
Throughout the dissection, care should be taken to avoid injury to the genitofemoral nerve which courses along the medial aspect of the psoas muscle and just lateral to the external iliac artery. Injury to this nerve can result in paresthesia of the medial aspect of the upper thigh. The size of the nerve is variable, as the genital and femoral branches may run separately.

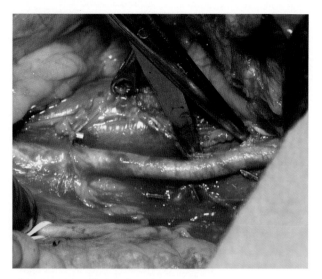

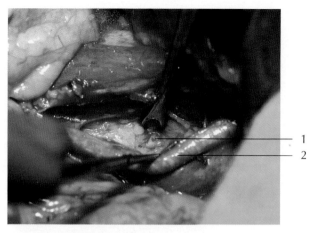

1 – Left obturator lymph nodes
2 – Left external iliac artery retracted medially

Figure 1.43. Entering the obturator space.
The obturator space may be entered either medially or
laterally to the external iliac vessels. For the lateral
approach, the space between the external iliac artery and
the psoas fascia is developed bluntly with scissors or a
similar instrument.

Figure 1.44. Obturator space.
Adequate exposure is obtained by retracting the psoas
laterally and the external iliac artery and vein medially
with a vein retractor or similar as shown in this figure.
The superior aspect of the obturator fossa is seen with
abundant lymphatic tissue.

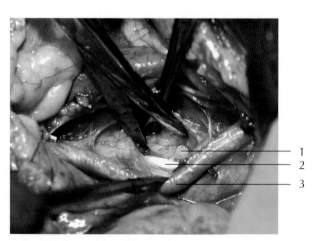

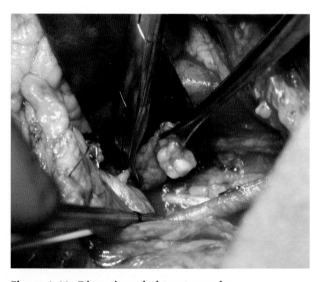

1 – Left obturator lymph nodes
2 – Left obturator nerve
3 – Left external iliac artery retracted medially

Figure 1.45. Identifying the obturator nerve.
Prior to performing the obturator lymph node dissection,
the obturator nerve should be clearly identified. This
should be done before removing any lymphatic tissue.
The obturator nodal tissue can be dissected bluntly with
scissors or a clamp. The nerve is identified using slightly
opened Metzenbaum scissors to separate it from the
obturator fat-pad as shown here.

Figure 1.46. Dissection of obturator nodes.
The obturator lymph nodes are often easily detached
from the surrounding tissues. In areas where the nodes
do not easily come free, a vessel or lymphatic channel is
most likely present and a hemostatic clip should be
placed. A combination of blunt dissection with clips as
needed usually renders this portion of the procedure
relatively bloodless.

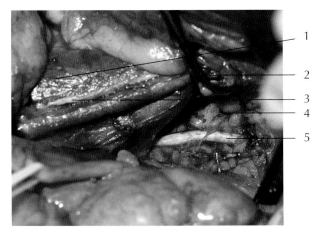

1 – Psoas muscle
2 – Left external iliac vessels retracted laterally
3 – Genitofemoral nerve
4 – Left obturator lymph nodes
5 – Left obturator nerve

Figure 1.47. Medial view.
The external iliac vessels are now retracted laterally, and much of the lymphatic tissue above the obturator nerve has been removed. If possible, one should continue to remove additional lymphatic tissue beneath the obturator nerve. If it is not possible to remove all the nodal tissue from a lateral approach, the medial approach will provide additional exposure.

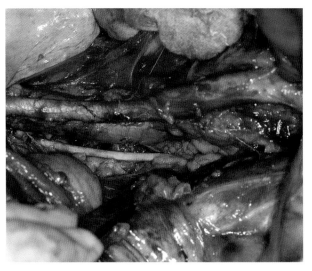

Figure 1.48. Obturator space.
After further dissection, the obturator space is mostly cleared of lymph-node-bearing tissue. While this should provide an adequate sampling of the lymph node basin, it has not yet removed all lymphatic tissue. Certain practitioners believe that it is prudent to remove as many lymph nodes as possible, even during a staging procedure, as some recent data support survival advantages in patients with more extensive lymph node dissection at the time of surgical staging for both endometrial and ovarian cancers. Occasionally, it may be necessary to ligate the obturator vein and artery during the dissection in order to control or prevent hemorrhage. This does not lead to any clinically significant sequelae.

Figure 1.49. Medial extent.
The obturator lymph nodes have been almost completely cleared at this point. Medially the obturator lymph node dissection should not extend beyond the superior vesical artery or the obliterated umbilical artery.

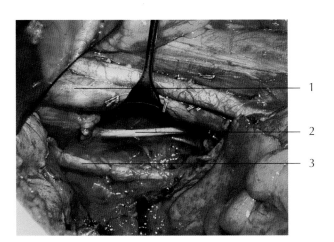

1 – Left external iliac vein
2 – Left obturator nerve
3 – Left superior vesical artery

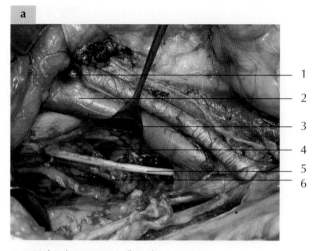

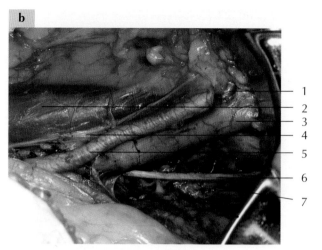

1 – Right deep circumflex iliac vein
2 – Right external iliac vein
3 – Right anastomotic pelvic vein
4 – Right obturator internus muscle
5 – Right obturator nerve
6 – Right obturator vein

1 – Left deep circumflex iliac vein
2 – Psoas muscle
3 – Left external iliac vein
4 – Genitofemoral nerve
5 – Left external iliac artery
6 – Left obturator nerve
7 – Left obturator vein

Figure 1.50. Extent of dissection.
The lateral extent of dissection is the psoas muscle, with care taken to preserve the genitofemoral nerve. Distally, the lateral dissection should also be conducted with care, as the superficial epigastric vessels can be encountered here. Proximally, the pelvic nodes are removed up to the bifurcation of the common iliac artery at this point. The formal common iliac artery nodes can either be removed with the pelvic node dissection or the paraaortic node dissection. Internal iliac nodes are sampled but usually run into the proximal extent of the obturator lymph node dissection. The distal extent of the dissection for lymph node sampling or complete lymphadenectomy is the deep circumflex iliac vein, a branch of the external iliac vein. In general, the obturator fossa will yield a greater number of lymph nodes than will the external iliac chain. (**a**) Fully dissected right obturator fossa; (**b**) fully dissected left obturator fossa. The anastomotic pelvic vein is quite variable in course and can originate from the external iliac vein or the obturator vein. It usually travels toward the pubic symphysis to join the contralateral pelvic vein and/or the inferior epigastric vein.

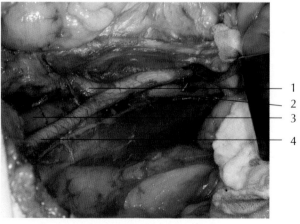

1 – Left internal iliac artery
2 – Left inferior vena cava
3 – Left external iliac vein
4 – Left external iliac artery

Figure 1.51. Vascular anomalies.
When operating in close proximity to major blood vessels, it is important to be cognizant of potential vascular anomalies. Shown here is an interesting patient who had a duplicated inferior vena cava. The common iliac artery is dissected to the level of the aortic bifurcation, but the left external iliac vein drains into the left inferior vena cava. Within the obturator fossa a plethora of vascular anomalies can be present. Most commonly, the anastomotic pelvic vein can be inconsistent in course and frequently not present at all. The deep circumflex iliac vein can also be found passing beneath the external iliac artery.

Paraaortic lymph node dissection

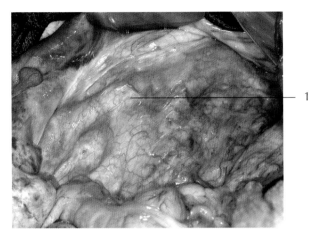

1 – Peritoneum overlying the right common iliac artery

Figure 1.52. Right peritoneal incision.
On the right side, the paraaortic node dissection begins by incising the peritoneum overlying the right common iliac artery. Alternatively, the incision used for the pelvic lymph node dissection can be extended over the common iliac artery to the aortic bifurcation. Care should be taken to identify the ureter as it crosses over the common iliac artery to minimize injury during the peritoneal opening.

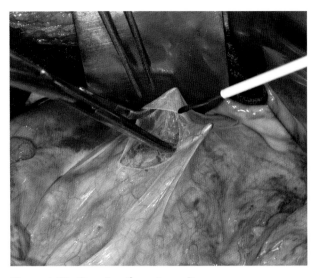

Figure 1.53. Opening the retroperitoneum.
A right angle clamp or forceps can be used to separate the peritoneum from the underlying areolar tissue while electrocautery or scissors are used to transect it.

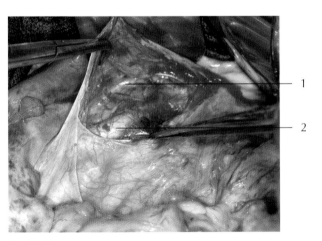

1 – Right ureter
2 – Right common iliac artery

Figure 1.54. Common iliac node dissection.
The ureter is identified lateral to the vena cava and common iliac artery. Next, the nodes overlying the common iliac vessels are removed. Pedicles are ligated with small clips if vessels or lymphatics are encountered.

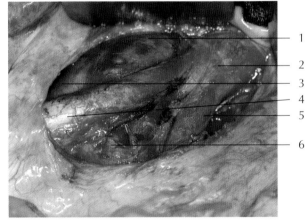

1 – Inferior vena cava
2 – Aortic bifurcation
3 – Right common iliac vein
4 – Right common iliac artery
5 – Left common iliac artery
6 – Left common iliac vein

Figure 1.55. Additional dissection.
Once the common iliac vein is encountered, a nodal sheath is removed longitudinally along the vessel up to the vena cava. The lymph nodes overlying the distal portion of the bifurcation can be removed at this point, as illustrated.

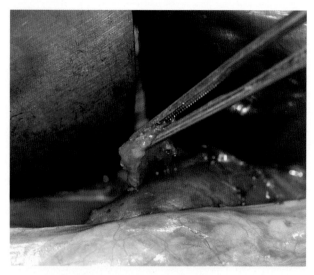

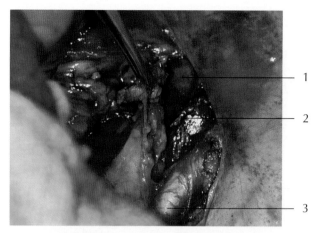

1 – Inferior vena cava
2 – Ligated 'fellow's vein'
3 – Right common iliac artery

Figure 1.56. Right paracaval dissection.
Dissection is then continued from the bifurcation of the vena cava superiorly. Node removal continues in a systematic fashion either from lateral to medial or vice versa, but not directly over the vena cava. Unlike other vascular structures, small perforating vessels can branch directly off the anterior surface of the vena cava. Hemostatic clips are placed on the lateral and medial borders of the nodal tissues, and the two edges of the dissection are approximated.

Figure 1.57. Vascular pitfalls.
When dissecting the distal vena cava, a constant small perforating vein is often encountered anteriorly and is affectionately referred to as the 'fellow's vein'. Careful dissection will allow this vein to be clipped prior to causing bothersome hemorrhage. More proximally, one must look out for an accessory renal artery, which may cross the vena cava anteriorly. The intervening aortocaval tissue is removed as well, sparing the lumbar vessels.

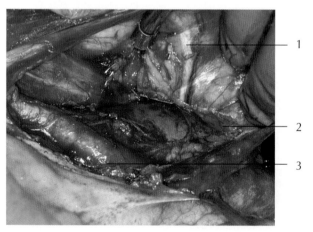

1 – Right ureter
2 – Inferior vena cava
3 – Right common iliac artery

Figure 1.58. Low paraaortic nodal dissection.
The lower right paraaortic nodes have been removed to the level of the inferior mesenteric artery (seen later). This level of dissection provides an adequate sampling for patients with endometrial cancer. For ovarian cancer, the lymphatic drainage follows the course of the ovarian veins and nodal sampling needs to be continued to the renal vessels. The ureter is retracted laterally from the vena cava and aorta.

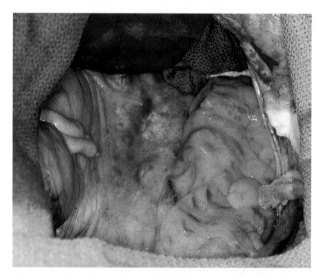

Figure 1.59. Left peritoneal incision.
The left paraaortic lymph nodes can be approached laterally or medially. More commonly in laparoscopy, the left side is approached by extending the peritoneal incision for the right-sided dissection across the midline, superiorly and inferiorly. During laparotomy, a lateral approach is often simpler due to the origin of the inferior mesenteric artery from the left anterior aspect of the aorta. The lateral approach can be performed as a continuation of the left-sided pelvic node dissection or de novo lateral to the sigmoid colon.

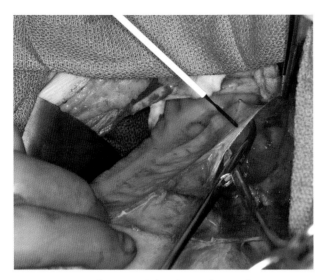

Figure 1.60. Reflection of the descending colon.
The peritoneum is opened using the electrocautery along the white line of Toldt in order to reflect the colon medially. This incision is carried up as high as possible, usually limited by the abdominal incision; otherwise it could be continued to the tip of the spleen, although this is usually unnecessary.

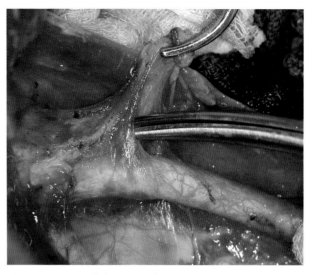

Figure 1.61. Medial approach.
As mentioned previously, left paraaortic lymph nodes can be obtained by crossing over the aorta after completing the right-sided dissection. Lymphatic tissue can be freed from the aorta with sharp and blunt dissection. Shown here is lymphatic tissue being gently separated from the aorta with Metzenbaum scissors. All pedicles in this region are clipped prior to transection with the scissors. The scissors are mostly used in an opening and closing fashion to free the lymph nodes from the vessel.

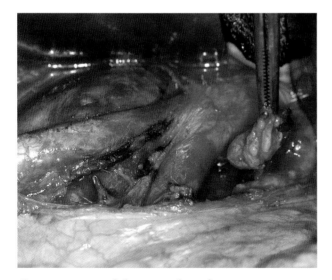

Figure 1.62. Low, left paraaortic nodes.
Low, left paraaortic nodes can readily be obtained in the region between the inferior mesenteric artery and the left aspect of the aorta. Shown here are lymph nodes being removed from this area.

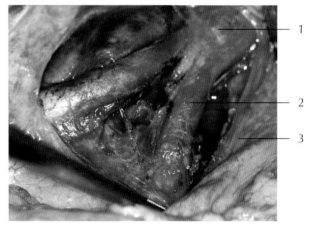

1 – Aorta
2 – Left common iliac artery
3 – Inferior mesenteric artery

Figure 1.63. Low, left nodal basin.
After removal of the lymph node package, the boundaries of this particular dissection can be seen, including the inferior mesenteric artery. The region can also be easily reached from a lateral approach as described above. Often, the lateral approach will be used to dissect the lower left paraaortic nodes and the medial approach will be used to dissect the higher paraaortic nodes.

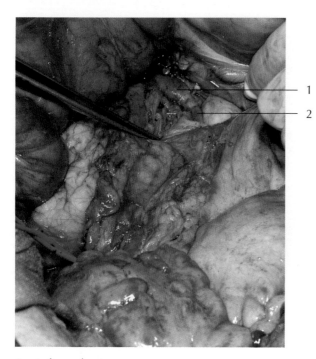

1 – Left renal vein
2 – Left ovarian vein

Figure 1.64. High-left paraaortic dissection.
Many practitioners will perform the low paraaortic dissections first, using the standard approach for the right side and the lateral approach for the left side, and then perform both sides of the higher paraaortic nodes sequentially. To sample fully the lymph node basins for ovarian cancer, the dissection needs to extend to the renal veins. As mentioned previously, the right ovarian vein drains directly into the vena cava and the left ovarian vein drains into the left renal vein. It is sometimes more logical to begin the dissection at the level of the renal veins and work downwards, depending on the approach used for the lower paraaortic nodes, the size of the abdominal incision and the patient's body habitus. Here, the left ovarian vein is seen joining the left renal vein. If desired, it can be ligated at its origin to minimize bleeding should injury occur during the dissection. Care must be taken to identify the ovarian vein definitively since its insertion can be confused with an accessory renal vein in certain patients.

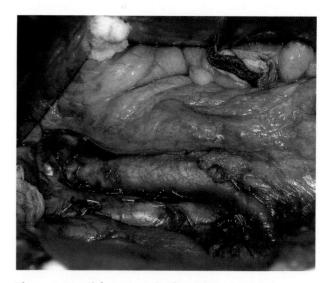

Figure 1.65. High paraaortic dissection.
The nodal tissue surrounding the vena cava and the aorta has been almost completely removed. The left renal vein can clearly be seen crossing over the aorta. This is the proximal extent of the dissection.

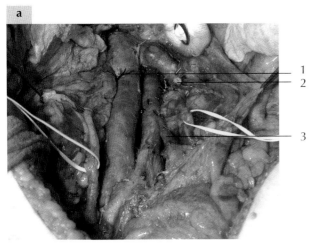

1 – Ligated right ovarian vein
2 – Ligated left ovarian vein
3 – Inferior mesenteric artery

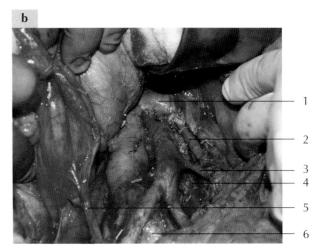

1 – Left renal vein
2 – Left ovarian vein
3 – Inferior mesenteric artery
4 – Low, left paraaortic nodal basin
5 – Right ureter
6 – Left common iliac vein

Figure 1.66. Completed paraaortic dissection.
The paraaortic nodal dissection has now been completed. (**a**) Both ureters are tagged with yellow vessel loops and both ovarian veins have been ligated at their origin. The inferior mesenteric artery and the bifurcation of the aorta are also demonstrated. (**b**) Many of the same structures seen in (**a**) are shown but, in addition, the left common iliac vein can be found passing just distal to the aortic bifurcation. When removing subaortic nodes, this anatomical relationship must be noted to prevent laceration of the left common iliac vein. When this vein is injured, troublesome bleeding is the rule. The course of the left ovarian vein is well delineated, as it has not been ligated. The ovarian veins always appear engorged during this procedure due to the fact that they have been transected and ligated within the infundibulopelvic ligament. This results in increased hemostatic pressure within an already low-pressure venous system. The low, left paraaortic basin is found between the inferior mesenteric artery and the aorta. The inferior mesenteric artery can be ligated at its origin if injured or if additional exposure to the left side of the aorta is needed. Clinically significant sequelae usually do not occur, except in patients who either have had previous colonic surgery or who have vascular disease that may compromise collateral flow to the descending and sigmoid colon.

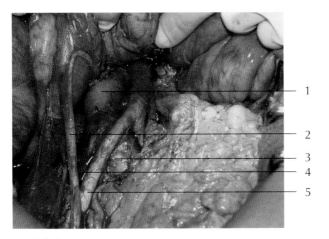

Figure 1.67. Course of the right ureter.
This figure is included to demonstrate the course of the right ureter. It can be seen traveling through the retroperitoneum and then crossing over the right common iliac artery. It is important to be cognizant of the ureters throughout the paraaortic lymph node dissection.

1 – Inferior vena cava
2 – Right ureter
3 – Left common iliac vein
4 – Right common iliac vein
5 – Right common iliac artery

Omentectomy and biopsies

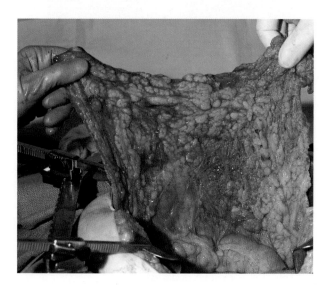

Figure 1.68. Infracolic omentum.
The omentum is elevated and spread out both to determine the interface with the transverse colon and to evaluate the normal anatomical relationships. The entire infracolic omentum will be removed.

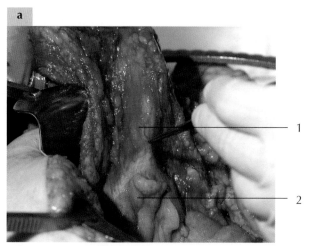

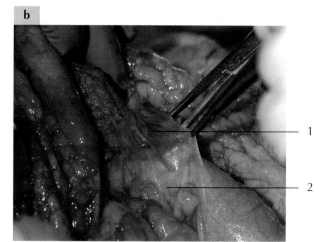

1 – Posterior leaf of omentum
2 – Transverse colon

1 – Posterior leaf of omentum
2 – Transverse colon

Figure 1.69. Infracolic omentectomy.
(**a**) An avascular area between the posterior leaf of the omentum and the colon is identified. (**b**) It is then entered sharply with the tip of a clamp (as shown) or with scissors. For the surgical staging of early-stage ovarian cancer or high-risk endometrial cancer, an infracolic omentectomy provides sufficient material to determine whether or not microscopic seeding has occurred.

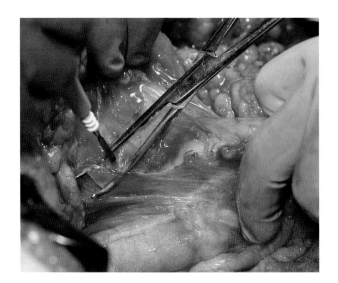

Figure 1.70. Dissecting the omentum.
Electrocautery is used to divide the posterior leaf of the omentum from the transverse colon. To perform a complete infracolic omentectomy, the omentum should be divided close to the transverse colon. Nonetheless, sufficient distance should be maintained to prevent lateral thermal spread from the electrocautery onto the colon. By dissecting between the posterior leaf and anterior leaf of the omentum, the lesser sac is entered. Care should be taken to avoid carrying the anterior dissection onto the mesentery of the transverse colon, as the middle colic artery can be easily injured. The dissection should be carried out from the hepatic flexure to the splenic flexure.

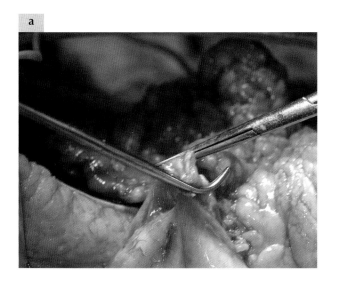

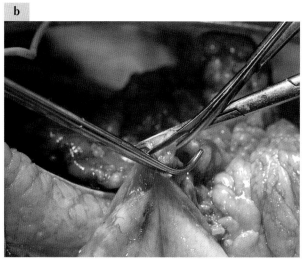

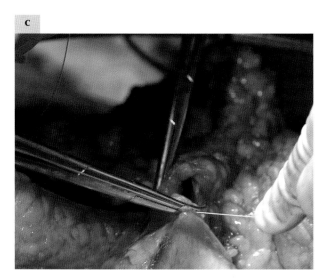

Figure 1.71. Clamping pedicles.
Once the omentum has been mobilized off the transverse colon, the gastrocolic ligament is incised. Avascular areas are incised with electrocautery or scissors. (**a**) Vascular pedicles are doubly clamped with right-angle Kelly or Halstead, or similar clamps. (**b**) A series of clamps is placed with each set being transected at the time of placement. (**c**) Ligation with free ties is done successively after several clamps have been placed in order to conduct the procedure as efficiently as possible. Recent advances in surgical instrumentation have provided a wide array of alternative instruments with which to perform the omentectomy. Currently, options include the use of the endoscopic stapler, the handheld harmonic scalpel, handheld LigaSure (Valleylab, Boulder, CO), the argon-beam coagulator, and the ligate and dividing powered stapler. Operator experience will dictate which device is most suitable for a particular patient or procedure.

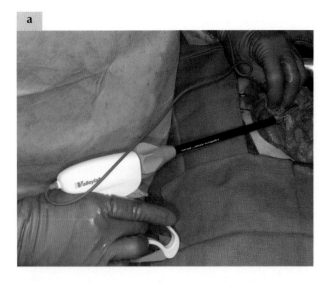

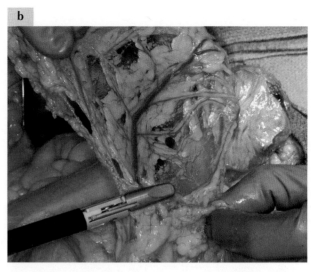

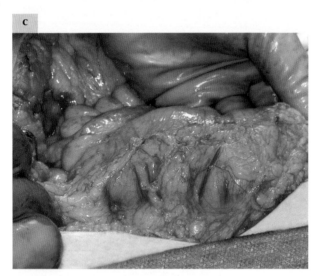

Figure 1.72. LigaSure.
The LigaSure is a device that can coagulate and transect tissue in a rapid manner. (**a**) The short handheld LigaSure Atlas. The jaws are closed by squeezing the handle until it locks. A foot pedal is then depressed to activate the bipolar electrocautery, which effectively seals the tissue and/or vessels up to 7 mm in diameter. The lever just above the handle is then depressed to activate a blade within the device that will transect the cauterized tissue. Squeezing the handle once again then opens the jaws. (**b**) The gastroepiploic artery, which is the main blood supply to the omentum, can easily be cauterized with the LigaSure. (**c**) Thermal spread is minimal and the resulting resection leaves a hemostatic, uninjured segment of transverse colon.

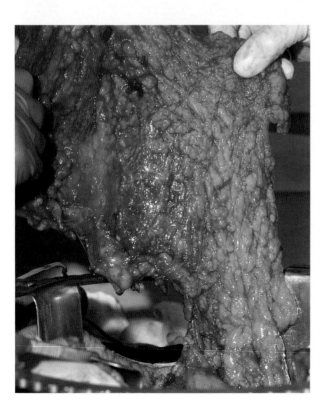

Figure 1.73. Omentectomy specimen.
The entire omentum is displayed. It has been almost completely separated from its surrounding attachments. Once the dissection is finished, it will be sent for routine pathologic evaluation. If clinically suspicious areas are noted during the procedure, the specimen should be sent for immediate intraoperative frozen section if the findings would alter the remainder of the operation.

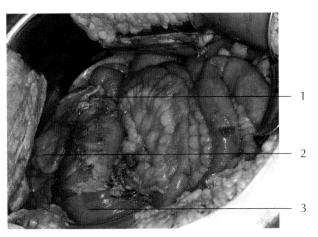

Figure 1.74. Transverse colon.
The entire infracolic omentum has been removed and the transverse colon can be seen cleared from the hepatic to the splenic flexure.

1 – Splenic flexure
2 – Supracolic omentum
3 – Hepatic flexure

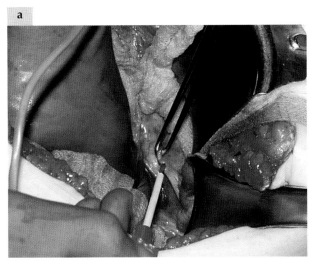 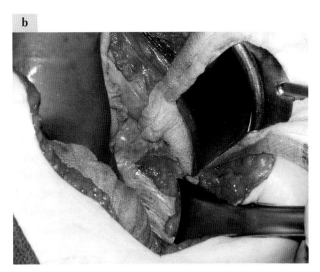

Figure 1.75 (a and b). Random biopsies.
If disease is not found outside of the pelvis at laparotomy, random biopsies are taken to search for microscopic disease. Multiple sites within the abdomen and pelvis should be sampled. These include the diaphragm bilaterally, the paracolic gutters bilaterally, the right pelvis, the left pelvis, and the anterior and posterior cul-de-sacs; any suspicious areas should also be biopsied. The biopsy specimens should be 2–3 cm in diameter to provide an adequate specimen for pathologic analysis. Shown is a biopsy from the right paracolic gutter.

Appendectomy

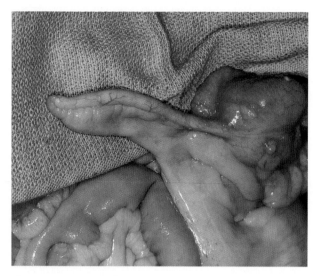

Figure 1.76. Appendix.
The appendix may be removed at the time of staging laparotomy for a variety of reasons. An inflamed, erythematous, or suppurative appendix should be removed. If it is thought to be involved with tumor, it should be removed as well. Importantly, an appendectomy should be performed whenever a mucinous ovarian neoplasm is diagnosed or suspected. All too frequently, mucinous ovarian tumors, particularly borderline tumors, are thought to be primarily from the ovary when in fact they are metastases from primary appendiceal tumors or other gastrointestinal tumors.

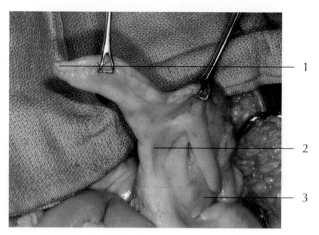

1 – Appendix
2 – Appendiceal mesentery
3 – Cecum

Figure 1.77. Traction.
One or two Babcock clamps are placed on the appendix to provide traction and mobility throughout the procedure. These particular clamps are useful since they are atraumatic when used in the manner demonstrated.

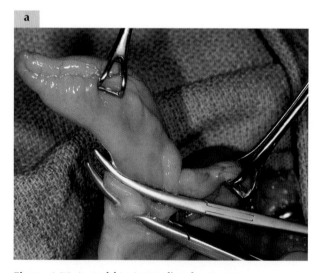

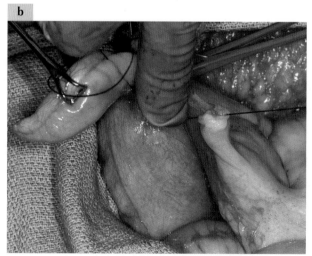

Figure 1.78 (a and b). Appendiceal mesentery.
The mesentery of the appendix contains small branches of the appendiceal artery. It should be doubly clamped, transected and suture ligated. By initially transecting the mesentery of the appendix, mobility will be gained, which is useful later in the procedure.

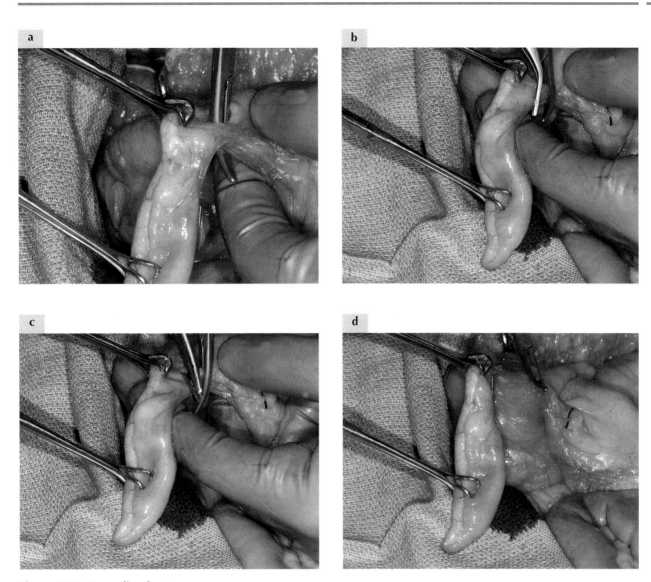

Figure 1.79. Appendiceal artery.

The main blood supply to the appendix is the appendiceal artery. The appendiceal artery usually enters the mesentery of the appendix near its base. As mentioned, small branches travel through the mesentery of the appendix. (**a**) The appendiceal artery is isolated with blunt dissection using the tip of a fine clamp. (**b** and **c**) It is then clamped and transected. A hemostatic clip may be placed on the distal side, since it will be removed with the specimen. (**d**) The proximal end is securely ligated with a permanent or delayed absorbable suture.

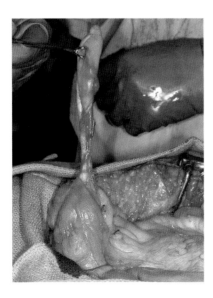

Figure 1.80. Specimen.

Once the mesentery and artery have been dissected free from the appendix itself, and securely ligated, the specimen is ready for removal. It is elevated perpendicular to the cecum in order to determine the level at which it should be transected.

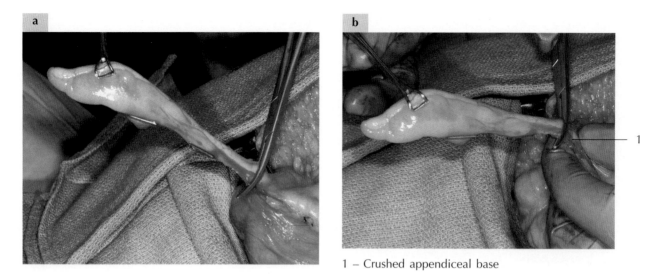

1 – Crushed appendiceal base

Figure 1.81. Crushing the base.
(**a**) The base of the appendix is clamped with a Halsted clamp or similar. Care should be taken to excise the appendix in its entirety while not compromising the cecum. If too much appendix is left attached to the cecum, not only will this portion be unavailable for pathologic evaluation, but it could also be the site of future inflammation. (**b**) Once the base of the appendix is crushed, the clamp is moved upwards several millimeters.

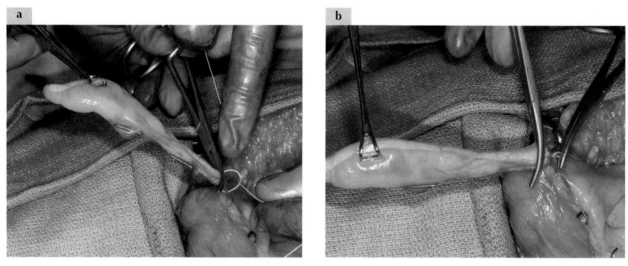

Figure 1.82. Ligating the appendix.
The appendix is ligated with a permanent or delayed absorbable free tie. (**a**) The tie is placed around the base of the appendix at the site where it was previously crushed. (**b**) Once the suture is cut, a small clamp is placed on the end of the suture, which will be used to bury the appendiceal stump.

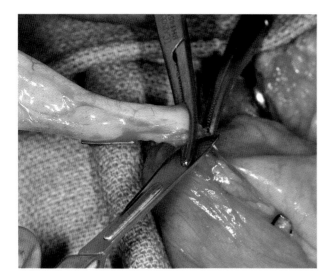

Figure 1.83. Transecting the appendix.
A small space is now present between the ligated base of the appendix and the small clamp that remains on the appendix. A scalpel is used to transect the appendix just **below** the clamp. The clamp will prevent spillage from the specimen, and the tie secures the cecum.

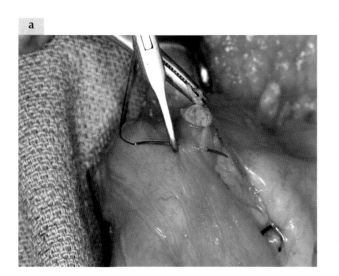
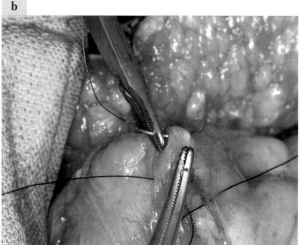

Figure 1.84 (a and b). Burying the stump.
The appendiceal stump is then buried by placing either a purse-string or a Z-stitch with nonabsorbable material. Any technique that will bury the stump is sufficient. Some practitioners do not bury the appendiceal stump and some will cauterize the cut end of the appendix. Neither technique has been shown to reduce postoperative complications in well-designed studies.

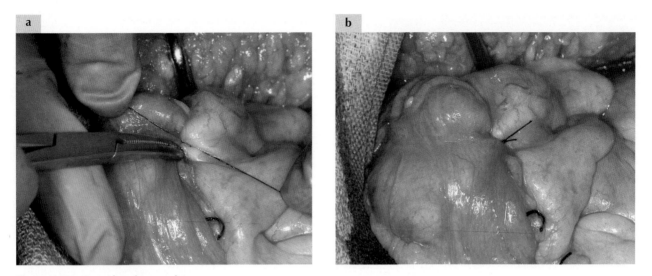

Figure 1.85. Completed procedure.
(**a**) The suture is tied down as the assistant inverts the appendiceal stump into the cecum. (**b**) The cecum as it appears after completing the appendectomy.

2 Radical abdominal hysterectomy

Mario M Leitao Jr and Carol L Brown

Radical abdominal hysterectomy has been the standard of care for surgical management of early-stage cervical carcinoma since its development and refinement in the late 1800s and early 1900s.[1] It is a procedure that was initially fraught with significant morbidity and mortality. However, developments in the use of antibiotics, surgical techniques, anesthesia, and pre- and postoperative care have significantly reduced the morbidity and mortality associated with this procedure.[1-3]

The most common indication for radical hysterectomy is early-stage [International Federation of Gynecology and Obstetrics (FIGO) Stages IA2–IIA] invasive cervical carcinoma. Radical hysterectomy may sometimes be indicated in patients with Stage IA1 invasive cervical cancers that have lymph–vascular space invasion. Further indications include selected cases of early-stage (FIGO Stages I and II) invasive vaginal cancer limited to the upper third of the vagina, selected cases of endometrial cancer with cervical stromal invasion (FIGO Stage IIB), and selected cases of persistent or recurrent cervical cancers, which after radiation therapy are limited to the cervix or proximal vaginal fornix.[1,4,5] Radiation therapy has always been considered equivalent to surgery for the definitive treatment of early-stage cervical carcinoma. However, the combination of radical surgery and radiation therapy is associated with significant morbidity.[3] Surgery offers the possibility of primary tumor removal, a shorter treatment time, more limited tissue injury, a specimen for pathological evaluation from which to tailor adjuvant treatments, the potential to preserve ovarian function, and, in certain cases, the potential to maintain reproductive function (see Chapter 11).[1,2,5] Patients with Stages IIB–IVA are best treated with concurrent chemoradiation.[6-8] Recent reports have suggested that patients with Stage IB2 and IIA cervical carcinoma also benefit most from chemoradiation;[9] however, this approach has never been directly compared to radical hysterectomy followed by appropriate adjuvant therapies and is, therefore, the subject of upcoming prospective randomized trials.

In 1974, Piver et al described five classes, or types, of hysterectomy (Table 2.1).[10] The Class III hysterectomy, or radical hysterectomy, is the most commonly performed, although some authors feel that a Class II hysterectomy, or modified radical hysterectomy, is as effective.[11] The main difference between these two types of hysterectomy is the amount of parametrial tissue taken along with the hysterectomy specimen and the degree of ureteral dissection. Complete bowel preparation is prescribed prior to the procedure. The choice of abdominal incision is based on the patient habitus and desire for cosmesis. Low transverse incisions (Maylard, Cherney, or Pfannenstiel) may provide sufficient exposure in certain cases.[1,12] Abdominopelvic washings are not needed, since they provide little information in the setting of cervical carcinoma.[13] Upon opening the abdomen, the paraaortic nodal region is inspected and palpated. Gross paraaortic nodal disease usually requires abandonment of the procedure, although some benefit from complete resection of grossly involved nodes has been reported.[14] Involved pelvic nodes are not an absolute contraindication to the procedure if they can be completely resected. The two most crucial initial steps of the procedure are the development of the pelvic spaces and mobilization of the bladder. Opening the pelvic spaces permits inspection and palpation of the parametria. Mobilization of the bladder confirms that disease has not penetrated anteriorly through the cervix, and that an adequate parametrial and vaginal resection should be possible. Unresectable parametrial disease, or an inability to sufficiently mobilize the bladder, are indications to abandon the procedure.

Table 2.1 **Five classes of hysterectomy.**[10]

Type	Name	Vagina	Bladder	Ureter	Uterine artery	Parametria	Uterosacral ligament
I	Extrafascial	Minimal tissue removed	Partially mobilized	Not mobilized	Ligated at uterus	Resected at uterus	Transected at uterus
II	Modified radical	Upper 1–2 cm removed	Partially mobilized	Unroofed in parametrial tunnel	Ligated medial to ureter	Resected medial to ureter	Transected at midpoint of ligament
III	Radical	Upper 1/3 to 1/2 removed	Completely mobilized	Completely dissected until entry into bladder	Ligated at origin from hypogastric artery	Resected at pelvic sidewall	Transected at distal attachment
IV	Extended radical	Same as Class III	Completely mobilized but not resected	All periureteral tissue removed	Ligation at origin and ligation of superior vesical artery	Same as Class III	Same as Class III
V	Partial exenteration	Same as Class III	Portion of bladder resected	Distal ureter removed	Same as Class IV	Same as Class III	Same as Class III

The radical hysterectomy involves removal of the uterus, cervix, and upper one third to one half of the vagina along with the parametrial tissue. The uterine artery is divided at its origin from the anterior division of the internal iliac artery, and the ureter is completely unroofed to its insertion into the bladder, allowing for resection of the entire parametrial tissue. Resection of the uterosacral ligaments near their distal-most attachments is also performed. Removal of uninvolved ovaries is not a required part of the procedure and should be performed based upon independent considerations. If adjuvant radiation therapy is anticipated, the ovaries can be transposed above the iliac crests to help reduce the risk of radiation-induced menopause. This procedure is typically accompanied by a bilateral pelvic lymphadenectomy, which may be performed before or after the hysterectomy. Leaving the uterus in place facilitates the nodal dissection, since the pelvic spaces and anatomy are well preserved. Additionally, unresectable pelvic nodes, a contraindication to the procedure, would be encountered at this point. Reasons to perform the hysterectomy prior to the lymphadenectomy are to accomplish removal of the primary lesion at the outset of the procedure. Although some practitioners place pelvic drains at the conclusion of the procedure, this has not been shown to decrease the incidence of postoperative lymphocyst formation or febrile morbidity.[15] A suprapubic catheter can be placed to assist with the postoperative assessment of bladder function. The abdomen is closed in a fashion appropriate to the chosen type of incision.

The extent of dissection associated with a Class III radical hysterectomy results in greater morbidity as compared to a Class II hysterectomy. The most common morbidities include bladder and rectal dysfunction, vesicovaginal fistulae, ureteral obstruction, hemorrhage, infection, and nerve injury. Improvements in antibiotics and surgical techniques have greatly reduced the incidence of these complications.

New surgical approaches are emerging that may become acceptable alternatives to the radical abdominal hysterectomy in select patients. Among these are the radical vaginal hysterectomy (Schauta–Amreich procedure) and the laparoscopic radical hysterectomy, both described in other sections of this text. Also, radical vaginal trachelectomy can offer the potential to preserve fertility in very select groups of patients.[16] Nonetheless, abdominal radical hysterectomy remains the current gold standard to which all other techniques should be compared.

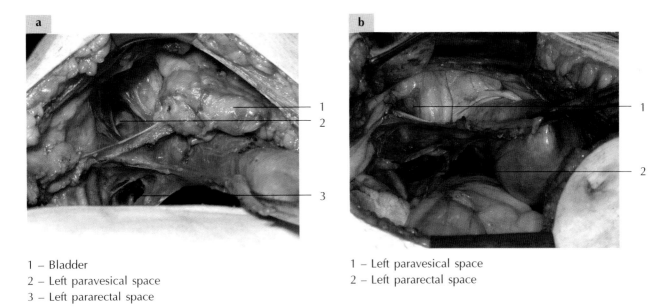

a

1 ─────── 1
        2

3 ─────── 3

b

1 ─────── 1

2 ─────── 2

1 – Bladder
2 – Left paravesical space
3 – Left pararectal space

1 – Left paravesical space
2 – Left pararectal space

Figure 2.1 (a and b). Entering the retroperitoneal spaces.
The procedure begins by opening the pelvic spaces. The round ligament is grasped, ligated and divided close to the pelvic sidewall. The peritoneum is incised, exposing the retroperitoneal spaces. At this time, a salpingo-oophorectomy may be performed if indicated. The paravesical and pararectal spaces are then developed.

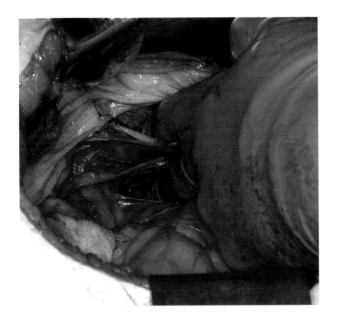

Figure 2.2. Developing the paravesical and pararectal spaces.
The paravesical and pararectal spaces are developed with blunt dissection using a finger, scissors, or clamp. Here, the surgeon's gloved fingers are within the paravesical space anteriorly and the pararectal space posteriorly. This permits palpation of the parametrium, which lies between the surgeon's fingers, in order to assess for possible tumor involvement.

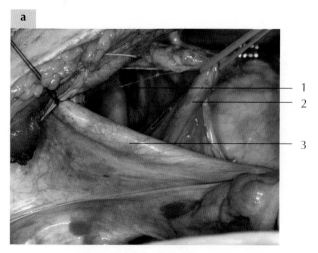

1 – Left paravesical space
2 – Left obliterated umbilical artery
3 – Left round ligament

1 – Cut end of left round ligament
2 – Left superior vesical artery
3 – Left ureter inserting into base of bladder

Figure 2.3. Paravesical space.
Alternatively, the paravesical space can be developed prior to transection of the round ligament. Here, the left round ligament is ligated close to the pelvic sidewall but not yet transected. The paravesical space is entered and developed bluntly anterior to the round ligament. (**a**) The boundaries of the paravesical space are the bladder and obliterated umbilical artery medially (blue vessel loop), the ventral aspect of the cardinal ligament posteriorly, the obturator fossa and muscle inferiorly, and the external iliac vessels laterally. (**b**) Visualization of the base of the left paravesical space after extensive dissection.

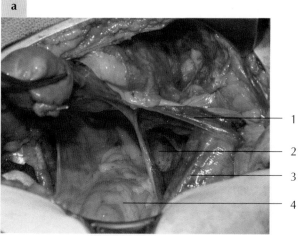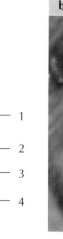

1 – Right cardinal ligament
2 – Right pararectal space
3 – Right external iliac vessels
4 – Rectum

1 – Left cardinal ligament
2 – Left uterine artery
3 – Left ureter

Figure 2.4. Pararectal space.
The pararectal space is bounded medially by the rectum and ureter, ventrally by the sacrum, laterally by the pelvic sidewall and internal iliac vessels, and anteriorly by the cardinal ligament. (**a**) Right pararectal space after blunt dissection; (**b**) left pararectal space with the uterine artery arising from the anterior division of the internal iliac artery and the ureter, which has not yet been completely unroofed.

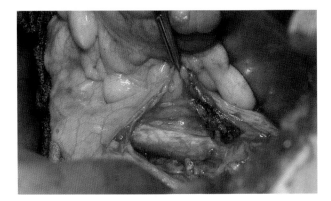

Figure 2.5. Pelvic lymphdenectomy.
The pelvic lymphadenectomy may be performed before or after the radical hysterectomy (this part of the procedure is described in more detail elsewhere in this text – see Chapter 1). The pelvic lymphadenectomy begins by incising the peritoneum overlying the external iliac artery. It proceeds with complete removal of all visible lymphatic tissue. This is considered a diagnostic and therapeutic procedure.

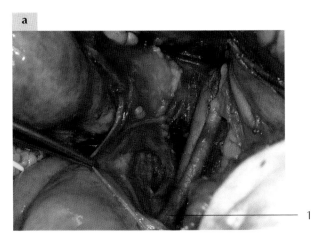

1 – Right common iliac artery bifurcation

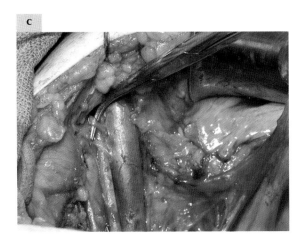

1 – Right deep circumflex iliac vein
2 – Right genitofemoral nerve
3 – Right external iliac vein

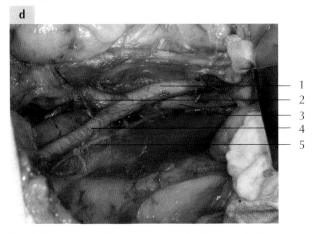

1 – Left common iliac artery
2 – Left internal iliac artery
3 – Left inferior vena cava
4 – Left external iliac artery
5 – Left genitofemoral nerve

Figure 2.6. Extent of dissection.
The lymphadenectomy begins proximally at the common iliac artery and proceeds distally until the deep circumflex iliac vein crosses over (or under in certain cases) the external iliac artery. (a) Bifurcation of the right common iliac artery into the external and internal (hypogastric) arteries is demonstrated. (b) Distal extent of the dissection, where the right external iliac vein gives off the deep circumflex iliac vein that crosses over the right external iliac artery. (c) The left deep circumflex iliac vein is seen crossing over the left external iliac artery. All visible lymphatic tissue surrounding these vessels has been removed. Care is taken to preserve the genitofemoral nerve, which runs in close proximity to the lateral aspect of the external iliac artery. (d) The proximal extent of dissection: here, the dissection is carried up to the top of the left common iliac artery. Care should be taken during any lymphadenectomy, as many patients may have vascular anomalies. This particular patient had the unusual anomaly of a duplicated inferior vena cava (IVC). Thus, the left IVC is seen lateral to the aortic bifurcation.

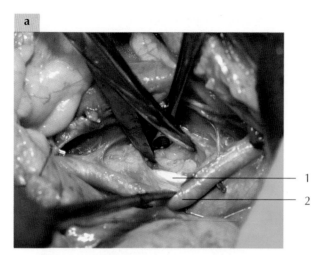

1 – Right obturator nerve
2 – Right external iliac artery

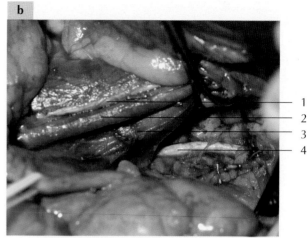

1 – Left genitofemoral nerve
2 – Left external iliac artery
3 – Left external iliac vein
4 – Left obturator nerve

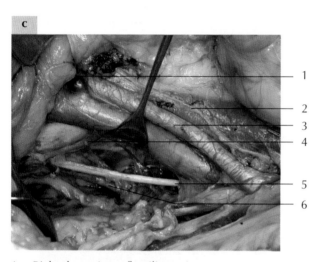

1 – Right deep circumflex iliac vein
2 – Right genitofemoral nerve
3 – Right external iliac artery
4 – Anastomotic pelvic vein
5 – Right obturator nerve
6 – Right obturator vein

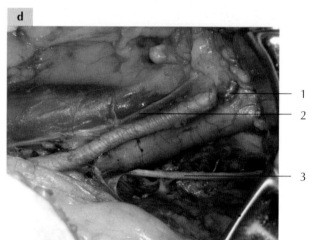

1 – Left deep circumflex iliac vein
2 – Left genitofemoral nerve
3 – Left obturator nerve

Figure 2.7. Obturator lymphadenectomy.
The obturator space can be entered laterally or medially to the external iliac vessels. (**a**) The right obturator nerve is identified laterally to the right external iliac artery, which is being retracted medially. Care should be taken to always locate the obturator nerve prior to excising any obturator lymph nodes. Transection of the obturator nerve will lead to some sensory loss of the upper medial aspect of the thigh and difficulty adducting the leg, which is often first noted getting into a bed or into a car. (**b**) The obturator nerve is now seen laterally to the external iliac artery and some obturator lymph nodes have been removed: further dissection will remove additional lymphatic tissue. Typically, all lymphatic tissue is removed superiorly to the obturator nerve, although many practitioners will clean out the entire obturator fossa, removing all visible nodal tissue and exposing the obturator internus muscle. The right (**c**) and left (**d**) obturator fossae are shown after removal of all lymph-node-bearing tissue. Both the obturator vein and the anastomotic pelvic vein can be seen in the right obturator dissection.

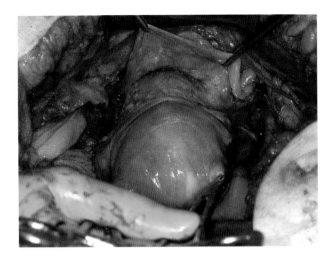

Figure 2.8. Bladder dissection.
After developing the pelvic spaces and transecting the round ligament, the vesicouterine peritoneum is incised in order to mobilize the bladder off of the uterus, cervix, and upper vagina. This dissection can be accomplished sharply with either scissors or electrocautery. Blunt dissection with sponges should be avoided, since this may increase the risk of vesicovaginal fistulae. The dissection is carried down so as to incorporate the upper 1–2 cm of the vagina. Dissection of this space also allows for assessment of possible tumor extension anteriorly. Here, the vesicouterine peritoneum is elevated and the bladder, with associated adipose tissue, has been dissected from the uterus, cervix, and vagina.

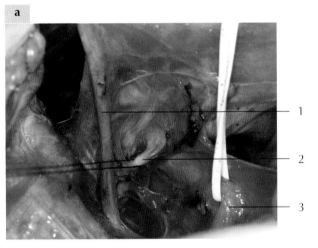

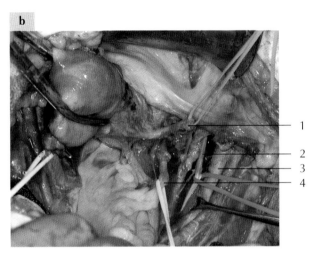

1 – Left superior vesical artery
2 – Left uterine artery
3 – Left ureter

1 – Right uterine artery
2 – Right obturator nerve
3 – Right external iliac vessels
4 – Right ureter

Figure 2.9. Uterine artery.
The uterine artery is dissected to its origin from the anterior division of the internal iliac artery. Although the uterine artery arises independently from the anterior division of the internal iliac artery in the majority of cases, anomalous origins may be seen. The uterine artery may arise from the internal iliac artery prior to its division or it may have common origin with the inferior vesical, middle rectal, internal pudendal, or vaginal arteries. It is important to note that the ureter courses inferior to the uterine artery in close proximity. (a) The left uterine artery, with a suture around it, is skeletonized to its origin. The ureter is illustrated by a yellow vessel loop and can be clearly seen heading beneath the uterine artery. (b) The right uterine artery (red vessel loop) has been further dissected to show its course toward the lateral aspect of the uterus. The ureter (yellow vessel loop) is again seen traveling directly underneath the artery. The lymphadenectomy has been completed and the obturator nerve (blue vessel loop) is seen in this image medially to the external iliac vessels and laterally to the internal iliac artery.

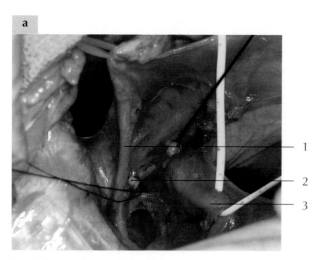

1 – Left superior vesical artery
2 – Transected left uterine artery
3 – Left ureter

1 – Left uterine artery
2 – Left ureter

Figure 2.10. Uterine artery divided.
(**a**) The left uterine artery is divided at its origin from the internal iliac artery with 3-0 silk sutures. In a simple hysterectomy, the artery would be taken at its insertion into the uterus instead of at its origin. Division of the uterine artery at its origin will allow the parametrium to be completely dissected. The uterine artery may be ligated by a variety of techniques including sutures, clamps, hemoclips, stapling devices, or bipolar coagulators. The ureter (yellow vessel loop) is again seen in its normal anatomic location beneath the uterine artery; the superior vesical artery has been identified with a blue vessel loop. (**b**) The left uterine artery is illustrated by a red vessel loop and a hemoclip can be seen being applied at the origin from the internal iliac artery. Usually, two to three hemoclips are placed proximally and one hemoclip is placed distally. The ureter is again illustrated with a yellow vessel loop.

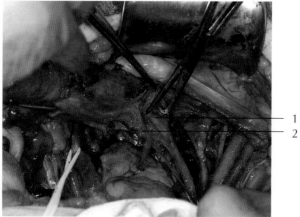

1 – Right ureter
2 – Right parametrium

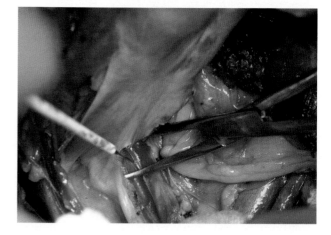

Figure 2.11. Unroofing the ureter.
The ureter is unroofed through the parametrial tunnel to its insertion into the bladder. This is accomplished with blunt and sharp dissection using a right-angled clamp and suture ligatures as needed. Unroofing the ureter allows complete mobilization of the parametrium toward the specimen; the parametrial tissue can be seen attached to the cervix. Care should be taken during this dissection: small vessels should be ligated with suture ligatures or hemoclips, since significant blood loss can occur during this part of the procedure. Electrocautery should be avoided, since the dissection is in such close proximity to the ureter.

Figure 2.12. Dissection of the rectovaginal space.
The rectovaginal peritoneum is incised with electrocautery and the rectovaginal space is developed with sharp or blunt dissection. Care should be taken to avoid injury to the rectum. Once the peritoneum is incised, the vagina is separated from the rectum.

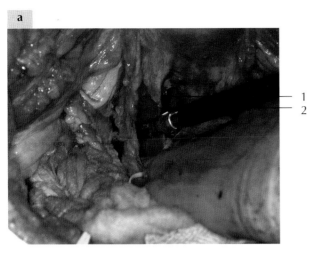

1 – Rectovaginal space
2 – Left uterosacral ligament

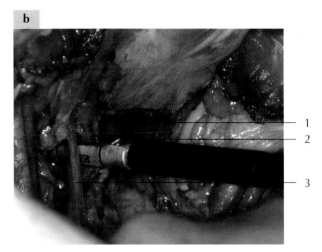

1 – Rectovaginal space
2 – Left uterosacral ligament
3 – Left ureter

Figure 2.13. Transection of the uterosacral ligaments.
(**a**) The surgeon's hands are in the developed rectovaginal space, and the rectum is retracted posteriorly toward the sacrum and medially toward the opposite side of the pelvis. The ureter has been mobilized from the medial aspect of the broad ligament and separated from the uterosacral ligament. The uterosacral ligament is seen between the surgeon's fingers with an endoscopic stapler applied. The uterosacral ligament can be transected with stapling devices, clamps, suture ligatures, or cautery. The uterosacral ligaments are transected close to their distal attachments in a Class III hysterectomy. In a Class II hysterectomy, the uterosacral ligaments would be transected more proximally. (**b**) The rectovaginal space has been further developed and the ureter has been cleaned off to show its relationship to the uterosacral ligament (grasped with the endoscopic stapler).

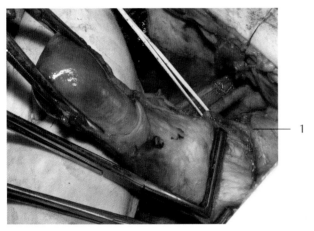

1 – Left ureteral insertion into bladder

Figure 2.14. Dividing the vagina (clamp technique).
After the uterosacral ligaments are transected and the bladder is adequately mobilized off the anterior vagina, the vagina is transected. This is typically accomplished by placing a Wertheim clamp, as shown here, to incorporate the upper 1–2 cm of the vagina and to ensure that the tumor is contained with the specimen. Zeppelin clamps or similar are used to secure the vaginal angles. Care should be taken when applying the Wertheim or Zeppelin clamps to avoid clamping, ligating, or transecting the ureter, which lies in close proximity as it enters the bladder. The vagina is then incised with a scalpel, scissors, or electrocautery.

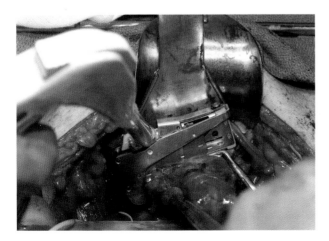

Figure 2.15. Dividing the vagina (stapler technique).
The vagina may also be divided with a thoracoabdominal stapling device, which divides the vagina and also staples the cut ends with synthetic absorbable staples. The use of stapling devices for transecting the vagina and the uterosacral ligaments can reduce blood loss and operative time.

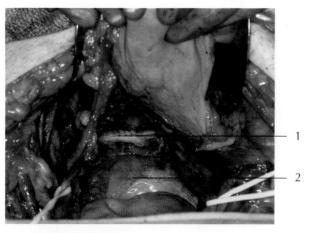

Figure 2.16. Pelvis after specimen removal.
The specimen (uterus, cervix, parametria, and upper vagina) has been removed. The ureters (yellow vessel loops) can be seen along their course into the bladder, which is lifted out of the pelvis and retracted anteriorly. The vaginal cuff has been approximated with the thoracoabdominal stapler. If a stapling device is not used, the vaginal cuff is approximated with hemostatic sutures. Hemostasis at all sites should be ensured prior to completion of the procedure. Pelvic drains and closure of the pelvic peritoneum is not required. The abdomen is closed in standard fashion.

1 – Stapled vaginal cuff
2 – Rectum

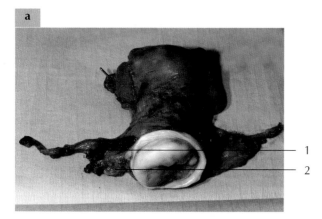

1 – Right uterine artery
2 – Right parametrium

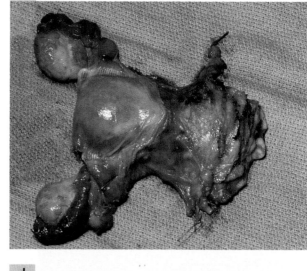

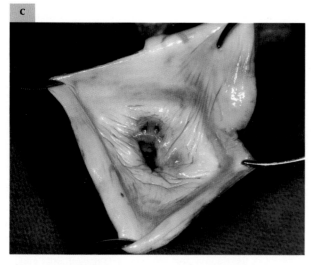

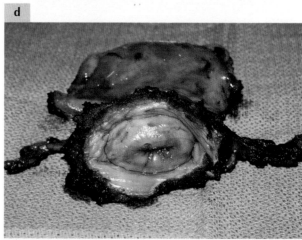

Figure 2.17. Radical hysterectomy specimens.
(**a**) The entire uterine artery is shown, as well as substantial parametrial tissue; the upper 1–2 cm of the vagina can also be seen; the ovaries were not removed in this case. (**b**) A specimen is shown with ovaries and tubes attached; adequate parametrial tissue is also seen in this specimen. (**c**) The vaginal cuff is splayed open to demonstrate adequate margins of resection; the lesion can be seen at the anterior cervicovaginal junction. (**d**) A specimen with the vaginal cuff transected by electrocautery: sufficient vaginal tissue was obtained and cautery artifact is evident. Were the lesion to be in the upper vagina, the cautery could obscure delineation of surgical margins.

References

1. Abu-Rustum NR, Hoskins WJ. Radical abdominal hysterectomy. *Surg Clin North Am* 2001; **52**:815–28.

2. Chi DS, Lanciano RM, Kudelka AP. Cervical cancer. In: (Pazdur R, Coia LR, Hoskins WJ, Wagman LD, eds) *Cancer Management: A Multidisciplinary Approach*, 5th edn. (PRR: Melville, NY, 2001) 359–84.

3. Landoni F, Maneo A, Colombo A et al. Randomised study of radical surgery versus radiotherapy for stage Ib–IIa cervical cancer. *Lancet* 1997; **350**:535–40.

4. Hoskins WJ, Perez CA, Young RC (eds). *Principles and Practice of Gynecologic Oncology*, 3rd edn. (Lippincott, Williams & Wilkins: Philadelphia, 2000).

5. Chi DS, Gemignani ML, Curtin JP, Hoskins WJ. Long-term experience in the surgical management of cancer of the uterine cervix. *Semin Surg Oncol* 1999; **17**:161–7.

6. Rose PG, Bundy BN, Watkins EB et al. Concurrent cisplatin-based radiotherapy and chemotherapy for locally advanced cervical cancer. *N Engl J Med* 1999; **340**:1144–53.

7. Morris M, Eifel PJ, Lu J et al. Pelvic radiation with concurrent chemotherapy compared with pelvic and paraaortic radiation for high-risk cervical cancer. *N Engl J Med* 1999; **340**:1137–43.

8. Whitney CW, Sause W, Bundy BN et al. Randomized comparison of fluorouracil plus cisplatin versus hydroxyurea as an adjunct to radiation therapy in stage IIB–IVA carcinoma of the cervix with negative paraaortic lymph nodes: a Gynecologic Oncology Group and Southwest Oncology Group study. *J Clin Oncol* 1999; **17**:1339–48.

9. Keys HM, Bundy BN, Stehman FB et al. Cisplatin, radiation, and adjuvant hysterectomy for bulky stage IB cervical carcinoma. *N Engl J Med* 1999; **340**:1154–61.

10. Piver SM, Rutledge F, Smith JP. Five classes of extended hysterectomy for women with cervical cancer. *Obstet Gynecol* 1974; **44**:265–72.

11. Landoni F, Maneo A, Cormio G et al. Class II versus class III radical hysterectomy in stage IB–IIA cervical cancer: a prospective randomized study. *Gynecol Oncol* 2001; **80**:3–12.

12. Scribner DR, Kamelle SA, Gould N et al. A retrospective analysis of radical hysterectomies done for cervical cancer: is there a role for the Pfannenstiel incision? *Gynecol Oncol* 2001; **81**:481–4.

13. Estape R, Angioli R, Wagman F et al. Significance of intraperitoneal cytology in patients undergoing radical hysterectomy. *Gynecol Oncol* 1998; **68**:169–71.

14. Potish RA, Downey GO, Adcock LL et al. The role of surgical debulking in cancer of the uterine cervix. *Int J Radiat Oncol Biol Phys* 1989; **17**:979–84.

15. Jensen JK, Lucci 3rd JA, DiSaia PJ et al. To drain or not to drain: a retrospective study of closed-suction drainage following radical hysterectomy with pelvic lymphadenectomy. *Gynecol Oncol* 1993; **51**:46–9.

16. Dargent D, Martin X, Sacchetoni A, Mathevet P. Laparoscopic vaginal radical trachelectomy: a treatment to preserve the fertility of cervical carcinoma patients. *Cancer* 2000; **88**:1877–82.

3 Surgical cytoreduction

Mario M Leitao Jr and William J Hoskins

Ovarian cancer is the fifth most common malignancy in women and the second most common gynecologic malignancy, but it is the leading cause of death of all gynecologic malignancies in the USA.[1] It is estimated that there will be 25,400 new cases of ovarian cancer in 2003 and an estimated 14,300 deaths in the USA.[1] Early-stage ovarian cancer has a high cure rate with surgery and chemotherapy. Unfortunately, 75% of patients will present with disease that is no longer confined to the ovary (FIGO Stage II–IV), in which long-term survival is worse.[2] Ovarian cancer can be thought of as a 'chronic' disease in the sense that many patients develop multiple recurrences that can often be induced into remission with further surgery and/or chemotherapy. Also, complications such as bowel obstruction are often a result of advanced, persistent, or recurrent ovarian cancer. Surgery is an essential modality in the treatment of ovarian cancer. Its role may be either therapeutic or palliative.

Advanced ovarian cancer is initially treated with a combination of surgery and chemotherapy. Surgery is most often performed prior to the initiation of chemotherapy. The goal of surgery in this setting should be to achieve a complete gross resection (complete cytoreduction) of all visible disease. Griffiths[3] first reported the value of surgical cytoreduction in 1975. Many retrospective studies and reviews since have confirmed that the amount of residual tumor strongly correlates with survival.[4–10] The adequacy of surgical cytoreduction is based on the maximum diameter of the largest residual tumor after cytoreduction and has been defined by specific cut-off levels. Cytoreduction to < 2 cm has been shown to provide a significant survival advantage.[4] Some authors have reported that cytoreduction to no visible disease offers an even greater benefit.[5,11] Cytoreductive surgery offers no benefit, except possibly for palliation of symptoms, if the tumor cannot be reduced to < 2 cm.[4] Based on more recent analyses, the Gynecologic Oncology Group (GOG) currently defines optimal cytoreduction as that in which the maximum diameter of residual tumor is ≤ 1 cm. The benefit of optimal cytoreduction has also been reported for patients with Stage IV disease (i.e. parenchymal liver metastases, distant metastases, and/or malignant pleural effusions).[12–15] Currently, there are no accurate or validated methods of preoperatively predicting optimal cytoreduction. Active research endeavors include using a combination of computerized tomography (CT) scanning, CA-125 levels, and physical examination to determine if the success of surgical cytoreduction can be predicted.

The rate of optimal cytoreduction varies between institutions, and to some degree depends on specialty training, philosophy and surgical aggressiveness.[16,17] It is essential that the surgeon is able to make a reasonable judgment as to the feasibility that any aggressive procedure will lead to optimal cytoreduction. The surgical morbidities must always be considered. Most often for the gynecologic oncologist, the extent of upper abdominal disease will limit the ability to perform optimal cytoreduction. Aggressive attempts at tumor resection may require radical hysterectomy, omentectomy, resection of either small or large intestine, splenectomy, diaphragmatic stripping, hepatic resection, or other related procedures. Splenectomy, diaphragmatic stripping, and hepatectomy, as well as elimination of peritoneal implants, can be safely performed in carefully selected patients with upper abdominal disease.[11,16,18–20] These procedures should be considered if they would result in an optimal cytoreduction. Bowel resection is often necessary, is safe to perform, and will offer a survival benefit if the end result is optimal cytoreduction.[9,21] Ovarian cancer rarely progresses below the pelvic peritoneal reflection and therefore it is possible to safely perform low colorectal anastomoses in the majority of cases.[21]

Patients who develop recurrent disease, or those with disease noted at the time of surgical reassessment procedures, will also benefit from cytoreduction.[6,18,22–25] These secondary cytoreductions offer the best survival benefits in patients with long disease-free intervals, solitary lesions, initial optimal cytoreduction, and who have responded well to prior chemotherapy.[23–25] In carefully selected patients, complete cytoreduction may be possible and appears to offer the best survival benefit if performed prior to the initiation of salvage chemotherapy.[25] The degree to which tumor must be cytoreduced to offer a benefit varies among reports. The goal in this setting should be to resect to no gross disease, but cytoreduction to < 2 cm may also be beneficial. Surgical cytoreduction has also been shown to benefit patients with advanced or recurrent endometrial cancer.[26–28] Therefore, the techniques and theories behind the procedures described in this chapter apply to properly selected patients with ovarian or endometrial cancer.

The role of palliative surgery for patients with persistent or recurrent ovarian cancer is not as well defined. A common manifestation of persistent or recurrent ovarian cancer is intestinal obstruction. These patients often have few remaining chemotherapy options. Patients should be thoroughly counseled that surgery in this setting will not be curative. Palliative surgery for intestinal obstruction has been shown to provide patients with symptomatic relief, prolonged survival, and the ability to ingest liquids and solids.[6] Since surgical morbidity can be high, patients should understand that the benefits of palliative surgery are not realized in all patients. The option of placing a percutaneous gastrostomy tube and receiving intravenous hydration should be discussed.

Successful surgical cytoreduction requires thorough knowledge of pelvic and abdominal anatomy. Normal anatomical structures and relations are often distorted in advanced ovarian cancer. The patient can be placed in the supine position if preoperative imaging and physical examination indicate the bulk of disease to be in the upper abdomen and radical pelvic surgery is unlikely. More commonly, radical pelvic and colorectal surgery must be anticipated, and the patient should be placed in the low lithotomy position. The skin should be antiseptically prepared from the breasts to the mid-thigh and perineum. A Foley catheter is placed in the urinary bladder. Rectal irrigation and suction may be considered in patients expected to undergo a colorectal anastomosis. All patients undergoing abdominal or pelvic surgery for gynecologic cancer should have pneumatic compression devices placed on the calves prior to the induction of anesthesia and should receive postoperative deep venous thrombosis prophylaxis with subcutaneous low-molecular-weight or unfractionated heparin.

A large vertical midline incision is critical. The peritoneal cavity is then entered carefully and any ascites suctioned. Omental tumor is generally removed first to aid visualization. Then, resection of the pelvic and abdominal disease is performed. Retroperitoneal nodal disease is usually assessed and resected after gross pelvic and abdominal disease has been removed. Entering the retroperitoneum and identifying the ureters and aortoiliac vessels early is essential in accomplishing successful cytoreduction and minimizing complications. If isolated disease is the target of resection, this is carried out after thorough evaluation of the abdomen and pelvis to identify unexpected sites of disease. A thorough mechanical and antibiotic bowel preparation is often prescribed prior to a planned surgical cytoreduction. Some data have suggested that such a vigorous preoperative bowel regimen may not actually decrease postoperative morbidity.

In this section, after a brief overview of advanced ovarian cancer, the procedures commonly performed for surgical cytoreduction of advanced and recurrent ovarian and endometrial cancers will be presented. Some procedures such as radical hysterectomy, omentectomy, and lymphadenectomy are described elsewhere in this *Atlas* and will therefore only be briefly touched upon in this section. Other specific procedures, such as partial hepatectomy, will not be presented here and may be found in general surgical atlases and texts. Most procedures are equally applicable to widely disseminated advanced disease and to isolated recurrences.

Advanced ovarian cancer

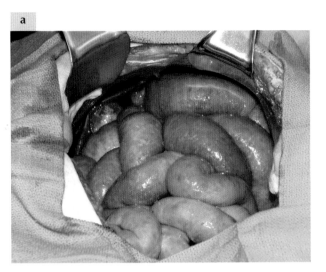

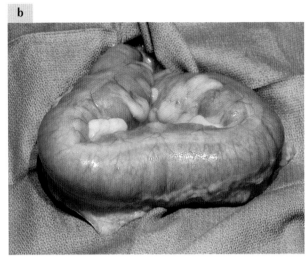

Figure 3.1. Bowel distention.
Patients with advanced or recurrent ovarian cancer often develop signs and symptoms of intestinal obstruction. This may be a result of tumor causing a point obstruction, diffuse mesenteric carcinomatosis, or adhesive disease. The patient may present with diffuse small bowel (**a**) or large bowel (**b**) distention depending on the point of obstruction. An intestinal resection and/or bypass may be required in order to relieve the obstruction.

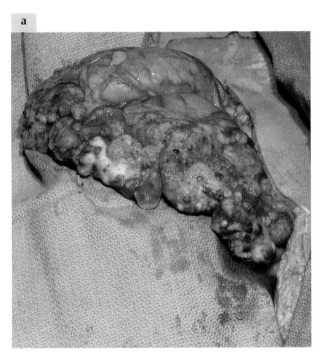

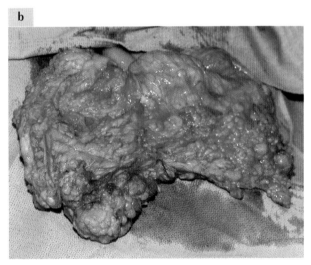

Figure 3.2 (a and b). Nodular omental tumor.
Extensive involvement of the omentum is common in advanced ovarian cancer. Here, diffuse nodular involvement of the omentum is observed. This is often referred to as an omental 'cake'. A gastrocolic omentectomy is necessary in such patients to remove all omental disease. If the omental disease is not growing onto the transverse colon or stomach, the removal is relatively straightforward. This type of omentectomy is described in the chapter on staging laparotomy (Chapter 1).

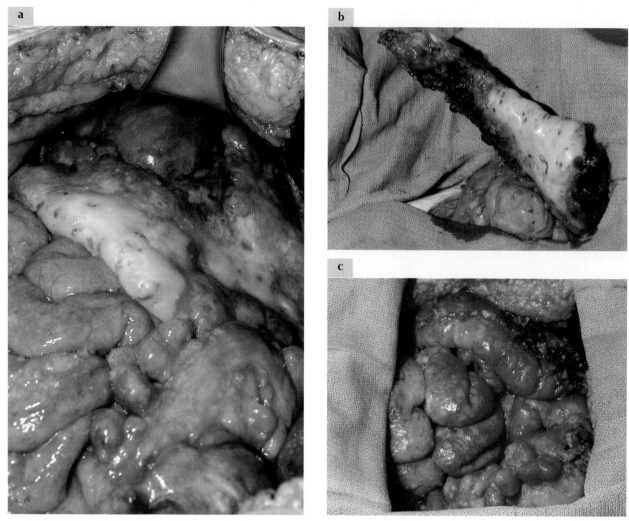

Figure 3.3. Solid omental tumor.
Some ovarian cancers form more solid and sheet-like masses. These tumors are not as easily resected off the transverse colon and stomach. Careful dissection is mandated to avoid injury to the transverse colon, and segmental bowel resection may occasionally be required. This solid omental 'cake' is seen in situ (**a**), after partial removal (**b**) and after complete resection (**c**). Residual tumor remains in the gastrocolic ligament and will be excised subsequently. Additionally, tumor nodules can be seen along the sigmoid colon in this patient, who ultimately required a low anterior resection to accomplish optimal cytoreduction.

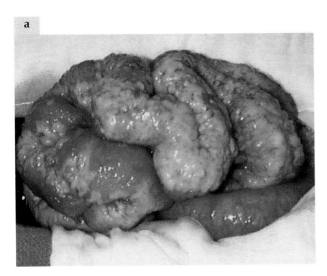
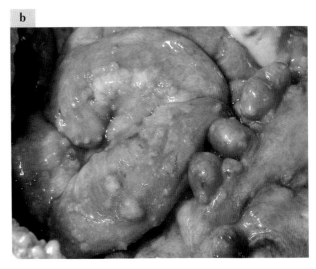

Figure 3.4. Intestinal carcinomatosis.

(**a**) Diffuse carcinomatosis of the small intestine may be seen in advanced ovarian cancer; (**b**) the large intestine may also be involved in a similar fashion – this frequently leads to obstructive symptoms. Resection of involved portions of the small or large intestine may be necessary to relieve the obstruction or to achieve an optimal cytoreduction. Judgment must be used to prevent the removal of excessive small intestine, which may lead to short bowel syndrome. In certain settings, more extensive bowel resection is appropriate. Factors to consider are the potential for prolonged disease-free survival, chemotherapy options available for a given patient, and the extent of intraabdominal disease. These factors guide the surgeon in determining the appropriate level of aggressiveness.

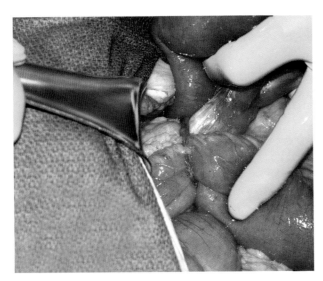

Figure 3.5. Adhesive disease.

Adhesive disease is often seen in the setting of advanced or recurrent ovarian cancer. Adhesive bands may be formed from inflammatory processes stimulated by the cancer itself or after surgery; simply releasing these bands may relieve the obstruction. The small bowel should be carefully inspected to ensure its integrity and viability. Necrotic or unhealthy appearing intestine should be resected. Occasionally, intestinal obstruction is completely due to adhesive bands in the absence of suspected recurrent disease, and both the surgeon and patient are pleasantly surprised. It can be difficult to determine from preoperative imaging whether the blockage is from adhesions or small-volume disease. Usually, carcinomatosis or large-volume disease is readily detectable from radiographic studies.

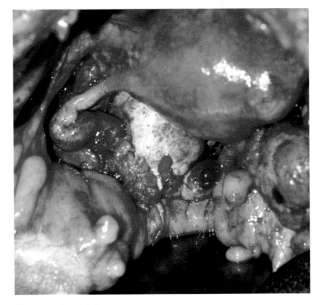

Figure 3.6. Pelvic tumor.

The primary ovarian mass seen here completely encompasses the posterior cul-de-sac. A radical hysterectomy and oophorectomy is needed to remove pelvic disease that is adherent to the cul-de-sac and pelvic sidewall. The procedure for standard radical hysterectomy is described elsewhere in this text. A radical pelvic resection usually requires techniques from radical hysterectomy and low anterior resection combined into a modified posterior exenteration, which is discussed later in this chapter.

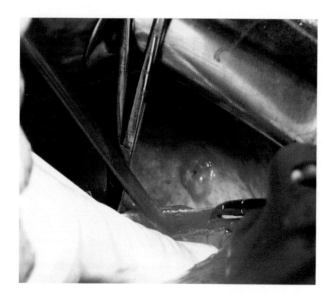

Figure 3.7. Diaphragmatic tumor.
Nodular or plaque-like implants may be encountered on the diaphragmatic surfaces. The peristaltic action of the intestines and the motion of the diaphragm accounts for finding disease more often on the right hemidiaphragm as opposed to the left. Removal of diaphragmatic nodules may be accomplished by using electrocautery, argon-beam coagulation, or a Cavitron ultrasonic surgical aspirator. Diaphragmatic stripping is required for extensive involvement of the diaphragm and is discussed in detail in this chapter.

Entering the abdomen

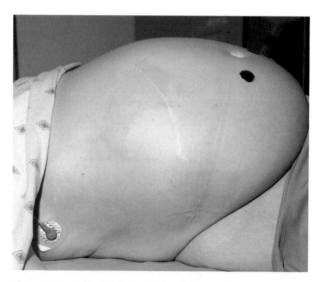

Figure 3.8. Advanced ovarian cancer.
Patients with advanced ovarian cancer often present with significant abdominal distention secondary to massive ascites. Shown is a patient with marked abdominal distention. It is prudent to drain the ascites slowly to avoid sudden hemodynamic changes. This patient has been marked in both lower quadrants for possible colostomy or ileostomy. The main reason preoperatively marking a patient for potential colostomy is to ensure that the colostomy is not placed directly at the waistline or in a subcutaneous fold, which would lead to compression when the patient flexes at the hip.

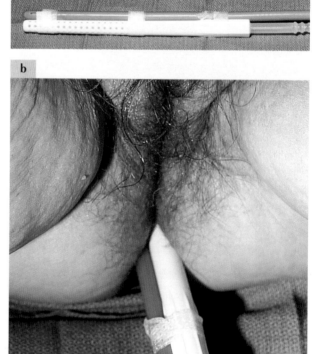

Figure 3.9. Rectal irrigation.
The use of a rectal irrigation/suction system may be considered if the preoperative bowel preparation is inadequate or if a rectal resection is likely. (**a**) To set up the system, a pool suction tip is attached to a large-bore Foley catheter with surgical tape or Steri-Strips. (**b**) This is then placed into the rectum and 1 l of sterile saline solution, with or without dilute Betadine, is introduced through the Foley catheter via gravity and suctioned with the pool suction tip.

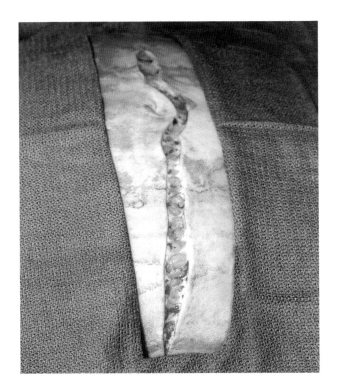

Figure 3.10. Abdominal incision.
A large vertical midline incision is necessary. If large-volume disease is not expected, the initial abdominal incision can be less generous and extended later in the procedure if needed. The amount of abdominal distention and ascites in this patient was consistent with the patient's preoperative imaging studies; therefore, a fairly large incision extending from the symphysis pubis to around and superior to the umbilicus was made. Rarely, it may be necessary to excise the umbilicus if it is infiltrated with tumor.

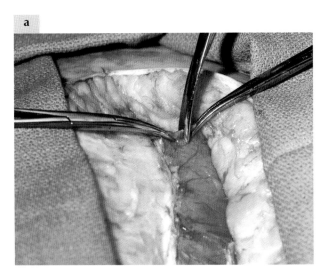
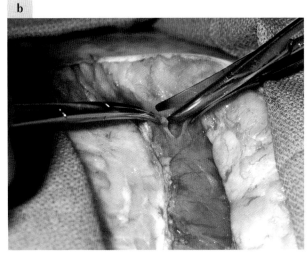

Figure 3.11. Entering the peritoneum.
The peritoneal cavity is entered carefully to prevent spillage of ascites. In this figure, the abdominal incision has been taken down to the level of the peritoneum. (**a**) A hyperemic peritoneum is grasped with clamps in the midline and incised using Metzenbaum scissors. (**b**) The clamps are left in place to provide gentle traction on the peritoneum to prevent spillage during aspiration of the ascites. This peritoneal incision is then extended just enough to allow entry of a pool suction tip.

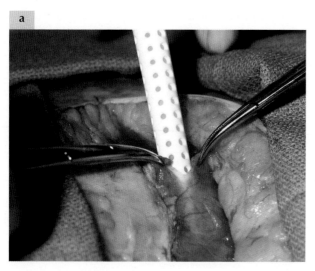
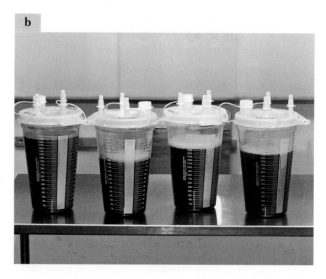

Figure 3.12. Drainage of ascites.
(**a**) The pool suction tip is passed through the newly created peritoneal incision while still grasping the peritoneum with clamps. The peritoneum is then sharply incised, using either scissors or electrocautery, along the full length of the abdominal incision after all the ascites has been drained. In cases with large-volume ascites, two suction apparatuses set-up prior to entering the peritoneum is useful in preventing spillage and in preventing delays when changing the suction canisters. (**b**) Nearly 8 l of ascites were drained from this patient. The color of the ascitic fluid can vary from clear to straw-colored or blood-tinged. Occasionally, the ascites will contain frank blood, which is usually due to recent bleeding from tumor implants.

Diaphragmatic stripping

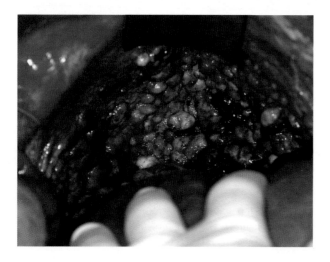

Figure 3.13. Diaphragmatic plaque.
The right diaphragm is most often involved with nodular or plaque-like metastatic tumor implants, as can be seen in this image. Initially, the liver is mobilized solely by the surgeon's hands. This is adequate for focal, limited, superficial anterior nodules, or for small plaques. The midline abdominal incision usually needs to be extended to the xiphoid process in order to reach the diaphragm. It may be necessary to extensively mobilize the liver in order to completely strip all disease off the diaphragm. The falciform ligament should be transected all the way to the coronary ligament and held for traction. The triangular ligament can provide additional medial mobilization and access to the posterior aspect of the diaphragm. Fixed retraction can also be invaluable during this part of the procedure. A well-positioned Bookwalter retractor is often sufficient; however, the Goligher retractor, with or without a Balfour retractor, provides excellent retraction.

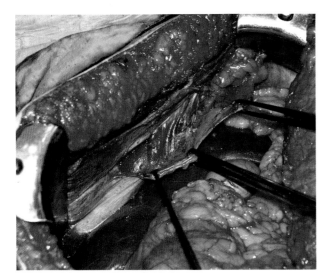

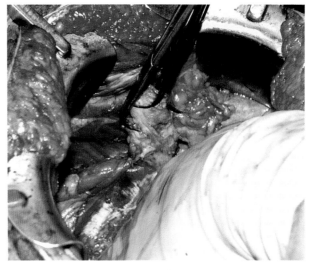

Figure 3.14. Entering the retroperitoneum.
The peritoneum overlying the anterior diaphragm is incised along the costal margin or more proximally if necessary. Allis clamps are then used to grasp the free peritoneal edge, and the plane between the peritoneum and diaphragm is developed sharply with electrocautery or scissors. This dissection can occasionally be accomplished with blunt dissection using a free hand, while traction on the peritoneum is maintained with the other hand. This may not be possible if the tumor has extended into or through the diaphragm.

Figure 3.15. Stripping the diaphragm.
The involved peritoneum is excised once it is completely dissected off the diaphragm: care should be taken to ensure hemostasis. Allis clamps or right-angled clamps help to maintain traction on the specimen during dissection. The specimen can be removed en-bloc if feasible; however, segmental resection is appropriate to improve visualization. A partially resected specimen may impair access to the remainder of the diaphragmatic disease.

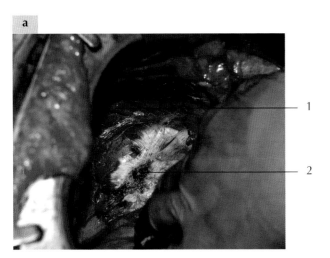

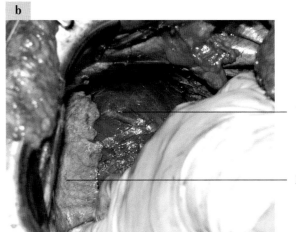

1 – Diaphragm
2 – Central tendon

1 – Diaphragm
2 – Residual peritoneum

Figure 3.16. Stripped diaphragm.
(a) After the involved diaphragmatic peritoneum is completely removed, the muscular and tendinous portions of the diaphragm can be seen. The white portion is the central tendon of the diaphragm and is the most common area of perforation into the chest. (b) A partial peritoneal resection is appropriate for more limited disease. The integrity of the diaphragm can be checked visually for any obvious defects. Furthermore, saline placed in the area of dissection will help check for air bubbles during inspiration. If a hole is detected, a #14 Red Robinson or Foley catheter can be placed through the hole and a purse-string suture applied. The purse string is tied down as the catheter is removed. Chest tube placement is rarely necessary, except for large defects that require mesh closure. Hemostasis of the liver should be assured prior to completion of the procedure.

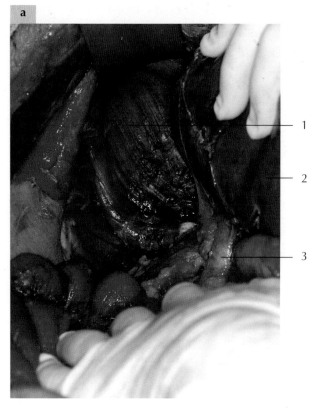

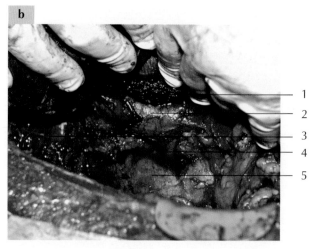

1 – Liver retracted medially
2 – Inferior vena cava
3 – Diaphragm
4 – Right renal vein
5 – Right kidney

Figure 3.17. Hepatorenal recess.
(**a**) The liver has undergone extensive mobilization in order to reach the most posterior and lateral aspect of the diaphragm. The inferior vena cava can be seen entering the posterior aspect of the liver. (**b**) The dissection has been carried through Gerota's fascia and the right renal vein can be seen entering the hilum of the right kidney. This patient had tumor extending from the diaphragmatic peritoneum onto Gerota's fascia. At the conclusion of the procedure the patient had no gross residual disease.

1 – Diaphragm
2 – Liver retracted medially
3 – Inferior vena cava

Figure 3.18. Specimen removed.
The involved diaphragmatic peritoneum is sent for routine pathologic analysis.

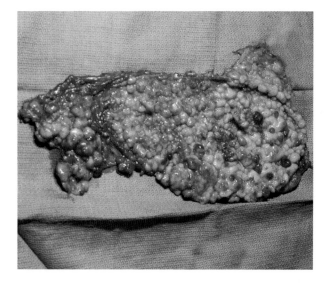

Low anterior resection and modified posterior exenteration

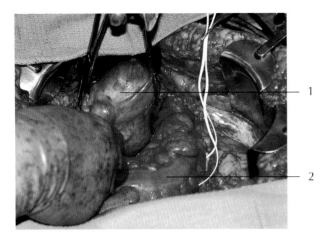

1 – Uterus
2 – Sigmoid

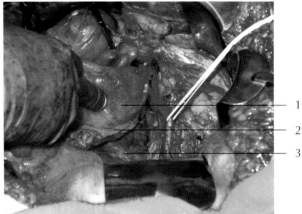

1 – Sigmoid
2 – Peritoneal reflection
3 – Presacral space

Figure 3.19. Initiating the resection.
The uterus and rectosigmoid are targeted for removal. Removal of the uterus en-bloc with the rectosigmoid is referred to as a modified posterior exenteration. Removal of the rectosigmoid by itself is a low anterior resection. If the resection does not progress below the peritoneal reflection, then it is simply an anterior resection. In ovarian cancer, the resection is almost always limited to above the pelvic diaphragm, resulting in sufficient rectal length to perform a stapled low rectal anastomosis. The development of the retroperitoneal space is this first part of the procedure. After entering the retroperitoneum, the ureters are identified and the infundibulopelvic ligaments are divided if the ovaries have not been previously removed.

Figure 3.20. Developing the presacral space.
The presacral space is then developed with care to mobilize the sigmoid colon. Sharp dissection is used to ensure that the dissection takes place in the proper plane and the risk of presacral bleeding is minimized. If the dissection proceeds above Waldeyer's fascia, presacral bleeding can easily be avoided. Bleeding from the sacral vessels is difficult to manage, as the vessels tend to retract. Sterile tacks or bone cement may be used to control such bleeding. Here, the rectosigmoid is seen being retracted anteriorly with the ureter identified with a white vessel loop and the presacral space developed.

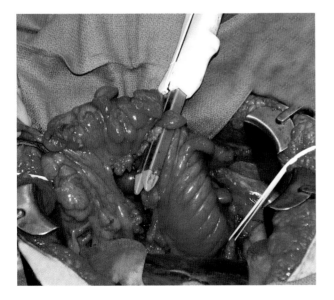

Figure 3.21. Transecting the bowel.
Usually, the vascular supply to the rectosigmoid is ligated and transected prior to dividing the colon. The inferior mesenteric artery can be ligated; however, it is appropriate to ligate only the sigmoid branches and the superior hemorrhoidal artery, while leaving the left colic artery patent. If tumor is obscuring the sigmoid mesentery this may not be possible. The sigmoid colon is freed of its peritoneal attachments and transected using a disposable stapling device. The point of transection should be proximal to the pelvic tumor and free of disease itself.

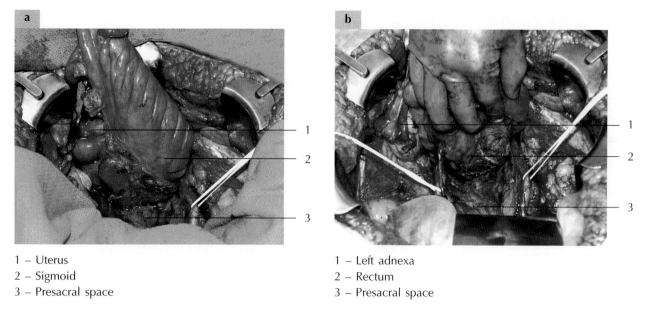

1 – Uterus
2 – Sigmoid
3 – Presacral space

1 – Left adnexa
2 – Rectum
3 – Presacral space

Figure 3.22. Presacral space.
Mobilizing the rectum from the sacral hollow further develops the presacral space. Once the major vascular pedicles have been ligated in the sigmoid mesentery the presacral dissection is relatively bloodless if the correct plane has been found. The lateral rectal pillars do not contain perforating blood vessels. Continuing the dissection with electrocautery is sufficient, as only rarely will a vessel be encountered. (**a**) Elevating the sigmoid sharply will locate the areolar tissue to keep the dissection in the proper plane. (**b**) The ureters can serve as a guide for dissection as they should continually be released laterally.

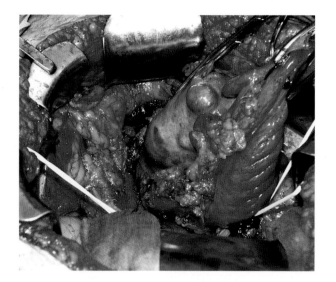

Figure 3.23. En-bloc resection.
The uterus and colon are treated as a single unit. The uterus is freed from its surrounding attachments as described previously. When performing a modified posterior exenteration the uterine arteries are usually encountered as they traverse the ureters; they can be clamped, ligated, and transected at this level. The vesicouterine peritoneum is incised in the usual fashion and the bladder is mobilized as far caudally as possible.

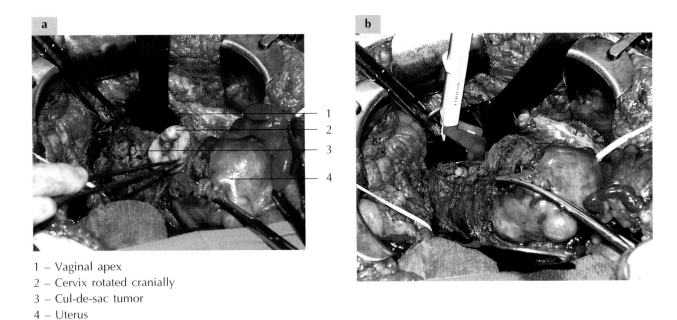

1 – Vaginal apex
2 – Cervix rotated cranially
3 – Cul-de-sac tumor
4 – Uterus

Figure 3.24. Modified posterior exenteration.
Once the bladder has been mobilized off the vagina, and the rectum has been dissected below the tumor, the specimen can be removed. The rectal tube should be cleared of its mesenteric fat to allow for easier placement of the stapler. The rectal transection is the last part of the specimen removal and therefore a retrograde hysterectomy is performed. (**a**) The vagina is entered and the cervix is brought into the pelvis. Straight clamps are placed on the vaginal mucosa, which can be closed at this point or after the entire specimen is removed. (**b**) The rectum is then divided above the pelvic diaphragm with a linear stapler.

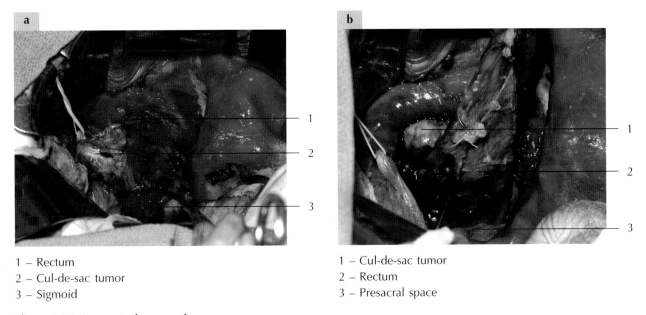

1 – Rectum
2 – Cul-de-sac tumor
3 – Sigmoid

1 – Cul-de-sac tumor
2 – Rectum
3 – Presacral space

Figure 3.25. Low anterior resection.
If the rectosigmoid resection is being performed for recurrent disease, the uterus and adnexa will have been removed previously. Shown here are anterior (**a**) and posterior (**b**) views of recurrent cul-de-sac tumor that is invading the rectosigmoid colon.

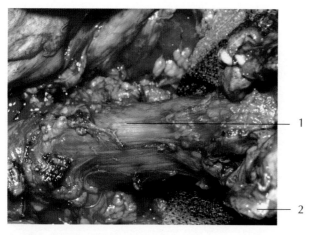

Figure 3.26. Prepared rectum.
The rectum is cleared of its mesenteric fat so that a stapler will fit across it without difficulty.

1 – Rectum
2 – Recurrent tumor

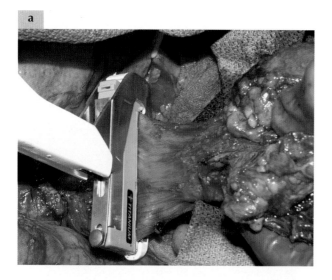

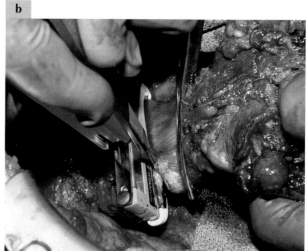

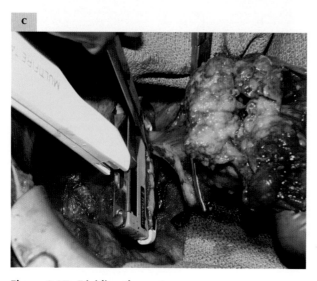

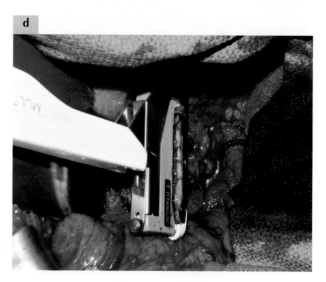

Figure 3.27. Dividing the rectum.
(**a**) The linear stapler is placed across the rectum and closed. (**b**) A large Kocher clamp or similar is placed across the proximal rectum to prevent spillage. The stapler is fired but not released. (**c**) The rectum is then incised using a scalpel along the superior edge of the stapler. The specimen is removed and placed off the operative field. (**d**) The stapler can then be released.

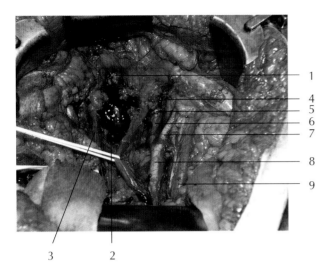

Figure 3.28. Pelvis.
Here, the pelvis is seen as it appears after removal of the specimen. The ureter is retracted medially and the normal pelvic anatomy is exposed.

1 – Vaginal apex
2 – Sacral hollow
3 – Left ureter
4 – Right external iliac vein
5 – Ligated right uterine artery
6 – Right internal iliac artery
7 – Right external iliac artery
8 – Right common iliac artery
9 – Psoas muscle

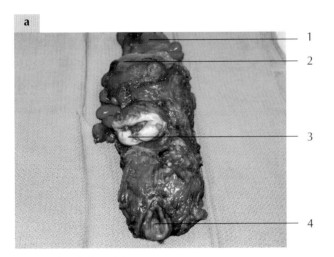

1 – Proximal sigmoid
2 – Uterine body
3 – Cervix
4 – Distal rectum

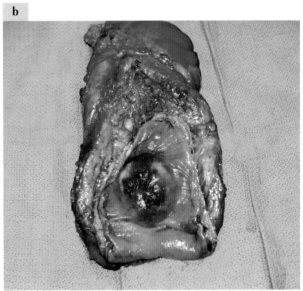

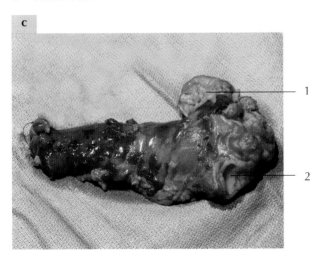

1 – Recurrent tumor
2 – Distal rectum

Figure 3.29. Modified posterior exenteration and low anterior resection specimens.
(a) Shown is the en-bloc modified posterior exenteration specimen consisting of the uterus and rectosigmoid. (b) The distal rectum opened with tumor invading from the posterior cul-de-sac through the rectal mucosa. (c) In a low anterior resection, the uterus has been previously removed and the tumor can be seen within the diseased rectosigmoid.

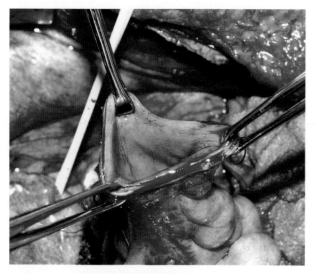

Figure 3.30. Opening the bowel.
The previously stapled end of the sigmoid is opened by excising the staple line with a knife or scissors. The opened bowel should be healthy appearing with viable mucosal tissue.

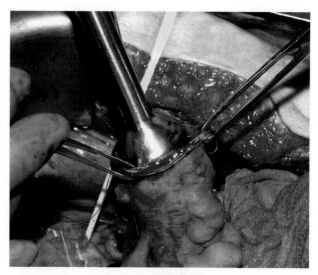

Figure 3.31. Rectal sizers.
A purse-string is placed around the open sigmoid with either a hand suture or an auto-purse-string device. A nonabsorbable 2-0 suture on a small needle should be used. Rectal sizers are then used to determine the proper stapler diameter. The largest sizer that will fit without difficulty should be used.

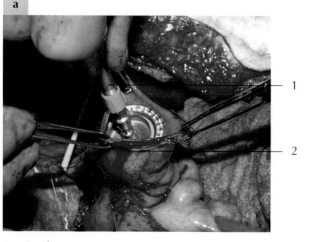

1 – Anvil
2 – Purse string

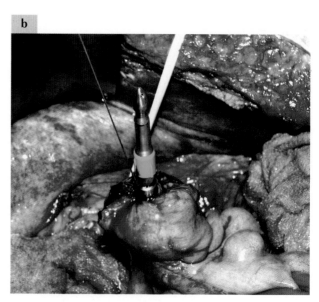

Figure 3.32. Placing the anvil.
(**a**) The anvil is placed into the open end of the sigmoid colon. (**b**) The previously placed purse string is securely tied to the shaft of the anvil to bring in the edges of the colon. If the suture is not tied tightly, the bowel edge may retract when compressed by the stapler leading to a defective anastomosis.

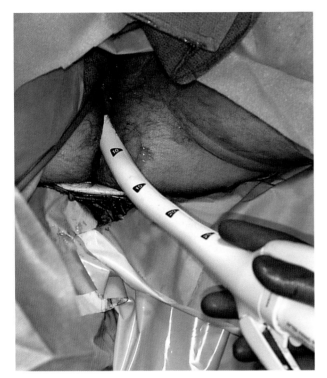

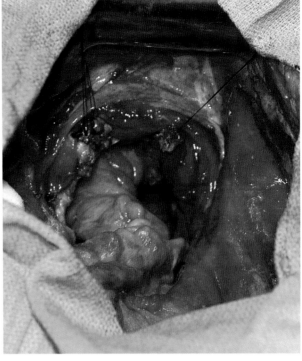

Figure 3.33. Transrectal stapler.

The shaft of the circular end-to-end anastomosis (EEA) stapler is lubricated after the removable trocar has been inserted into the cartridge head and fully retracted. It is then passed through the anus and advanced to the staple line of the distal rectum. The trocar is then advanced until it pierces through the rectal staple line. Once fully extended, the trocar is grasped and removed with a clamp through the abdomen. The trocar and clamp should be placed off the operative field as they are contaminated from their passage through the rectum.

Figure 3.34. Anastomosing the bowel.

The trocar is passed through the rectal staple line and engaged with the cartridge head. The stapler is then locked and fired, simultaneously stapling the anastomosis and removing the intraluminal tissue. Once the fired stapler is removed, the colorectal anastomosis is complete. The anastomosis can be examined with a rigid proctoscope and insufflated with air to check for leaks. If the pelvis is filled with saline, any air leak will result in bubbles through the saline.

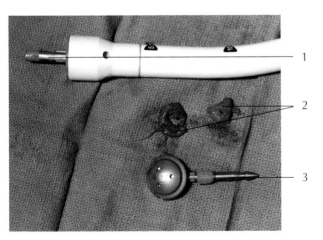

1 – Retractable stalk for disposable trocar
2 – Complete doughnuts
3 – Anvil

Figure 3.35. Colorectal anastomosis.

A colorectal anastomosis is commonly performed with a circular end-to-end anastomosis (EEA) stapler. The EEA stapler consists of a handle with a safety release (not shown), a cartridge head, and an anvil with a trocar. There are centimeter markings on the shaft to help determine the level of the anastomosis. The stapler simultaneously staples and excises excess tissue from the inverted anastomosis. The two excised specimens are referred to as 'doughnuts' and should be examined for completeness. If they are complete, it is unlikely that there is any unopposed tissue at the anastomosis site. The use of disposable stapling instruments has made performing such anastomoses more rapid and efficient. These benefits are particularly appreciated when they are conducted as one of several radical procedures in the surgical cytoreduction of an individual patient.

End colostomy

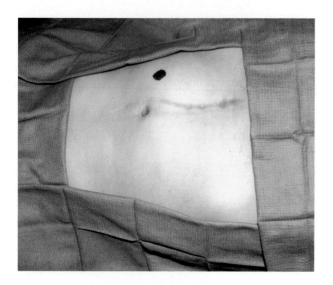

Figure 3.36. Stoma.
An enterostomal therapist preoperatively marks the patient to serve as a guide when creating the stoma. Generally, the stoma is placed midway between the umbilicus and the anterior superior iliac spine: it should come out through the rectus muscles. It is helpful to mark the patient prior to surgery with the patient in a variety of positions. This will allow the patient to participate in the location of the stoma and allow her to meet the enterostomal therapist prior to the procedure. If the patient does not have a prior midline incision that goes around the umbilicus, it is prudent to place the incision to the right of the umbilicus so that the left-sided colostomy is ultimately further away from the incision. If the patient has a previous high midline incision, it is not a good idea to create a second scar on the opposite side of the umbilicus.

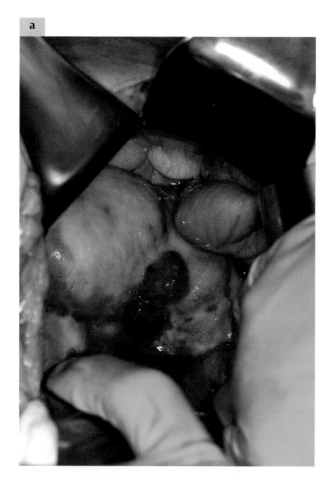

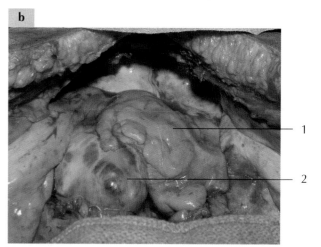

1 – Sigmoid
2 – Recurrent pelvic tumor

Figure 3.37 (a and b). Pelvic tumor.
In advanced ovarian cancer, an end colostomy is created when a low rectal anastomosis is not technically feasible. Reasons to create an end colostomy at the time of primary surgery would include inadequate mobilization of the sigmoid colon to allow for a tension-free anastomosis, inadequate bowel preparation, the need to limit operative time due to significant medical co-morbidities or instability under anesthesia, or poor vascular supply to the anastomosis. In recurrent ovarian cancer, an end colostomy is often created when a large unresectable pelvic tumor is the cause of a large bowel obstruction, as shown here. Thus, an end colostomy may be part of a modified posterior exenteration, a low anterior resection, secondary cytoreduction, or surgery for large bowel obstruction.

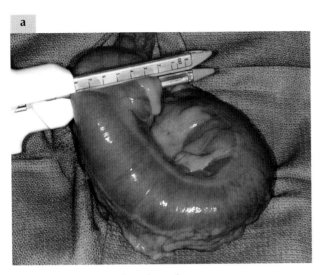 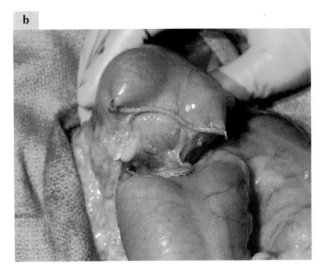

Figure 3.38. Transecting the colon.

A disease-free area for dividing the colon is chosen. A small defect is created in the mesentery close to the colon. Any excess fat or epiploicae can be removed at this point or prior to maturing the colostomy. The colon is then transected with a disposable stapler. This procedure can be easily accomplished with a scalpel to transect the bowel and a noncrushing clamp to prevent spillage. However, with current technology, a disposable stapler results in a faster and safer procedure for the patient and the surgeon. (**a**) An 80-mm gastrointestinal anastomosis (GIA) stapler is placed across the large intestine and then closed with the colon completely within the cut line on the instrument. The stapler is fired in a firm continuous motion, which simultaneously staples and divides the colon. (**b**) The divided ends are then inspected for defects and hemostasis.

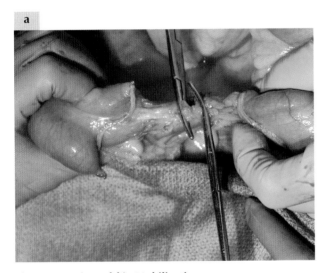 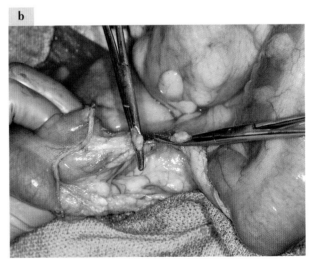

Figure 3.39 (a and b). Mobilization.

The mesentery is divided to reduce any tension on the portion of the colon that will be brought through the skin. Tension on the colostomy can lead to subsequent stomal retraction. Mobilization is accomplished by successively clamping, cutting, and ligating the colonic mesentery.

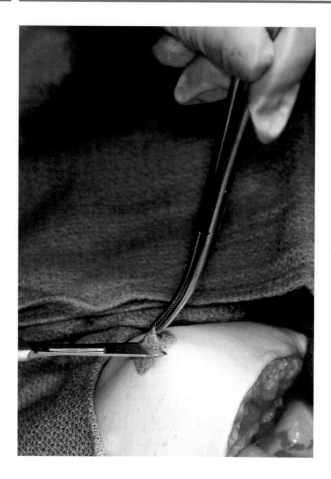

Figure 3.40. Making the stoma.
The skin is grasped with a Kocher or similar traumatic clamp. A 2–2.5 cm circle of skin in the center of the previously marked spot is excised using a knife. The scalpel is held parallel to the abdominal wall in order to create a symmetric ostomy. This site should overlie the rectus muscle so that the bowel can be brought out through the belly of the rectus. Often the preoperative marking is useful to determine the vertical positioning of the stoma to avoid placing it at the waistline or in body folds; however, the horizontal placement of the stoma should be determined at the time of the procedure so that it is through the rectus muscle and not too close to the incision. By placing the bowel through the rectus muscle, the risks of prolapse and herniation are minimized. The resulting defect should be about the size of a United States quarter, which is 2.5 cm in diameter. In general, the stoma site ends up being larger than expected. Should the site be too small to fit the colon through, it can always be enlarged, which is much easier than trying to taper a stoma site that is too large from the outset. Furthermore, the colon is usually edematous from handling and manipulation, so a snug ostomy is preferred to prevent subsequent prolapse when the edema resolves.

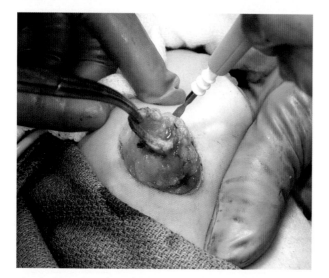

Figure 3.41. Removing the subcutaneous tissue.
The subcutaneous tissue and fat can be bluntly dissected, especially in thin patients. Here, the subcutaneous tissue is excised down to the anterior rectus fascia using electrocautery as traction is maintained with the clamp. Clearing the subcutaneous tissue is not absolutely necessary, but will help to mature the colostomy and facilitate suture placement.

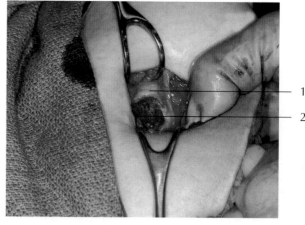

1 – Anterior rectus sheath
2 – Rectus abdominus

Figure 3.42. Incising the anterior rectus fascia.
A cruciate incision is made in the anterior rectus fascia. This incision should also be made conservatively, as it can easily be stretched with instruments or manually as needed to result in the proper size stoma. When completed, the rectus muscle is seen through the defect in the fascia.

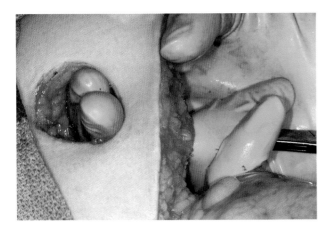

Figure 3.43. Sizing the stoma.

The rectus muscle is separated bluntly, and the posterior fascia (if present) and the peritoneum are incised sharply or bluntly. It is important to align the skin and fascia from the abdominal incision at the level of the stoma to prevent angulation of the colon as it traverses the anterior abdominal wall. The stoma site can be stretched bluntly until it accommodates two normal-sized fingers. If this is not possible to accomplish bluntly, additional fascia can be incised or additional skin can be excised.

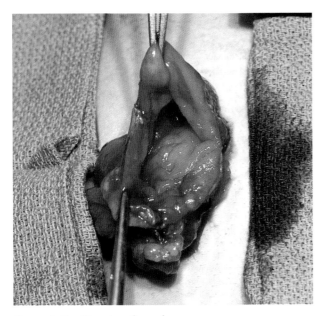

Figure 3.45. Opening the colon.

Towels or laparotomy pads are placed around the exteriorized colon. The entire staple line of the colon is excised sharply with a scalpel or scissors. Electrocautery is not used to open the colon due to the small risk of combustion from methane gas that can accumulate within the large intestine. A pool suction tip should be ready in case bowel contents begin to spill. They can be suctioned and/or collected with towels and pads. For this reason, the colon is opened only after the abdominal incision has been closed. The distal edge should be pink to ensure that the vascular supply has not been compromised. If a small portion is dusky, it can usually be excised; however, if a major portion is very dark, the entire colostomy may need to be revised.

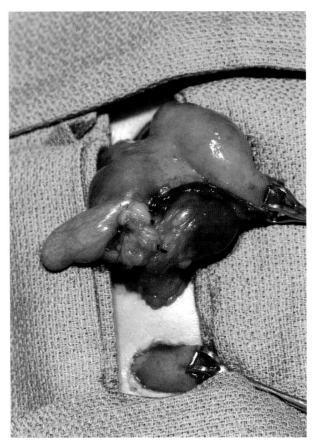

Figure 3.44. Exteriorizing the colon.

Using a Babcock clamp, the afferent limb of the divided colon is brought through the newly created abdominal passage. In general, the bowel should be pushed rather than pulled through the abdominal wall. If the bowel does not come through the stoma easily, the mesentery may be too short or the ostomy may be too small. If the bowel comes through the stoma too easily, tapering may be required to prevent subsequent prolapse or herniation. Excessively redundant fat or epiploicae can be excised, but it is important not to clean the bowel too much as this may lead to devascularization. If a small, unobstructed distal rectum is present it can be left closed as a Hartmann pouch. Usually, a nonabsorbable monofilament suture is placed at the apex of the rectal stump and left very long. This is helpful when searching for the rectal stump at the time of rectal reanastomosis. If operating for a large bowel obstruction, the distal rectosigmoid may be obstructed. In this case, a mucous fistula should be brought out through a very small circular incision in the lower quadrant. Only the corner of the distal bowel needs to come through the abdominal wall to create a mucous fistula.

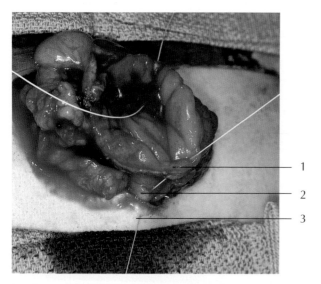

1 – Suture through full thickness of bowel
2 – Suture through seromuscular layer only
3 – Suture through full thickness of skin

Figure 3.46. Suturing the stoma.
The stoma can be secured using a 4–0 absorbable suture. The first sutures are used to evert the colostomy. The suture is passed through the full thickness of the distal colonic mucosa, a seromuscular portion of colon is then incorporated approximately 1–2 cm from the distal edge, and finally the suture is brought through the skin. The suture brought through the skin can be placed either subcuticularly or at full thickness. If it is placed through the full thickness of the skin, it should be very close to the stomal site. When tied, the colonic mucosa should overlie the skin edge. If the skin overlies the colonic mucosa, a fibrotic ridge may form. Typically, four everting sutures are placed in a circumferential manner at equal distances. Usually, one or two simple sutures are placed in between the everting sutures. These incorporate the full thickness of the bowel and the skin only. The deeper seromuscular portion that was included in the everting sutures is excluded at this point. If the full thickness of the bowel is not included, the peritoneum may sink into the stoma and lead to an uneven mucosal–cutaneous bridge. The final product has sutures that are each approximately 1 cm apart.

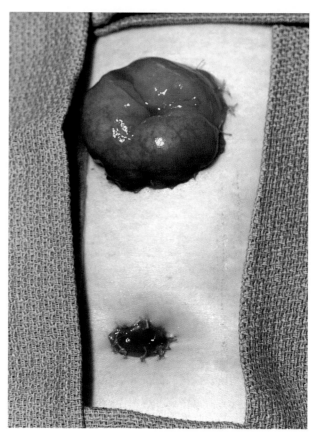

Figure 3.47. Completed stoma.
Placement of the sutures as described above leads to the formation of a protruding stoma often referred to as a 'rosebud'. The completed stoma is viable and patent. Patency should be assessed by gently introducing a small finger into the stoma. It should pass down to and through the level of the fascia. If it is constricted, the vascular supply may be compromised. The colonic mucosa should be pink. The mucous fistula is opened and sutured to the skin with simple sutures. No eversion of the mucous fistula is necessary. Usually, the mucous fistula has minimal output for several weeks and then will dry up and often close spontaneously. After several weeks, nothing more than a small adhesive bandage is required to cover the mucous fistula.

Small bowel resection and ileostomy

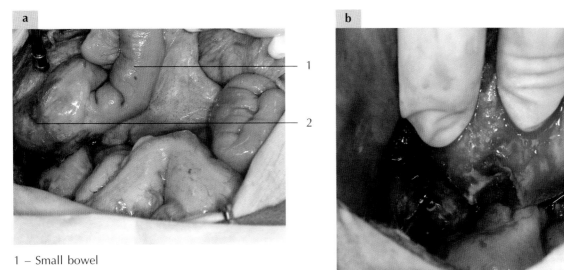

1 – Small bowel
2 – Recurrent tumor

Figure 3.48 (a and b). Small bowel tumor.
Tumor can be seen on the small bowel. In this patient it was causing a chronic partial small bowel obstruction, and extensive abdominal disease was also present. Choices for therapeutic intervention include small bowel resection with reanastomosis or end ileostomy. If the distal bowel is not obstructed, reanastomosis is usually the treatment of choice. Occasionally, with very advanced disease, an ileostomy needs to be created. If a distal small or large bowel is present, a mucous fistula should be made.

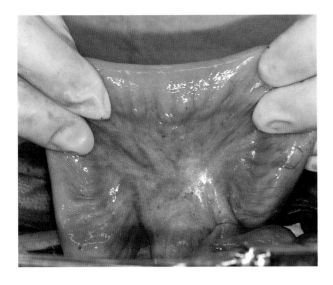

Figure 3.49. Selecting a site for transection.
A portion of small bowel proximal to the disease is selected for transection. The selected area should contain healthy bowel with sufficient mobility to reach the anterior abdominal wall without tension for the creation of an ileostomy or to allow the approximation of both bowel ends. These are more significant issues in obese patients.

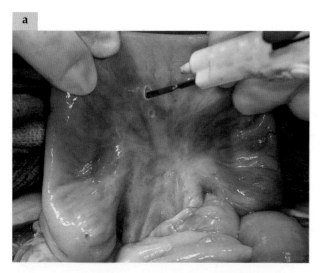
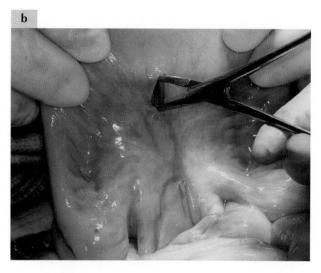

Figure 3.50. Creating an enteromesenterotomy.
(**a**) A defect is created in the mesentery just adjacent to the mesenteric border of the bowel. This can be accomplished using scissors, electrocautery, or a fine-tipped clamp. (**b**) The defect is then bluntly developed to allow introduction of a stapling device. To perform a bowel resection, a second site distal to the obstruction is created and the intervening bowel is then removed after resecting the mesentery.

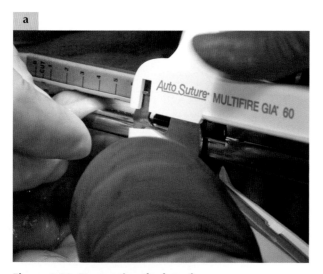
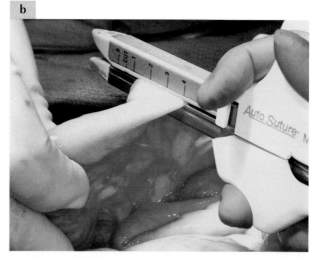

Figure 3.51. Transecting the bowel.
(**a**) A multifire stapling device can then be placed around the bowel through the newly developed mesenterotomy. Generally, a 60-mm device is sufficient to transect the small intestine. The standard staple height for small or large bowel is 3.8 mm. (**b**) The stapling device is then closed with the bowel lying within the cut line. The stapler is fired, which simultaneously divides and staples the bowel.

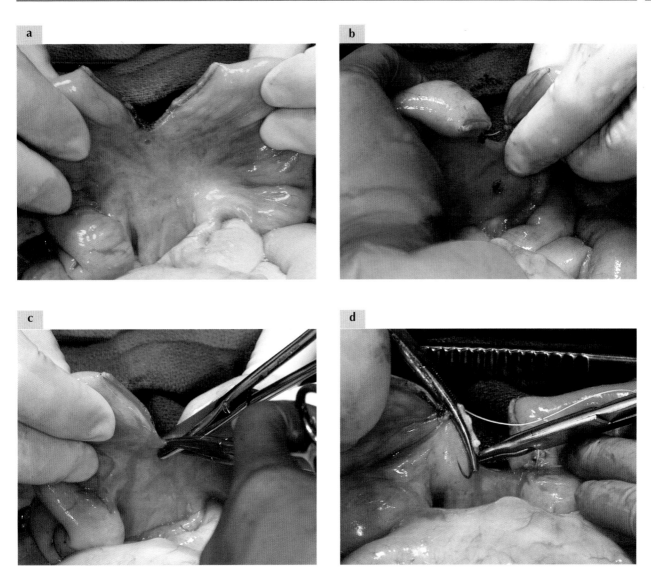

Figure 3.52. Dividing the mesentery.
(**a**) The stapled ends of the bowel are inspected for hemostasis and enterotomy. (**b**) Small windows are created in the mesentery to place clamps without causing bleeding. (**c**) The mesentery is sequentially doubly clamped and transected, as it has a rich vascular anastomosis. (**d**) The cut ends of the mesentery are suture ligated with absorbable synthetic suture. The division of the mesentery is continued until sufficient mobility is achieved to allow the stapled ends to reach each other or through the abdominal wall without tension. Successive clamping, cutting, and ligation are employed as needed.

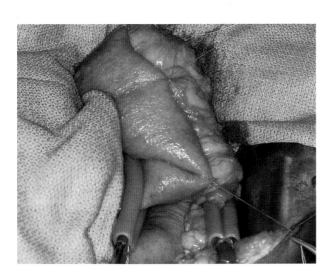

Figure 3.53. Approximating the bowel.
After resecting the diseased portion of small bowel, the stapled ends are approximated. Ultimately, the enteroenterostomy will be created along the antimesenteric edges of the small bowel. The bowel is aligned appropriately and one or two stay sutures are placed to maintain orientation. The small bowel is clamped with noncrushing clamps in order to prevent spillage of the small bowel contents when the bowel is opened.

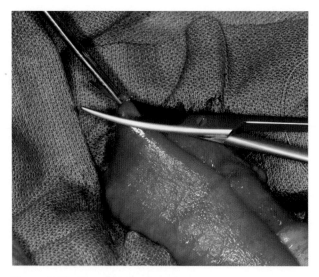

Figure 3.54. Opening the bowel.
The antimesenteric corners of the previous staple line are excised from each limb of the bowel. If too much tissue is excised, bowel contents may spill and the created enterotomy may be too large to close in the standard fashion.

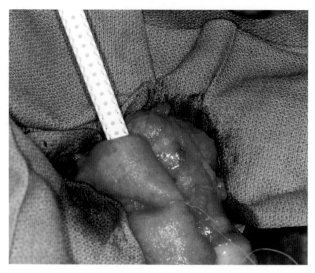

Figure 3.55. Decompressing the bowel.
Each limb is emptied with pool suction in order to prevent spillage of small intestinal contents. If bowel obstruction is present, the noncrushing clamp is slowly released to decompress the proximal bowel with the pool suction.

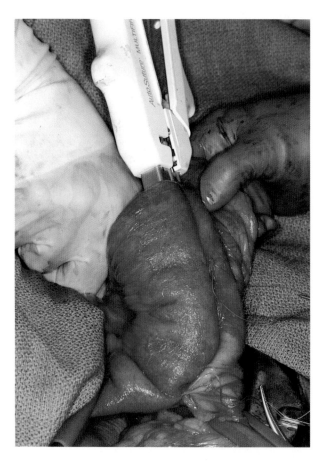

Figure 3.56. Creating the anastomosis.
A disposable linear cutting stapler is used to approximate and anastomose the two small bowel ends. One side of the stapler is inserted into each side of the bowel, it is then closed and fired. The lumen of the bowel is inspected for hemostasis while removing the stapler.

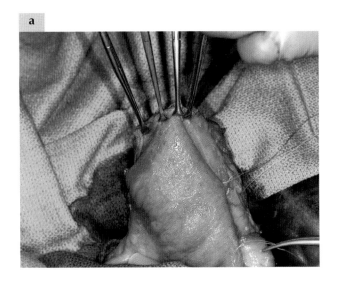

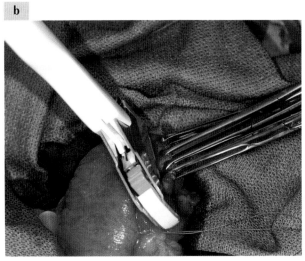

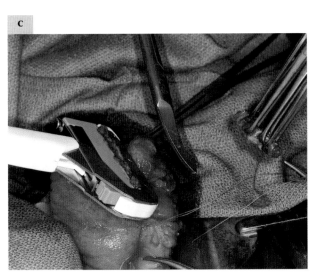

Figure 3.57. Closing the anastomosis.
Allis clamps are used to close the enterotomy. (**a**) After ensuring hemostasis, the clamps are placed equidistant across the lumen of the bowel. (**b**) A linear noncutting stapler is placed just beneath the clamps and fired. (**c**) The residual tissue is then excised with scissors or a scalpel. A portion of the previous staple line will be excised along with this tissue, and a scalpel is often inadequate for the resection.

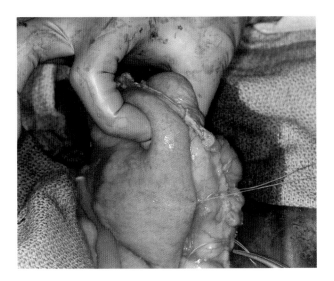

Figure 3.58. Assessing the lumen.
The lumen of the new anastomosis can be palpated and is usually much larger than the width of an index finger. Since small bowel contents are liquid, a particularly wide anastomosis is not required. The mesenteric defect should be closed with absorbable sutures; the stay sutures placed previously may be left in place or removed.

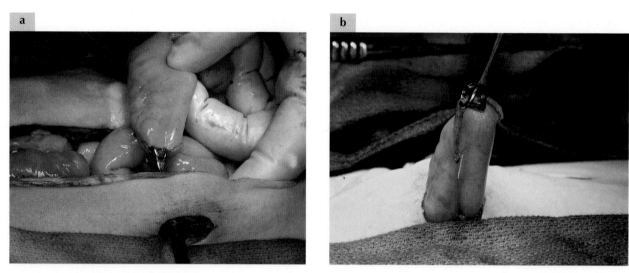

Figure 3.59. Exteriorizing the bowel.
If an end ileostomy is created, the stoma is approximately 2 cm in diameter. For an end ileostomy, the stoma is generally smaller than that of an end colostomy due to the smaller caliber intestine that will pass through the site. (**a**) A Babcock clamp is passed through the abdominal stoma site. The stapled line is then grasped with the Babcock clamp and brought through the abdominal wall. (**b**) An ileostomy should have sufficient length so that it will evert nicely. If insufficient bowel is brought through the abdominal wall, the stoma will not evert adequately.

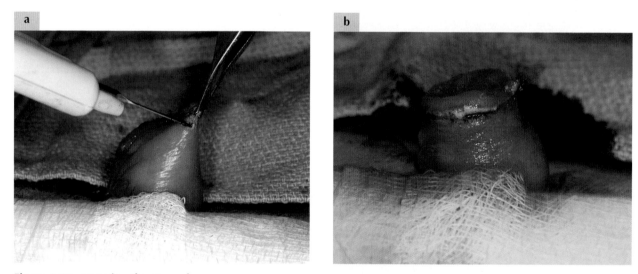

Figure 3.60. Maturing the stoma.
The abdominal incision is closed prior to maturing the stoma. (**a**) The line of staples is excised with scissors, a scalpel, or electrocautery. Small bowel contents are thought to be sterile and, if necessary, may be opened prior to abdominal closure. Electrocautery can provide good hemostasis. (**b**) The staple line needs to be excised in its entirety.

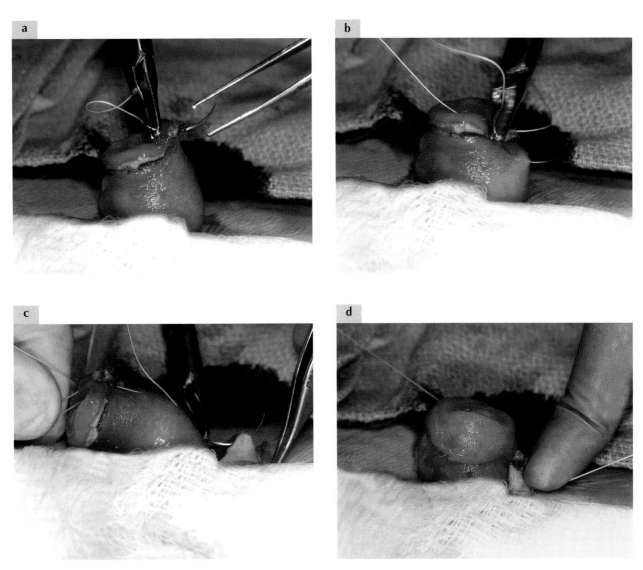

Figure 3.61. Securing the stoma.
The stoma is secured with 4-0 absorbable sutures. (**a**) The suture is first passed full thickness through the cut edge of the bowel; (**b**) it is then passed through the seromuscular layer approximately 1 cm from the opened edge of the bowel; (**c**) finally, it is passed through the skin. The skin suture may be placed subcuticularly or through the entire thickness of the skin. (**d**) The suture is then tied parallel to the skin. This creates a prominent 'rosebud' and offers the best likelihood that the small bowel mucosa will overlie the skin rather than vice versa.

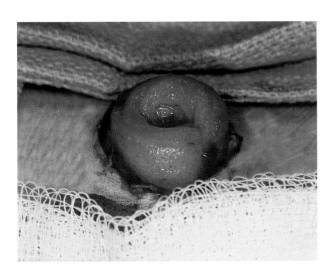

Figure 3.62. Completed stoma.
The completed stoma is protuberant and has healthy pink viable mucosa. The gauze seen in the foreground is used to protect the closed abdominal incision from potential contamination while maturing the ileostomy. Adhesive tape and a formal dressing may be placed prior to maturing the ileostomy.

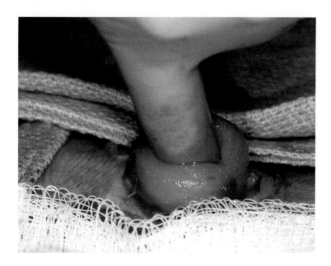

Figure 3.63. Checking stoma patency.
The patency of the stoma is checked by passing a small, gloved finger through the ostomy. There should be little resistance down to and through the fascia.

Recurrent nodal disease

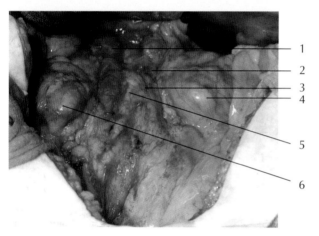

Figure 3.64. Recurrent paraaortic disease.
One of the most common sites of recurrent nodal disease in ovarian cancer patients is the high paraaortic region. It is hypothesized that if paraaortic nodes are systematically removed at the time of initial staging or debulking, recurrence in this area may be less likely. This emphasizes the importance of sampling or removing nodal tissue all the way up to the renal vessels due to the known lymphatic and venous drainage patterns.

1 – Inferior vena cava
2 – Left renal vein
3 – Left ovarian vein
4 – Left kidney
5 – Recurrent tumor
6 – Right kidney

a
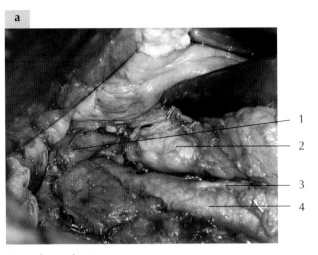

1 – Left renal vein
2 – Recurrent tumor
3 – Inferior mesenteric artery
4 – Aorta

b

Figure 3.65. Left paraaortic recurrence.
(**a**) After exposing the retroperitoneal vessels, the left paraaortic nodal recurrence can be seen. Left-sided recurrences are more common since the landing zone is higher on the left than the right due to venous and lymphatic drainage patterns. (**b**) After further dissection the node is ready for removal.

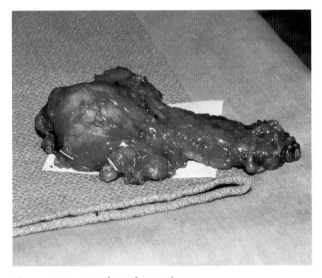

Figure 3.66. Lymph node specimen.
The enlarged lymph node has been completely removed and the tumor is well circumscribed; this node was approximately 5 × 3 cm at its maximum dimensions.

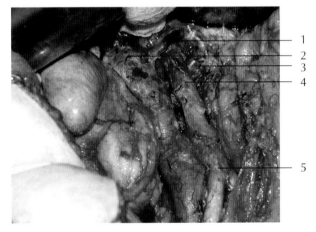

1 – Anterior limb of left renal vein
2 – Inferior vena cava
3 – Posterior limb of left renal vein
4 – Aorta
5 – Aortic bifurcation

Figure 3.67. Renal vein anomalies.
Vascular anomalies can occur anywhere along major blood vessels. Shown here is the passage of the left renal vein anterior and posterior to the aorta. This bifurcated renal vein can easily be detected on preoperative imaging and is a normal variant. It should be noted prior to embarking on a retroperitoneal lymph node dissection so that vascular injury does not occur.

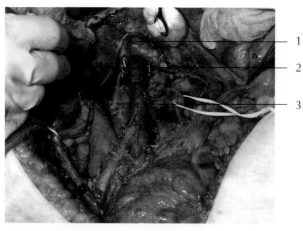

Figure 3.68. Anterior spinous ligament.
To remove interaortocaval lymph nodes the vena cava and aorta are separated. The resulting dissection will usually mandate ligating and transecting the lumbar arteries and veins. At the conclusion of this type of extensive dissection, the anterior spinous ligament overlying the vertebrae can be seen.

1 – Left renal vein
2 – Inferior vena cava
3 – Anterior spinous ligament

Splenectomy

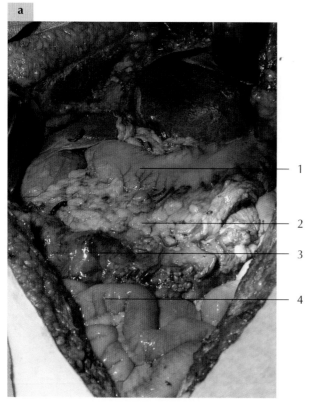

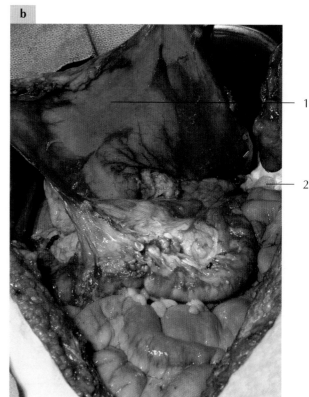

1 – Stomach
2 – Gastrocolic ligament
3 – Transverse colon
4 – Small intestine

1 – Stomach reflected cranially
2 – Laparotomy pad covering spleen

Figure 3.69 (a and b). Splenic tumor.
The spleen can be approached laterally from the left paracolic gutter, which will permit transection of the lateral ligamentous attachments. Once the spleen has been mobilized, the lesser sac is entered through the gastrocolic ligament to identify the pancreas and splenic vessels.

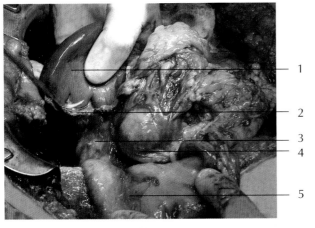

Figure 3.70. Splenic tumor.
The spleen has been freed of most of the surrounding ligamentous attachments. Typically, the splenophrenic ligament is transected first. The splenocolic and splenorenal ligaments are then transected. These are usually avascular and may be transected simply with electrocautery. The gastrosplenic ligament is then sequentially clamped, transected, and suture ligated. This ligament contains the short gastric vessels that need to be meticulously controlled. Shown here is a tumor in the hilum of the spleen; a portion of the gastrosplenic ligament remains.

1 – Spleen retracted laterally
2 – Transected gastrosplenic ligament
3 – Residual gastrosplenic ligament
4 – Tumor in splenic hilum
5 – Stomach retracted medially

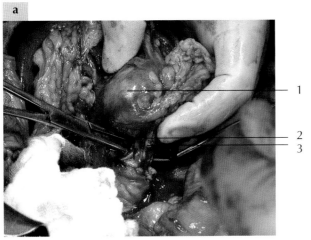
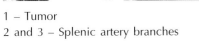
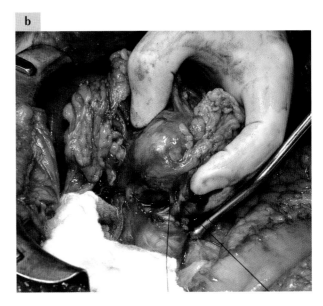

1 – Tumor
2 and 3 – Splenic artery branches

Figure 3.71. Splenic artery.
The splenic artery frequently branches as it gets close to the hilum of the spleen. Therefore, care should be taken to ligate it before it branches, or to secure each branch of the artery. The artery is ligated separately and before the splenic vein. This will reduce the pressure within the vein when it is ligated and will also allow additional blood sequestered within the spleen to return to the circulation. (**a**) The splenic artery is carefully isolated; (**b**) a permanent silk suture is passed around the vessel. Distally, the artery may be clipped or tied, as it will be removed with the specimen.

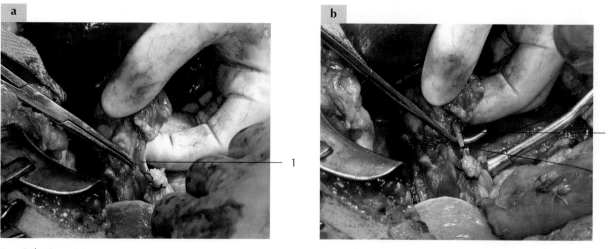

1 – Splenic vein   1 – Splenic vein

Figure 3.72. Splenic vein.
(**a**) The splenic vein is carefully isolated from the surrounding tissues. Often, the tail of the pancreas will be in close proximity to the splenic vein, and a distal pancreatectomy can be performed if it is involved with tumor. (**b**) The splenic vein is also ligated with a permanent suture. Again, distal control may be obtained with a tie or clip, as appropriate.

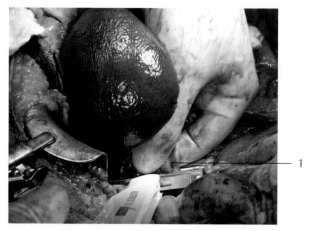

1 – Tail of pancreas

Figure 3.73. Distal pancreatectomy.
In this case, the tail of the pancreas was intimately involved with the hilum of the spleen since the recurrent tumor had altered the normal anatomic relationships. The tail of the pancreas is isolated and a linear stapler is placed across the distal pancreas. After it is fired, a scalpel is used to transect the pancreas on the outer edge of the stapler.

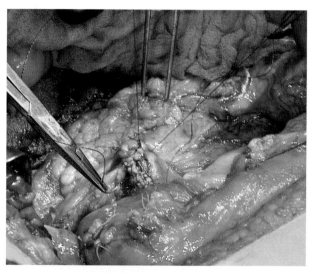

Figure 3.74. Securing the pancreas.
The staple line on the transected border of the pancreas is then oversewn with a small delayed absorbable suture. This will help to minimize the risk of postoperative pancreatic leak, which can lead to postoperative collection or abscess formation.

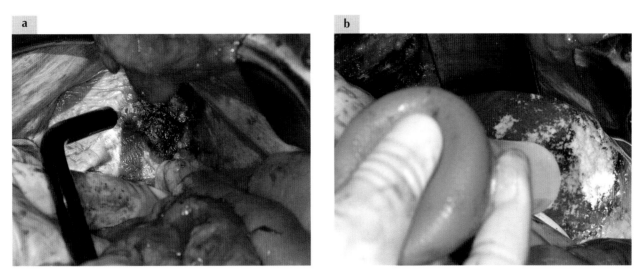

Figure 3.75. Hemostasis.
Large bleeding vessels need to be secured with sutures, ties or hemostatic clips. However, there can often be minimal oozing or small-vessel bleeding in the splenic bed. Once the spleen is removed, it is much easier to visualize the exact sites of bleeding. If not amenable to sutures or clips, they can be readily controlled by electrocautery, argon-beam coagulation (**a**) or with a synthetic hemostatic agent such as Avitene (**b**). Avitene is a microfibrillar collagen hemostat manufactured by Davol, Inc. (Cranston, RI).

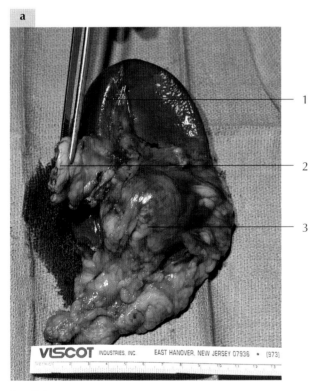

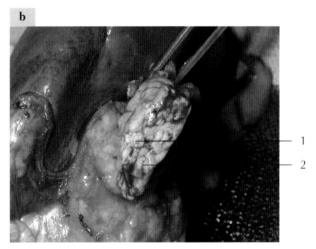

1 – Pancreatic duct
2 – Pancreatic parenchyma

Figure 3.76. Specimen.
(**a**) The recurrent tumor involving the splenic hilum is clearly visible. The forceps are grasping the tail of the pancreas, which was removed with the specimen. (**b**) A closer view of the pancreas shows the transected pancreatic duct.

1 – Spleen
2 – Resected distal pancreas
3 – Tumor in splenic hilum

References

1. Jemal A, Murray T, Samuels A, Ghafoor A, Ward E, Thun J. Cancer statistics. *CA Cancer J Clin* 2003; **53**:5–26.
2. Ozols RF, Rubin SC, Thomas GM et al. In: (Hoskins WJ, Perez CA, Young RC, eds) *Principles and Practice of Gynecologic Oncology*, 3rd edn. (Lippincott Williams & Wilkins: Philadelphia, 2000.)
3. Griffiths CT. Surgical resection of tumor bulk in the primary treatment of ovarian carcinoma. *Natl Cancer Inst Monogr* 1975; **42**:101–4.
4. Hoskins WJ, McGuire WP, Brady MF et al. The effect of diameter of largest residual disease on survival after primary cytoreductive surgery in patients with suboptimal residual epithelial ovarian carcinoma. *Am J Obstet Gynecol* 1994; **170**:974–80.
5. Eisenkop SM, Friedman RL, Wang HJ. Complete cytoreductive surgery is feasible and maximizes survival in patients with advanced epithelial ovarian cancer: a prospective study. *Gynecol Oncol* 1998; **69**:103–8.
6. Hoskins WJ, Chi DS, Boente MP, Rubin SC. State of the art surgical management of ovarian cancer. *Cancer Res Ther Control* 1999; **9**:373–82.
7. Marsden DE, Friedlander M, Hacker NF. Current management of epithelial ovarian carcinoma: a review. *Semin Surg Oncol* 2000; **19**:11–19.
8. Holschneider CH, Berek JS. Ovarian cancer: epidemiology, biology, and prognostic factors. *Semin Surg Oncol* 2000; **19**:3–10.
9. Scarabelli C, Gallo A, Franceshi S et al. Primary cytoreductive surgery with rectosigmoid colon resection for patients with advanced epithelial ovarian carcinoma. *Cancer* 2000; **88**:89–97.
10. Chi DS, Liao JB, Leon LF et al. Identification of prognostic factors in advanced epithelial ovarian carcinoma. *Gynecol Oncol* 2001; **82**:532–7.
11. Eisenkop SM, Nalick RH, Wang HJ, Teng NNH. Peritoneal implant elimination during cytoreductive surgery for ovarian cancer: impact on survival. *Gynecol Oncol* 1993; **51**:224–9.
12. Curtin JP, Malik R, Venkatramann ES et al. Stage IV ovarian cancer: impact of surgical debulking. *Gynecol Oncol* 1997; **64**:9–12.
13. Liu PC, Benjamin I, Morgan MA et al. Prognostic significance of residual disease in patients with stage IV epithelial ovarian cancer. *Gynecol Oncol* 1997; **64**:4–8.
14. Munkarah AR, Hallum AV, Morris M et al. Prognostic significance of residual disease in patients with stage IV epithelial ovarian cancer. *Gynecol Oncol* 1997; **64**:13–17.
15. Bristow RE, Montz FJ, Lagasse LD et al. Survival impact of surgical cytoreduction in stage IV epithelial ovarian cancer. *Gynecol Oncol* 1999; **72**:278–87.
16. Eisenkop SM, Spirtos NM. Procedures required to accomplish complete cytoreduction of ovarian cancer: is there a correlation with 'biological aggressiveness' and survival? *Gynecol Oncol* 2001; **82**:435–41.
17. Eisenkop SM, Spirtos NM. What are the current surgical objectives, strategies, and technical capabilities of gynecologic oncologists treating advanced epithelial ovarian cancer? *Gynecol Oncol* 2001; **82**:489–9.
18. Chen L, Leuchter RS, Lagasse LD, Karlan BY. Splenectomy and surgical cytoreduction for ovarian cancer. *Gynecol Oncol* 2000; **77**:362–8.
19. Chi DS, Fong Y, Venkatraman ES, Barakat RR. Hepatic resection for metastatic gynecologic carcinomas. *Gynecol Oncol* 1997; **66**:45–51.
20. van Dam PA, Tjalma W, Weyler J et al. Ultraradical debulking of epithelial ovarian cancer with the ultrasonic surgical aspirator: a prospective randomized trial. *Am J Obstet Gynecol* 1996; **174**:943–50.
21. Obermair A, Hagenauer S, Tamandl D et al. Safety and efficacy of low anterior en bloc resection as part of cytoreductive surgery for patients with ovarian cancer. *Gynecol Oncol* 2001; **83**:115–20.
22. Hoskins WJ, Rubin SC, Dulaney E et al. Influence of secondary cytoreduction at the time of second-look laparotomy on the survival of patients with epithelial ovarian carcinoma. *Gynecol Oncol* 1989; **34**:365–71.
23. Segna RA, Dottino PR, Mandeli JP et al. Secondary cytoreduction for ovarian cancer following cisplatin therapy. *J Clin Oncol* 1993; **11**:434–9.
24. Munkarah A, Levenback C, Wolf JK et al. Secondary cytoreductive surgery for localized intra-abdominal recurrences in epithelial ovarian cancer. *Gynecol Oncol* 2001; **81**:237–41.
25. Eisenkop SM, Friedman RL, Spirtos NM. The role of secondary cytoreductive surgery in the treatment of patients with recurrent epithelial ovarian carcinoma. *Cancer* 2000; **88**:144–53.
26. Bristow RE, Zerbe MJ, Rosenshein NB et al. Stage IVB endometrial carcinoma: the role of cytoreductive surgery and determinants of survival. *Gynecol Oncol* 2000; **78**:85–91.
27. Chi DS, Welshinger M, Venkatraman ES, Barakat RR. The role of surgical cytoreduction in Stage IV endometrial carcinoma. *Gynecol Oncol* 1997; **67**:56–60.
28. Scarabelli C, Campagnutta E, Giorda G et al. Maximal cytoreductive surgery as a reasonable therapeutic alternative for recurrent endometrial carcinoma. *Gynecol Oncol* 1998; **70**:90–3.

4 Pelvic exenteration

Douglas A Levine, Bernard H Bochner and Dennis S Chi

Pelvic exenteration is one of the most radical surgical procedures performed by gynecologic oncologists. The most common indication is a central pelvic recurrence of cervical cancer. Alexander Brunschwig first described the procedure in 1948 as 'the most radical surgical attack so far described for pelvic cancer'.[1] The initial report described the en-bloc removal of the pelvic organs with the creation of a 'wet colostomy' by implanting the ureters into the sigmoid colon, which was then brought out as an end colostomy. Today, reconstruction after a total pelvic exenteration consists of separate bowel and urinary conduits. A total pelvic exenteration consists of the en-bloc removal of the bladder, rectum, vagina, and tumor. In an anterior exenteration, the rectum is not removed. In a posterior exenteration, the bladder and ureters remain intact. In all cases the uterus and adnexa are removed if they have not been previously removed as part of primary therapy or for unrelated reasons. A pelvic exenteration may be further subclassified into a supralevator or infralevator exenteration, depending on whether or not the perineum is excised as part of the operation. At the conclusion of the procedure, the colon is either reanastomosed or brought out as an end colostomy. There are many techniques to create a neovagina, the most common being bilateral gracilis flaps or a rectus abdominus flap. The details of this reconstruction are beyond the scope of this text but are readily available elsewhere for the interested reader.

The urinary system may be reconstructed into a continent or noncontinent conduit. The most common noncontinent conduit is created from a segment of distal ileum into which the ureters are inserted and then brought out through a lower quadrant ostomy. Other segments of the intestinal tract may also be used as a conduit, the most common alternatives being a portion of the jejunum, transverse colon or sigmoid colon. Generally, the distal ileum is the easiest portion to use since it is usually not involved by tumor, has not been subject to previous surgery, has adequate mobility and a rich vascular supply. The major drawback of using the distal ileum is that it may have been included in a previous radiation field. A continent conduit is created by establishing an intestinal reservoir and an efferent limb, which is brought out through the abdominal wall. Depending on the type of continent conduit created, the ureters are either directly inserted into the intestinal reservoir or into an afferent limb that drains into this reservoir. The most commonly performed continent conduits are the Miami and the Indiana pouches. The ureters are inserted into a detubularized segment of ascending colon that serves as a low-pressure, high-capacity reservoir. The appendix is removed and the distal ileum is brought out as a urostomy. The reported incidence of early and late complications is approximately 60%, with the most common complications being ureteral obstruction, difficult catheterization, or pyelonephritis.[2,3] A modified Penn pouch offers certain attractive advantages over the more standard pouches and will be described in this chapter.

The most common indication for pelvic exenteration is a central recurrence of cervical cancer. The intent of the procedure is usually curative, although a palliative exenteration may be appropriate for selected patients with unmanageable symptoms, such as intractable pain, uncontrollable bleeding, or gross disfigurement. It can also be performed for selected recurrences of other pelvic malignancies including endometrial, vulvar, vaginal, and colorectal cancers. Current surgical practices, including the use of antibiotics, modern anesthesia, exceptional intensive care units, meticulous surgical technique, blood banking, and advances in interventional radiology, have all contributed to a reduction in perioperative morbidity and mortality. Surgical mortality in recent reports has ranged from 2 to 5% and postoperative major morbidity ranges from 30 to 60%.[4–6] In certain centers, a multidisciplinary approach, with a urologist, a radiation oncologist, a plastic surgeon, and a colorectal surgeon, may be useful in achieving optimal surgical outcomes. The 5-year survival for patients undergoing pelvic exenteration for recurrent cervical cancer is between 30 and 50%.[7,8] The largest review of exenterative surgery for recurrent endometrial cancer reported a 5-year survival of 20%.[9] In each of these series the patients undergoing these procedures are highly selected using various nonstandardized criteria.

Due to the radicality of the procedure, patients must be appropriately counseled regarding the chance of cure and the physical alterations that can be expected after surgery, as well as the extended postoperative recovery time. For these reasons, exenterative surgery is usually performed in patients who have had full pelvic irradiation either as part of initial treatment or for the management of recurrent disease. Unfortunately, the previous pelvic irradiation renders the surgery and recovery more difficult. For patients who have either suspected positive margins or confirmed positive margins on frozen section, intraoperative radiation therapy offers an attractive technique to help reduce the risk

of recurrence and is discussed in a later chapter within this text.[10] Typically, 1500–2000 cGy are given to the tumor bed with a linear accelerator or a high-dose-rate afterloader. Some practitioners believe that a laterally extended endopelvic resection is a reasonable treatment for recurrent disease that involves the pelvic sidewall.[11]

This chapter will highlight the major aspects of pelvic exenteration. it is not possible to illustrate all of the varied techniques available to the practicing surgeon, important differences will be highlighted. The authors have elected to illustrate the ileal conduit and a modified Penn pouch as techniques in urinary diversion, representing a common technique and a relatively novel technique for the gynecologic oncologist, respectively. Many of the technical aspects of pelvic exenteration overlap with the other radical surgical procedures presented in Chapter 3. Similar techniques will be referred to, but are not thoroughly illustrated to avoid repetition.

Exenteration

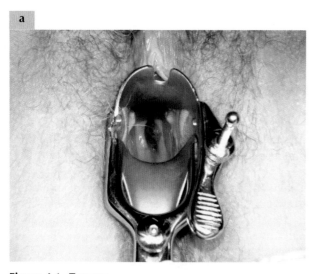 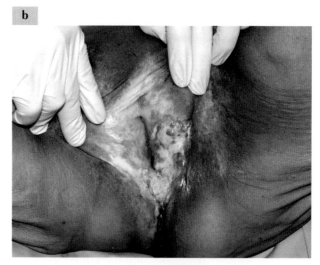

Figure 4.1. Tumors.
Most recurrent tumors are not visible prior to abdominal exploration due to their location deep within the central pelvis. (**a**) A view of a centrally recurrent cervical cancer that can be seen in the endocervical canal. (**b**) A recurrent vulvar cancer that was causing intractable perineal pain. Prior to beginning a total pelvic exenteration the rectum is sewn closed with a #0 permanent suture.

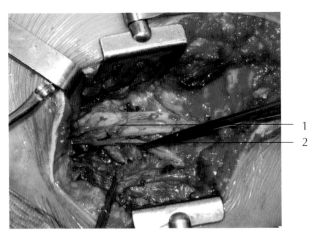

1 – Right sciatic nerve
2 – Right posterior femoral cutaneous nerve

Figure 4.2. Lateral approach.
For a patient with a sidewall recurrence a lateral approach may be considered. The patient shown here had a recurrent tumor involving the obturator internus muscle. In order to protect the sciatic nerve and to gain control of the gluteal vessels, a posterior thigh incision was made to perform a sciatic neuroplasty. After fully mobilizing the sciatic nerve, the thigh was closed and the patient was placed in the dorsal lithotomy position to perform the pelvic exenteration.

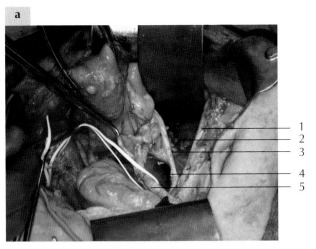

1 – Right external iliac vessels
2 – Right paravesical space
3 – Right internal iliac artery
4 – Right pararectal space
5 – Right ureter

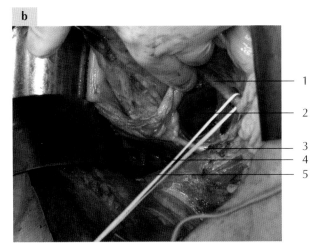

1 – Left ureter
2 – Left pararectal space
3 – Left internal iliac artery
4 – Left paravesical space
5 – Left external iliac vessels

Figure 4.3. Pelvic spaces.
After exploring the abdomen, both pelvic sidewalls are opened and the pelvic spaces developed, which aids in the dissection and resection of the pelvic tumor. Incising the peritoneum lateral to the medial umbilical ligament develops the paravesical space. Loose areolar tissue will be encountered, which can be gently dissected to arrive at the base of the paravesical space. The pararectal space is developed between the hypogastric artery and the ureter. The dissection is carried out inferiorly and dorsally along the curve of the sacrum. (**a**) The right paravesical and pararectal spaces; (**b**) the left paravesical and pararectal spaces. (**c**) The right pelvic sidewall has been opened and the deep circumflex iliac vein can be seen passing over the right external iliac artery. The paraaortic and/or common iliac lymph nodes are sampled prior to proceeding with the pelvic exenteration. The presence of metastases in these areas is suggestive of systemic disease making the possibility of cure after exenteration unlikely.

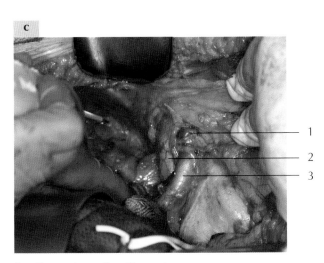

1 – Deep circumflex iliac vein
2 – Right external iliac vein
3 – Right external iliac artery

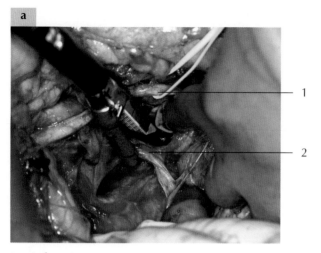

1 – Left ureter
2 – Left hypogastric vessels

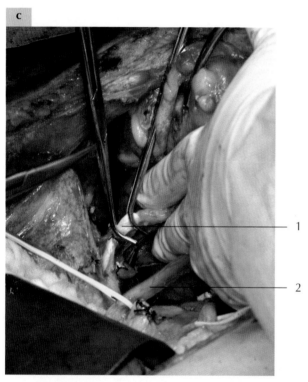

1 – Left hypogastric artery
2 – Left ureter

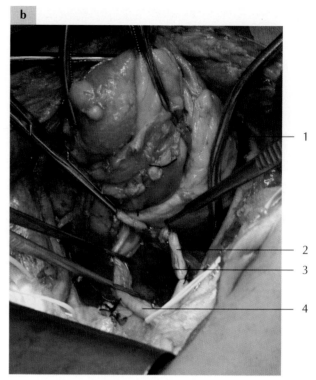

1 – Right paravesical space
2 – Ligated right hypogastric artery
3 – Right pararectal space
4 – Right ureter

Figure 4.4. Internal iliac vessels.
The anterior division of the internal iliac vessels are skeletonized and ligated to reduce blood flow to the pelvis and to minimize blood loss. The vessels may or may not be transected after they are ligated. (**a**) The endoscopic stapler is used to transect and ligate the left hypogastric artery and vein. The use of stapling devices helps to decrease operative time and reduce blood loss. (**b**) Alternatively, the vessels may be simply ligated and not transected. The hypogastric vessels may also be transected in the traditional fashion. (**c**) A proximal tie has been placed prior to introducing the right-angled clamps onto the vessel, which will subsequently be transected and ligated again.

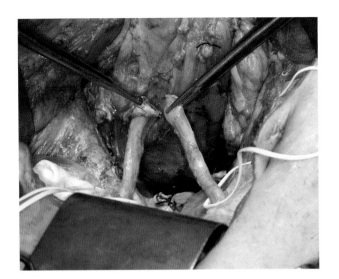

Figure 4.5. Transecting the ureters.
The ureters are transected close to the pelvic brim. They are examined closely and cut back to try to resect any portion that has been irradiated so that an unirradiated segment can be used for the ureteral anastomosis. In this picture the ureters have been transected but will be further trimmed prior to creating the uretero–ileal anastomosis.

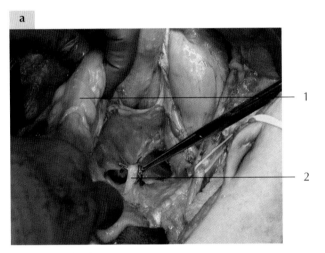

1 – Sigmoid colon
2 – Superior rectal artery

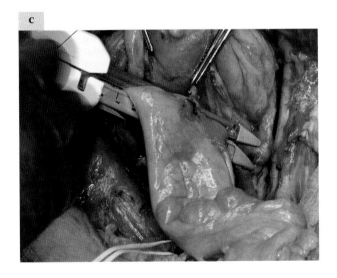

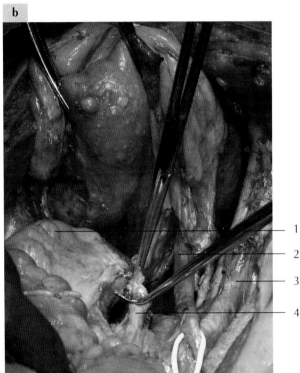

1 – Sigmoid colon
2 – Right ureter
3 – Right external iliac vessels
4 – Superior rectal artery

Figure 4.6. Dividing the colon.
(**a**) The colonic mesentery is incised to identify the superior rectal artery. (**b**) The artery is isolated and transected with right-angled clamps. Alternatively, the artery can be transected with the LigaSure vessel-sealing system (Valleylab, Boulder, CO) or a disposable stapler with vascular loads. (**c**) The colon is then transected at the pelvic brim so that most of the irradiated bowel will be included with the final specimen. Usually, the left colic artery and some sigmoid branches can be preserved.

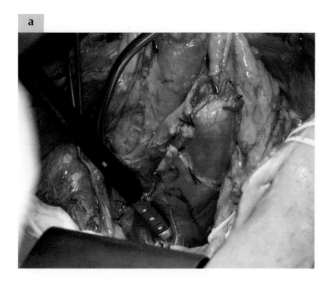

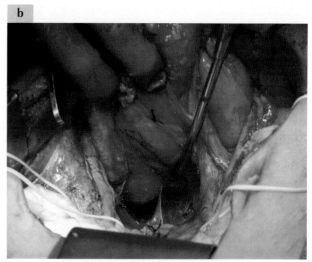

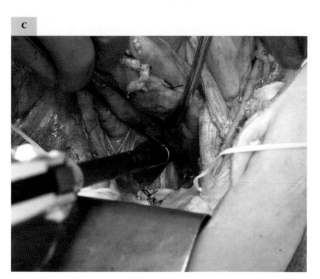

Figure 4.7. Mesorectal excision.
The distal colon is placed on traction and the presacral space is dissected. Areolar tissue can be incised with electrocautery and the endoscopic stapler is used to transect the mesorectum. Care must be taken not to injure the sacral veins when placing the stapler as this can lead to troublesome bleeding. (**a**) The sigmoid is elevated and the remaining mesenteric attachments are transected with the endoscopic stapler with vascular loads. (**b**) The rectosigmoid has been further mobilized and the hollow of the sacrum is now apparent. (**c**) Successive fires of the stapler are required to transect the mesorectum completely and gain access to the pelvic floor. The dissection from above should continue distal to the tip of the coccyx to facilitate the perineal dissection. If a supralevator exenteration is planned, the dissection must be continued far enough to resect the tumor with an adequate negative margin.

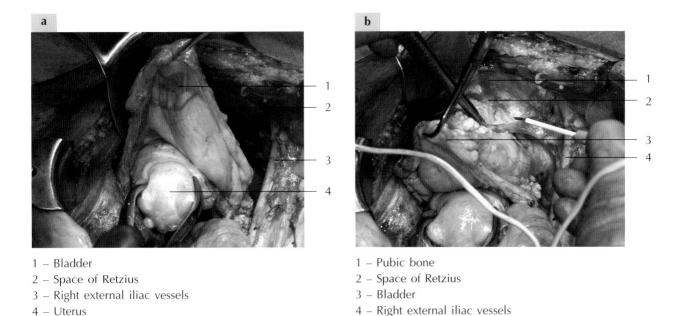

1 – Bladder
2 – Space of Retzius
3 – Right external iliac vessels
4 – Uterus

1 – Pubic bone
2 – Space of Retzius
3 – Bladder
4 – Right external iliac vessels

Figure 4.8. Space of Retzius.
(**a**) The lateral dissection is continued anteriorly until the bladder is reached. The bladder is then retracted posteriorly and the space of Retzius is entered. The anterior and lateral dissections are joined. (**b**) The space of Retzius is dissected along the undersurface of the pubic symphysis. Venous bleeding from the plexus of Santorini can be avoided if the dissection is performed close to the pubic bone. If a perineal phase is not performed, the urethra should be securely clamped prior to transection to avoid difficult bleeding. The transurethral urinary catheter should be removed prior to transecting the urethra. Otherwise, the dissection continues to the perineum with the urethra being dissected off the pubic bone as the last step, since bleeding can occur in this location and obscure the operative field.

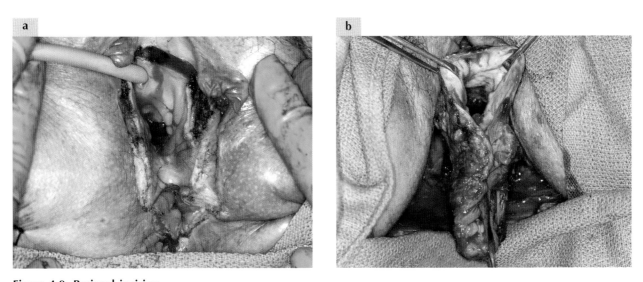

Figure 4.9. Perineal incision.
Once the pelvic dissection is complete, the surgeon or assistant moves between the patient's legs with a separate set of instruments to perform the perineal phase. (**a**) The perineum is incised circumferentially to delineate the portion that needs to be resected – in this case, the urethra, vagina, and rectum will all be removed. (**b**) The incision is then carried into the underlying subcutaneous tissues working from posterior to anterior to aid visualization.

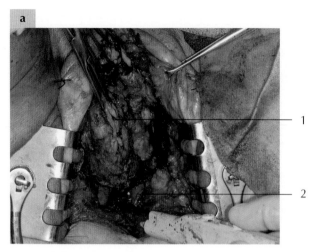

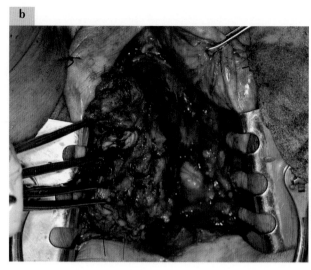

1 – Anal purse string suture
2 – Assistant's finger in the pelvis

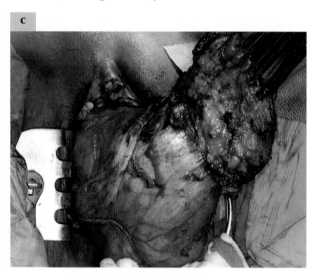

Figure 4.10. Perineal resection.
Allis clamps are used to evert the perineum. The labia majora can be temporarily sutured to the medial thigh to improve exposure if they do not need to be resected. The specimen is elevated and the posterior incision is continued until it meets the pelvic dissection. (**a**) A surgeon performing the perineal phase can work with an assistant whose hand is in the pelvis to serve as a guide for depth and orientation during the perineal dissection. (**b**) The specimen is then retracted laterally and the incision is continued circumferentially. A Lace self-retaining retractor is shown providing additional exposure. (**c**) Once the specimen is free it can be delivered through the perineum.

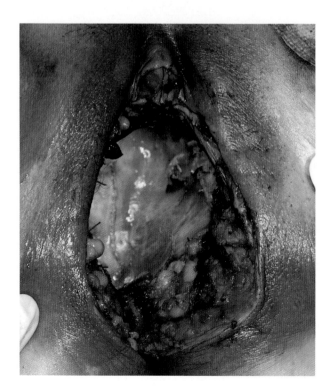

Figure 4.11. Perineal defect.
After removal of the specimen, a large perineal defect remains. Options for closing the defect include primary closure with interrupted delayed absorbable suture or one of a variety of vascular pedicle flaps. The most commonly used flaps are the gracilis and the rectus abdominus. The gracilis flap may be unilateral or bilateral depending on whether the intent is to fill the pelvis or to create a neovagina. The rectus abdominus flap provides a large amount of tissue to fill the pelvic defect and may also be used to create a neovagina. Since many of these patients have had prior surgery, one drawback with a rectus flap is that the main blood supply from the inferior epigastric vessels may have been previously interrupted.

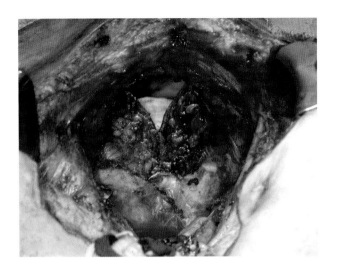

Figure 4.12. Pelvic defect.
After completing the exenterative procedure, all pelvic organs have been removed. The sidewall vessels and nerves remain, but the sacral hollow is empty and the perineal defect can be seen transabdominally. Often, many staple lines can be seen, reflecting the heavy use of the endoscopic stapler as a means of performing the exenteration in a more efficient manner.

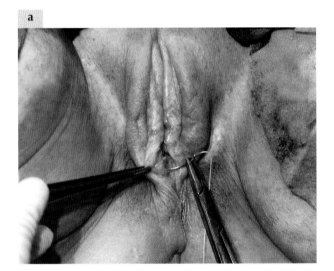

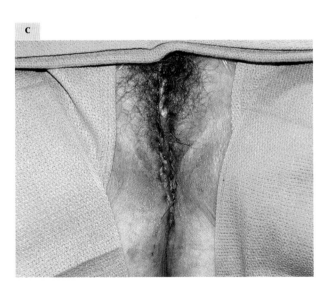

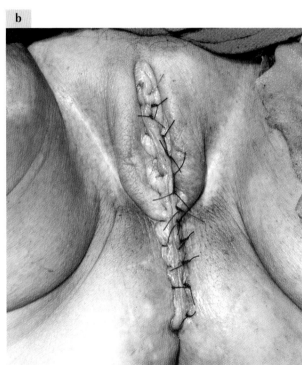

Figure 4.13. Perineum.
(**a**) The perineum is closed in multiple layers of interrupted delayed absorbable suture. Larger caliber suture is used in the deeper layers and a finer suture is used on the skin. The final appearance of the perineum will depend on the extent of perineal resection (contrast (**b**) and (**c**)). At the conclusion of the procedure a sterile dressing is placed on the perineum and held in position with a pelvic binder.

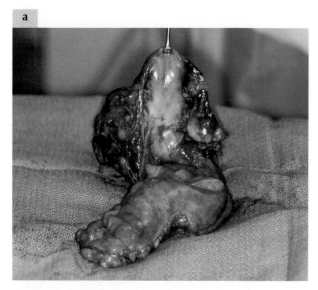

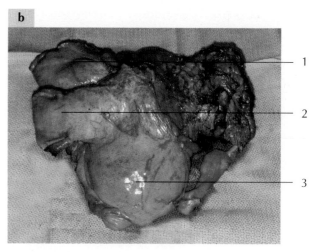

1 – Sigmoid
2 – Uterus
3 – Bladder

Figure 4.14. Specimen.
(**a**) The posterior view of the specimen shows the distal sigmoid in relation to the uterus, which is elevated with a clamp. (**b**) The superior view shows the bladder in relation to the uterus, with the sigmoid seen posteriorly. (**c**) The anterior view shows the relations within the perineum.

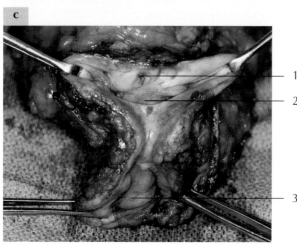

1 – Urethra
2 – Vagina
3 – Rectum

Noncontinent urinary conduit (ileal conduit)

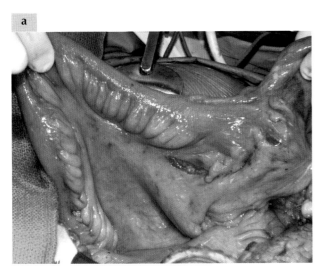
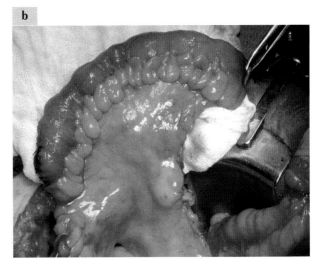

Figure 4.15. Dividing the bowel.
(**a**) An 8–10-cm segment of ileum is chosen approximately 10 cm proximal to the cecum. The ileum is manipulated to ensure that it will span from the ureters to the abdominal wall. If ureteral mobility is a problem, the conduit may be made longer to provide adequate length for a tension-free uretero–ileal anastomosis. (**b**) The bowel is transected in two sites to create a defunctionalized segment of ileum, taking care not to disrupt the mesenteric blood supply to this area. The proximal and distal ileum are reanastomosed in the usual fashion (described in Chapter 3). The butt-end of the ileal conduit may remain closed with the stapler or excluded with permanent silk suture.

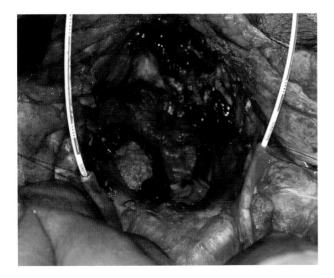

Figure 4.16. Ureters.
The ureters are transected at approximately the level of the pelvic brim to resect the distal portions that may have been previously irradiated, which reduces the likelihood of leakage and stricture from the uretero–ileal anastomosis. The ureters are mobilized only enough so that adequate length is obtained for a tension-free anastomosis. Aggressive mobilization or skeletonization of the periurethral tissues increases the risk of devascularization and subsequent stricture formation. It is prudent to intentionally leave some tissue attached to the ureters as the blood supply runs longitudinally. Single-J ureteral stents may be placed at the discretion of the operator to bridge the uretero–ileal anastomosis, though they are not required.

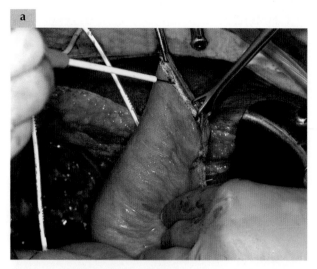
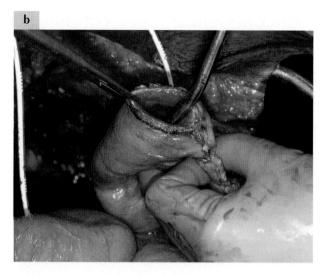

Figure 4.17. Opening the ileum.
(a) The distal end of the conduit is opened with electrocautery or scissors to completely excise the staple line. (b) The lumen is then suctioned to remove residual small bowel contents. If the noncontinent conduit is created with a different segment of intestine, such as the sigmoid or transverse colon, it too should be thoroughly cleaned prior to performing the anastomosis.

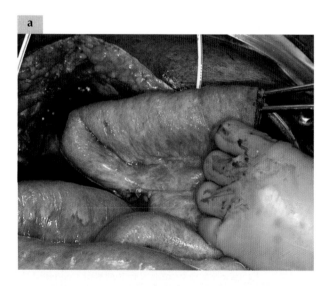
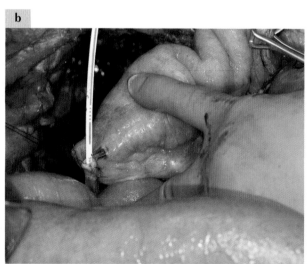

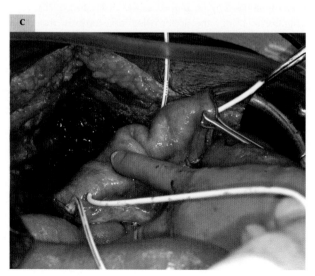

Figure 4.18. Enterotomy.
If a stent is used, it must be guided through the conduit. (a) A long fine-tipped clamp, such as a tonsil clamp, is placed through the conduit to a point a few centimeters from the staple line. (b) A small enterotomy is then made over the tip of the clamp with scissors, not electrocautery. (c) The stent is placed into the jaws of the clamp and removed through the conduit – it will later be brought out through a lower quadrant ostomy. Often, the first few ureteral sutures are placed prior to passing the stent to avoid visual obstruction from the stent while suturing.

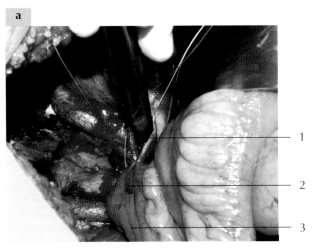

1 – Distal ureter
2 – Enterotomy in the small bowel
3 – Ileum

1 – Distal ureter
2 – Enterotomy in the small bowel
3 – Ileum

Figure 4.19. Beginning the anastomosis.
The uretero–ileal anastomosis begins from posterior to anterior. (**a**) The initial suture is placed at the most inferior part of the planned anastomosis. If a stent is used it is placed into the renal pelvis prior to beginning the anastomosis. Fluoroscopy is not necessary to place the stent; however, a postoperative radiograph should be obtained to confirm placement in the renal pelvis and to serve as a baseline for comparison against future films. In this case, the ureter was widely patent and a stent was not passed. If the ureter has not been subject to chronic dilation, it is spatulated with Potts–Smith scissors. The first few sutures are placed and tied. (**b**) The remaining sutures are laid into place and tied sequentially at the same time. The placement of sutures begins posteriorly and moves anteriorly; usually, six to eight sutures of 4-0 polyglactin are required to complete the anastomosis.

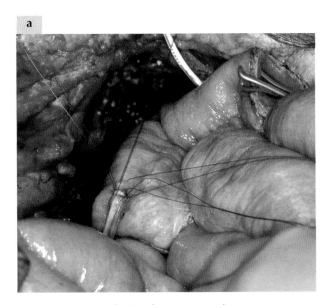

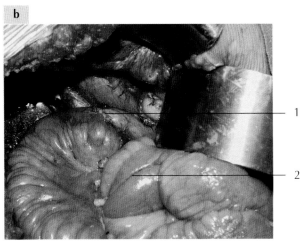

1 – Completed ureteral anastomosis
2 – Completed ileal anastomosis

Figure 4.20. Completing the anastomosis.
(**a**) The remaining sutures are placed and the ureter is seen in close approximation to the ileum; these sutures are then carefully tied. The procedure is repeated on the contralateral ureter. Again, if a stent is used, a clamp should be placed through the conduit to serve as a guide. If a stent is not used, the ileum may be opened directly over the site of anastomosis. (**b**) A completed right uretero–ileal anastomosis and the reanastomosed small bowel are seen. The distal portion of the ileum is then brought to the abdominal wall. It is the authors' practice not to suture the proximal end of the conduit to the sacral promontory.

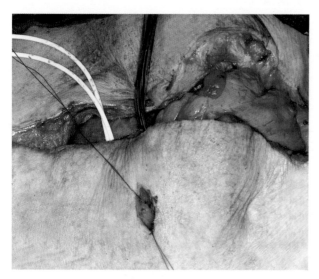

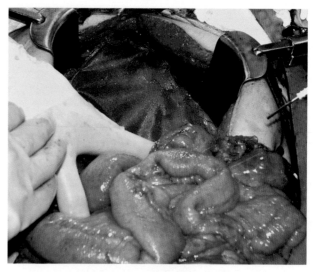

Figure 4.21. Creating the stoma.
An ostomy is created in the right lower quadrant. It is recommended that an enterostomal therapist evaluates the patient preoperatively and marks the appropriate ostomy sites. The site should be chosen in a location that will not be cumbersome for the patient to change the appliance or interfere with the normal position of clothing. If the site has not been previously marked, the ostomy should be placed two thirds from the anterior iliac spine toward the umbilicus. It is important that the ileum is brought through the rectus abdominus muscle to minimize the risk of stomal herniation.

Figure 4.22. Filling the pelvis.
Prior to closing the abdomen it is prudent to fill the pelvis with some sort of material. If a neovagina is created this will provide bulk in the pelvis. Otherwise, an omental pedicle flap may be placed to fill in the defect. A delayed absorbable mesh offers an attractive alternative to a tissue flap in the pelvis. It will keep the small bowel from prolapsing into the pelvis and will decrease the likelihood of small bowel obstruction and fistula formation. In comparison to a permanent mesh, it has a lower likelihood of resulting in a serious pelvic infection that would require mesh removal. Closed suction drains are placed in the pelvis and beneath the ureteral anastomoses.

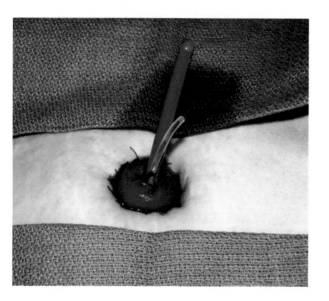

Figure 4.23. Completed conduit.
The completed ileal conduit is shown after closure of the abdomen and prior to placement of the stomal appliance. The rosebud is created with delayed absorbable suture (described in Chapter 3), and any catheters protruding through the conduit are sutured in place to prevent accidental dislodging or migration. An 18-French (Fr) fenestrated catheter is placed through the stoma and beyond the fascia to prevent obstruction of urine at the fascial level during initial healing. In this case, the anatomical circumstances dictated that only one ureter was stented. The stents are usually left in place for 7–10 days, and radiologic imaging is not required.

Continent urinary conduit (modified Penn pouch)

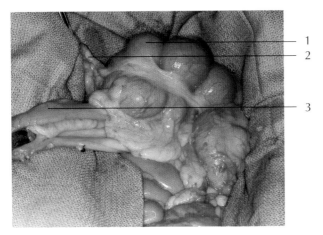

1 – Cecum
2 – Appendix
3 – Terminal ileum

Figure 4.24. Anatomy.
The appendix serves as the perfect source for the catheterizable limb of the continent urinary conduit if it has not been previously removed; it demonstrates no significant radiation damage; and it has an adequate lumen. If the appendix has been removed, alternative configurations should be considered, including the Miami or Indiana pouches. In this section, a modification of the Penn pouch will be described. For this technique, the ureters are implanted into a segment of distal ileum approximately 10 cm from the ileocecal valve; the appendix serves as the catheterizable limb and continence valve, and the ascending colon functions as the reservoir. A longer segment of terminal ileum can be used if additional length is needed to replace excised or irradiated ureters. The ureters are not tunneled, but implanting them proximal to the ileocecal valve prevents reflux, which is more likely to occur in a pouch that uses the ascending colon as both the reservoir and the site of ureteral implantation. The appendix is placed into a submucosal tunnel in situ to provide a short efferent limb that is easy to catheterize. Traditional ileocecal pouches that use the terminal ileum as the efferent limb have demonstrated higher revision rates for difficult catheterization or stomal incontinence.

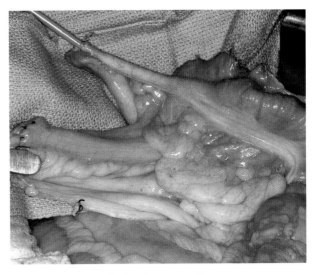

Figure 4.25. Cannulating the appendix.
The mesentery of the appendix is carefully mobilized taking care not to disrupt the appendiceal artery, as this will lead to subsequent ischemia and necrosis. The tip of the appendix is resected and the appendix is cannulated first with a fine probe or an 8-Fr pediatric feeding catheter. Subsequently, the appendix is dilated to accommodate a 12–14-Fr red rubber catheter.

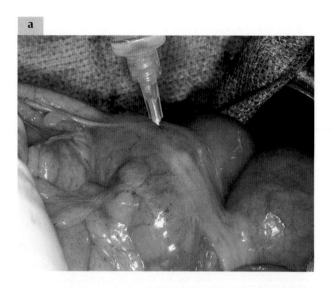

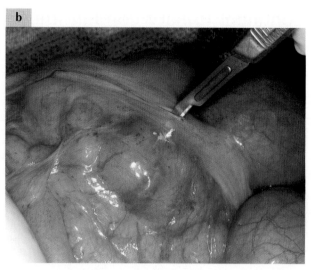

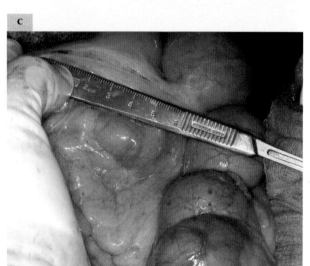

Figure 4.26. Incising the taenia.
(a) The taenia leading toward the appendix is injected with 1% lidocaine with 1:100,000 epinephrine to create a wheal from the appendix–cecal junction along the taenia for 4 cm. (b) The seromuscular layer of the cecum is incised with a #15 blade along the anterior taenia coli. (c) The length of the incision should be 4–5 cm. Care should be taken not to enter the cecal mucosa.

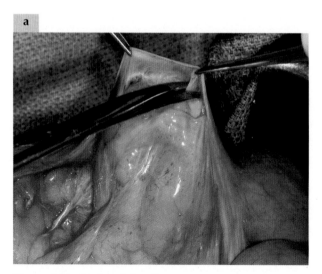

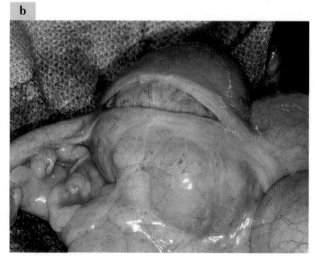

Figure 4.27. Undermining the cecum.
(a) The seromuscular incision is undermined with Metzenbaum scissors to create a trough for subsequent embedding of the appendix. (b) When complete, the mucosa of the cecum is readily apparent.

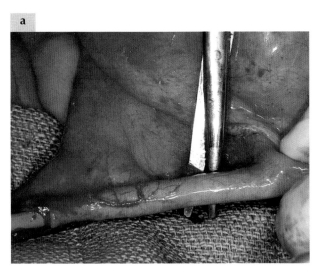
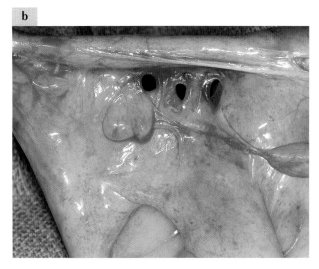

Figure 4.28 Creating windows of Deaver.
Several windows are created beneath the appendix, which will subsequently be used to tunnel and secure the appendix. (**a**) Scissors are used to carefully identify avascular windows of Deaver beneath the appendix. Again, care should be taken not to disrupt the appendiceal artery or its branches – staying very close to the appendix is useful in avoiding these vessels. (**b**) Usually, three windows will provide adequate ability to tunnel and secure the appendix.

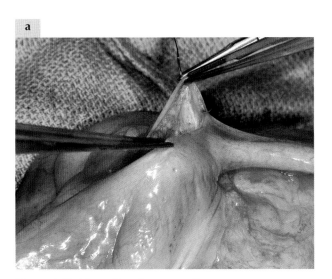
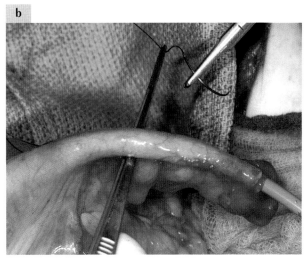

Figure 4.29. Tunneling the appendix.
Sutures of 3-0 silk are used to secure the appendix into the submucosal trough. The appendix is flipped into the trough created along the taenial incision. Initially, one side of the cecal seromuscular incision is grasped close to the base of the appendix. The tunnel is formed from the appendix–cecal junction and works towards the distal end of the appendix and along the cecal incision. (**a**) The suture is passed through the seromuscular layer, laterally to medially; (**b**) it is grasped with a fine forceps through the first window.

continued overleaf

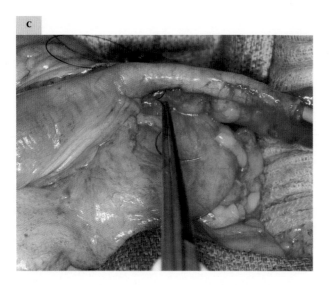

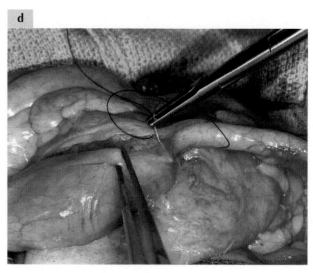

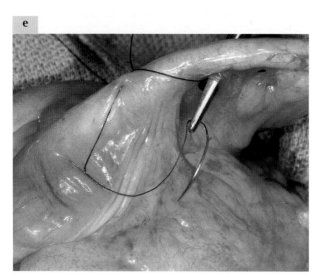

Figure 4.29. Continued.
(**c**) The suture itself, not the needle, is grasped to allow for easier mobility when it is brought through the window beneath the appendix. (**d**) The suture is then reloaded and passed through the seromuscular layer on the opposite side, medially to laterally; (**e**) it is then regrasped through the window to be brought back beneath the appendix in the opposite direction. The appendix is secured into the trough as this suture reopposes the serosa of the cecal flaps.

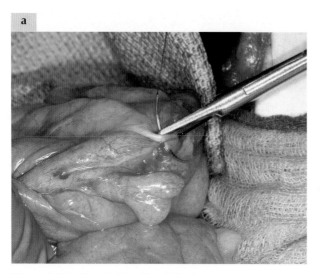

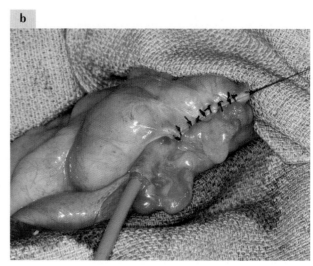

Figure 4.30. Completing the embedment.
(**a**) Additional sutures are placed from one seromuscular layer through the window to the other side, which is then sutured, passed back, and tied. The subsequent stitches are not quite as complex since the appendix has already been inverted. (**b**) After completing the suturing through the windows, the remainder of the undermined cecal serosa is re-approximated over the appendix with interrupted permanent silk sutures.

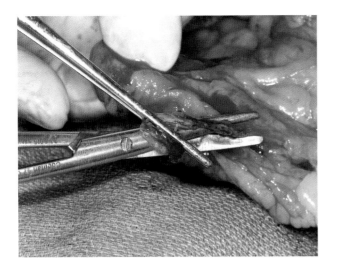

Figure 4.31. Creating the reservoir.
The reservoir is created from approximately 25 cm of ascending colon with care taken not to disrupt the middle colic vessels. The colon is divided with a disposable stapler (described in Chapter 3). The hepatic flexure needs to be mobilized to gain adequate length for the reservoir and mobility to perform the ileocolic anastomosis. The first step in creating the reservoir is to excise the entire staple line so that the colon can be opened and cleaned. The purpose of detubularizing the colon is to eliminate the normal peristaltic activity of the colon to provide a low-pressure, high-capacity reservoir.

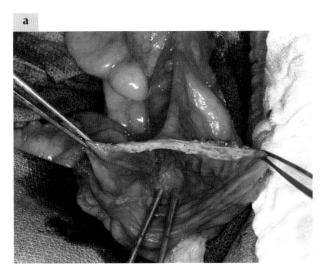
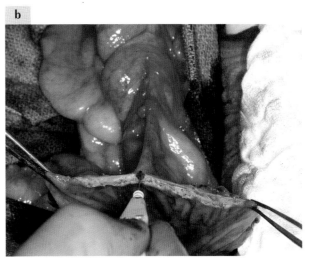

Figure 4.32 (a and b). Opening the colon.
The colon is grasped lateral to the anterior taenia coli. It is opened longitudinally along the taenia with electrocautery. A forceps or clamp can serve as a guide to assist in opening the colon, which is opened all the way to the cecum. When performing a modified Penn pouch the incision stops prior to reaching the base of the cecum near the appendiceal trough.

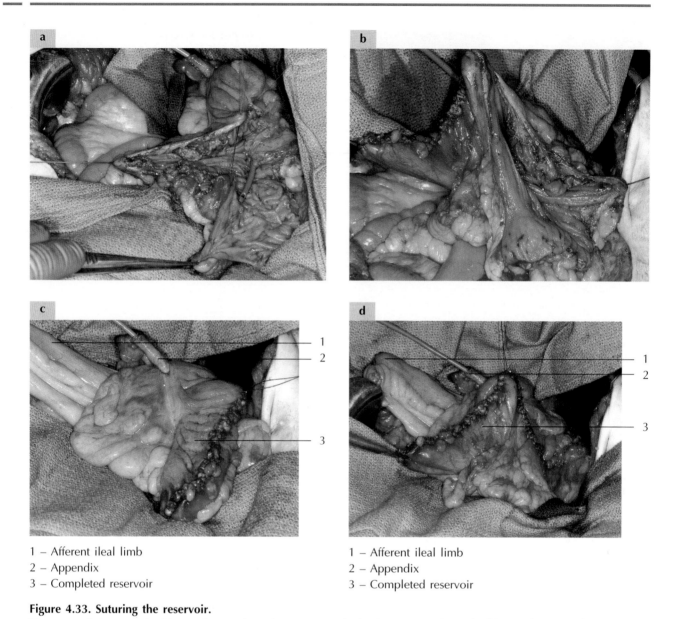

1 – Afferent ileal limb
2 – Appendix
3 – Completed reservoir

1 – Afferent ileal limb
2 – Appendix
3 – Completed reservoir

Figure 4.33. Suturing the reservoir.
The reservoir is created with two layers of continuous 3-0 polyglactin sutures. The red rubber catheter is adjusted to lie in the base of the pouch. (**a**) The entire ascending colon has been opened and thoroughly rinsed with normal saline to remove as much of the colonic contents as possible. A stay suture is placed to align the edges of the bowel. In this case, since the cecum has not been completely divided, the bowel will be closed with two adjoining suture lines. (**b**) One side of the reservoir has been closed but the lumen can still be seen on the other side. (**c**) The embedded in situ appendix as it protrudes from the reservoir. This is the posterior view of the appendiceal limb, whereas, previously, the anterior view was seen during its creation. (**d**) The completed pouch. The ureters are now inserted into the proximal end of the ileal afferent limb in the manner described above for the ileal conduit. The ureters are placed end to side into the terminal ileum without tunneling.

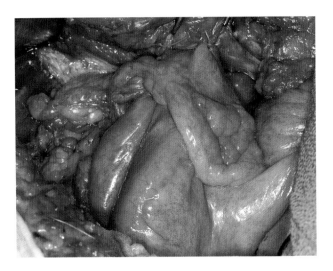

Figure 4.34. Fixation.
The appendiceal limb is usually anastomosed to the base of the umbilicus, though it may also come out through the right lower quadrant. The completed pouch is fixed to the anterior abdominal wall just lateral and superior to the umbilicus. When beginning the pelvic exenteration it is prudent to extend the skin and fascial incisions to the left side of the umbilicus so that a 2-cm edge of fascia is available for closure. Care is taken so that the pouch and appendix are not injured during the fascial closure. It is wise to use interrupted sutures through this area so that the pouch can be thoroughly examined prior to final abdominal closure.

References

1. Brunschwig A. Complete excision of pelvic viscera for advanced carcinoma. *Cancer* 1948; **1**:177–83.
2. Penalver MA, Angioli R, Mirhashemi R, Malik R. Management of early and late complications of ileocolonic continent urinary reservoir (Miami pouch). *Gynecol Oncol* 1998; **69**:185–91.
3. Ramirez PT, Modesitt SC, Morris M et al. Functional outcomes and complications of continent urinary diversions in patients with gynecologic malignancies. *Gynecol Oncol* 2002; **85**:285–91.
4. Crozier M, Morris M, Levenback C et al. Pelvic exenteration for adenocarcinoma of the uterine cervix. *Gynecol Oncol* 1995; **58**:74–8.
5. Matthews CM, Morris M, Burke TW et al. Pelvic exenteration in the elderly patient. *Obstet Gynecol* 1992; **79**:773–7.
6. Morley GW, Hopkins MP, Lindenauer SM, Roberts JA. Pelvic exenteration, University of Michigan: 100 patients at 5 years. *Obstet Gynecol* 1989; **74**:934–43.
7. Shingleton HM, Soong SJ, Gelder MS et al. Clinical and histopathologic factors predicting recurrence and survival after pelvic exenteration for cancer of the cervix. *Obstet Gynecol* 1989; **73**:1027–34.
8. Stanhope CR, Webb MJ, Podratz KC. Pelvic exenteration for recurrent cervical cancer. *Clin Obstet Gynecol* 1990; **33**:897–909.
9. Barakat RR, Goldman NA, Patel DA et al. Pelvic exenteration for recurrent endometrial cancer. *Gynecol Oncol* 1999; **75**:99–102.
10. Gemignani ML, Alektiar KM, Leitao M et al. Radical surgical resection and high-dose intraoperative radiation therapy (HDR-IORT) in patients with recurrent gynecologic cancers. *Int J Radiat Oncol Biol Phys* 2001; **50**:687–94.
11. Hockel M. Laterally extended endopelvic resection: surgical treatment of infrailiac pelvic wall recurrences of gynecologic malignancies. *Am J Obstet Gynecol* 1999; **180**:306–12.

5 Laparoscopic staging procedures

Yukio Sonoda and Richard R Barakat

Surgical staging remains the gold standard by which spread of disease is measured. The surgical staging of gynecologic malignancies relies heavily on the evaluation of the pelvic and paraaortic lymph nodes; however, the evaluation of these nodes can be technically challenging given their proximity to major vascular structures. The concept of decreasing the morbidity associated with the surgical staging procedure has given rise to the use of minimally invasive techniques for the surgical staging of gynecologic malignancies.

Laparoscopy has been used in the field of gynecology for many years. Only recently, with the evolution of laparoscopic skills and improvements in instrumentation, has operative laparoscopy expanded to the field of gynecologic oncology. In 1989, Dargent and Salvat reported on the use of laparoscopy to evaluate pelvic lymph nodes.[1] This concept was soon applied to the staging of gynecologic malignancies. Querleu et al described the use of laparoscopy as a means of staging patients with cervical cancer.[2] Reports of the use of laparoscopic staging for the management of endometrial cancer and ovarian cancer soon followed.[3,4] The use of minimally invasive surgery for the management of gynecologic malignancies seems ideal for surgical staging. Avoiding the morbidity associated with traditional laparotomy in the early-stage patient is the primary goal of the laparoscopic staging procedure. Yet, this must be performed without the loss of accuracy. The comparable precision of the two approaches to staging has been demonstrated in terms of lymph node counts in both humans and porcine models.[5,6] Additional benefits of the laparoscopic approach include decreased length of stay, overall costs and postoperative adhesions.[5–7]

The potential value of operative laparoscopy in the surgical staging of gynecologic malignancies has become obvious worldwide. Prospective randomized trials are ongoing to evaluate the role of operative laparoscopy compared to laparotomy in the management of gynecologic malignancies. If these two approaches prove to be equal, the skills required to perform laparoscopic staging should become part of the gynecologic oncologist's armamentarium. This chapter illustrates the different components of the laparoscopic staging procedures.

The procedures described in this chapter are used for the comprehensive staging of ovarian and endometrial cancers. Patients with cervical cancer are currently staged clinically, and the laparoscopic management for this disease is described elsewhere within this text. The techniques described in this chapter are intended for use in patients who have organ-confined disease. While laparoscopy may be appropriate in selected circumstances where disease has spread out of the pelvis, the procedures described within are not intended for those purposes. There are differences in the staging procedures performed for primary ovarian and endometrial cancers, but the overwhelming similarities warrant them to be presented together. The general outline of the chapter applies to the comprehensive laparoscopic staging of ovarian cancer. This laparoscopic staging procedure includes a thorough survey of the abdomen and pelvis, bilateral pelvic and paraaortic lymph node dissections, an infracolic omentectomy, pelvic and peritoneal washings, random biopsies, a hysterectomy, and bilateral salpingo-oophorectomy. For endometrial cancer, a similar procedure is conducted except that the paraaortic lymph node dissection is terminated at the level of the inferior mesenteric artery instead of continuing to the level of insertion of the ovarian veins, and an omentectomy is only performed in selected cases. An omentectomy is indicated for patients with serous or clear-cell histologic subtypes of endometrial cancer. Some practitioners also perform an omentectomy for high-grade endometrioid endometrial cancer, as these tumors are part of the spectrum of high-risk lesions that include serous and clear-cell histologies. The lymphadenectomy depicted in this chapter is the standard way that the authors perform a lymph node dissection for all early-stage ovarian and endometrial cancers. Some practitioners may elect to perform a more limited lymph node sampling; however, there are no specific criteria to determine the adequacy of lymph node sampling versus formal dissection. A number of reports in the peer-reviewed literature suggest a therapeutic advantage to performing a complete lymphadenectomy in patients with early-stage disease. Additionally, it is often less complicated to remove all lymphatic tissue, rather than only selected packages, since these nodal packets are frequently adherent and laden with small blood vessels. Thus, a formal lymphadenectomy is demonstrated in this chapter.

Entering the abdomen, survey and washings

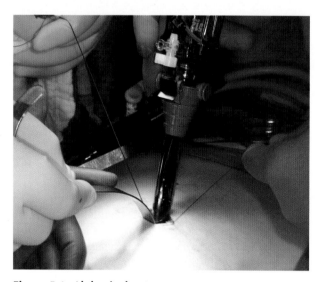

Figure 5.1. Abdominal entry.
The laparoscopic staging procedure begins with the introduction of the laparoscope. Techniques for placement of the initial trocar (open versus direct insertion versus pneumoperitoneum) vary depending on surgeon preference but, in general, the laparoscope is placed through an umbilical port. Some practitioners believe that the open laparoscopic technique can minimize the risk of injury to underlying tissues, particularly in the patient who has undergone prior abdominal or pelvic surgery.

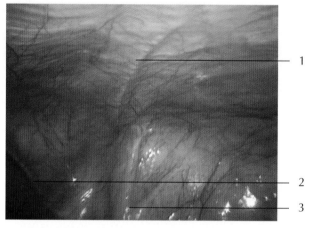

1 – Right inferior epigastric artery
2 – Right medial umbilical ligament
3 – Distal portion of right round ligament

Figure 5.2. Inferior epigastric vessels.
After the introduction of the laparoscope, accessory trocars must be placed. The placement of the lateral accessory trocars is crucial, since improper placement can make the procedure difficult. Given that the staging procedure requires access to both the abdomen and the pelvis, accessory trocars are usually placed in a position lateral to the inferior epigastric vessels and rectus muscles. These vessels should be visualized before introduction of the lateral trocars. Identification of the inferior epigastric vessels can be aided by simple external pressure applied in the inguinal region, which distends the vessels.

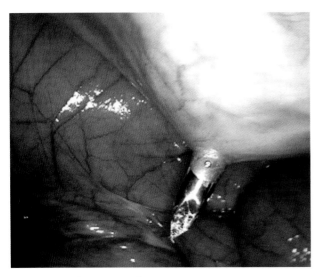

Figure 5.3. Placement of accessory trocars.
The size of the accessory trocar depends on the diameter of instruments that the surgeon prefers to use. Several fundamental principles should be adhered to when placing any sized trocar: the insertion should be under direct visualization and the direction of insertion should be perpendicular to the abdominal wall to avoid 'tunneling'.

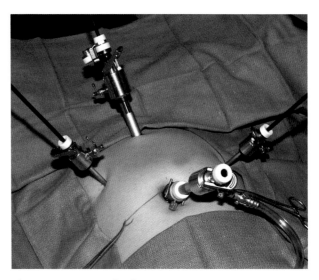

Figure 5.4. Trocars in situ.
One of several final trocar configurations is shown here. The staging procedure can be conducted through reusable or disposable trocars. The reusable trocars certainly provide cost savings over time; however, lymph node removal is often more efficient with disposable trocars that have superior vents and caps. Five millimeter lateral trocars, which can accommodate many instruments, are shown in this figure. When larger devices such as the argon-beam coagulator or the endoscopic stapler are used, these lateral trocars are replaced with larger diameter trocars.

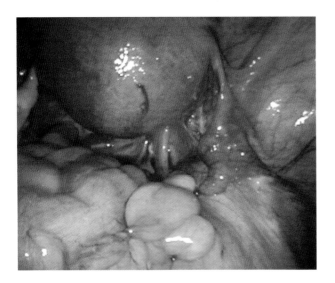

Figure 5.5. Laparoscopic inspection of the pelvis.
The staging procedure begins with a thorough exploration of the pelvic structures. The pelvic organs and peritoneal surfaces should be carefully examined. Laparoscopy is helpful in examining these surfaces since the surgeon's view is magnified. If the patient has had prior pelvic surgery, the adnexa may be densely adherent to the pelvic sidewall, resulting in a challenging dissection.

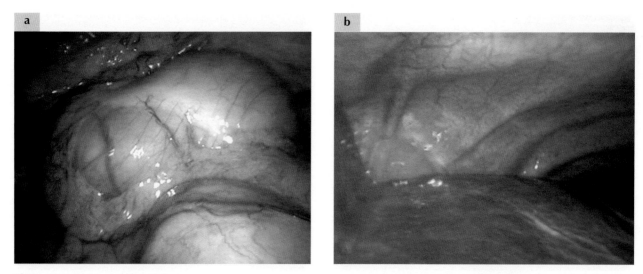

Figure 5.6. Survey of the abdomen.
Once the pelvic inspection is completed, the upper abdomen should be inspected for metastatic disease. This should be done systematically, usually starting from the cecum in the right lower quadrant and working up the paracolic gutter toward the hepatic flexure where the gallbladder can be inspected. Next, the transverse colon and omentum should be examined, followed by the descending colon, left paracolic gutter, and the sigmoid colon. The small bowel should also be inspected in its entirety. (**a**) The intestinal surfaces are examined closely. Both the right and left diaphragms and the liver surface should be scrutinized for evidence of disease. The laparoscopic view facilitates this portion of the exploration of the upper abdomen. (**b**) A magnified view of the left lobe of the liver and the left diaphragm.

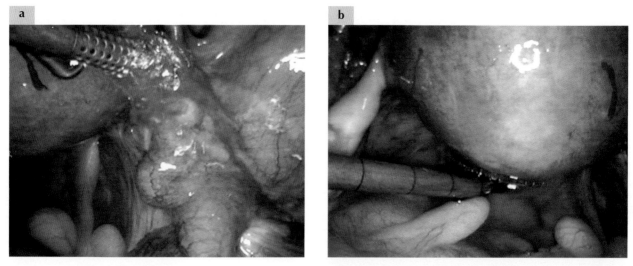

Figure 5.7. Peritoneal washings.
Prior to commencing any portion of the dissection, peritoneal cytology should be obtained. If peritoneal fluid is present, this can be aspirated. If there is no obvious peritoneal fluid, washings should be obtained by (**a**) irrigating the abdomen and pelvis, and (**b**) then aspirating the fluid. The fluid is aspirated from the most dependent portion of the pelvis in order to remove the irrigation completely and obtain a representative sample. Collection traps connected to the suction tubing can be used to accumulate the specimen while aspirating. The diaphragms, paracolic gutters and pelvic peritoneum should all be irrigated with heparinized saline (1 unit/ml).

Pelvic lymphadenectomy

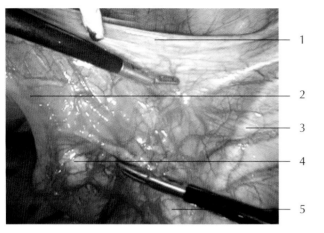

1 – Right round ligament
2 – Right fallopian tube
3 – Right external iliac artery
4 – Right ovary
5 – Right infundibulopelvic ligament

Figure 5.8. Beginning the pelvic lymph node dissection.
The dissection for the laparoscopic staging procedure begins with the pelvic lymph node dissection. The authors perform these staging procedures with the argon-beam coagulator; however, other forms of energy (bipolar, monopolar, and ultrasound) can be used. The pelvic lymph node dissection begins by identifying the round ligament. This is grasped with a forceps to tent the posterior leaf of the broad ligament. Alternatively, a uterine manipulator is used to create tension on the broad ligament.

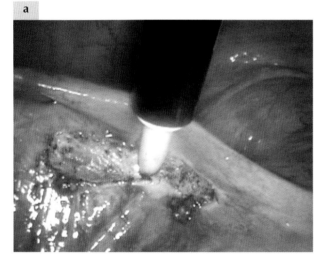

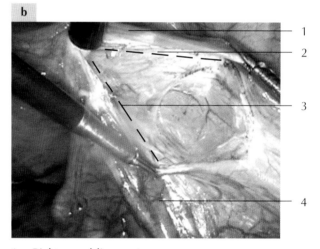

1 – Right round ligament
2 – Broken line indicating first incision parallel to round ligament
3 – Broken line indicating second incision parallel to infundibulopelvic ligament
4 – Right infundibulopelvic ligament

Figure 5.9. Opening the posterior leaf of the broad ligament.
(a) Making an incision parallel to the round ligament opens the posterior leaf of the broad ligament. This incision is started laterally and continued medially towards the uterus. (b) A second incision is made parallel to the infundibulopelvic (IP) ligament. This two-incision technique provides ample access to the retroperitoneum. (c) When complete, all intervening peritoneum has been dissected away from the round ligament and the IP ligament.

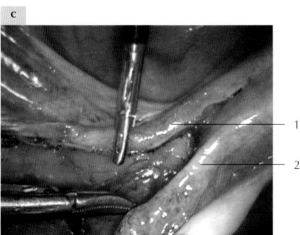

1 – Left round ligament
2 – Left fallopian tube

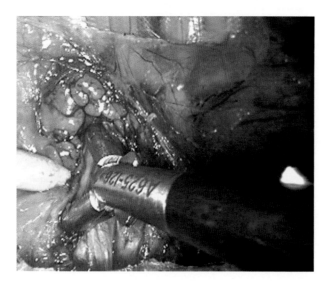

Figure 5.10. Identifying the external iliac artery.
Prior to removing the lymphatic tissue, the external iliac artery should be clearly identified. This can be done with gentle blunt dissection using atraumatic forceps or the tip of the argon-beam coagulator. Identifying normal anatomic structures is an important way of minimizing vascular complications during pelvic or paraaortic lymph node dissections.

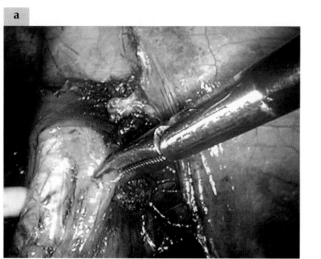
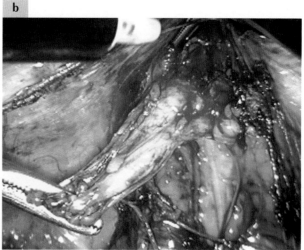

Figure 5.11. Dissecting the external iliac lymph nodes.
The lymphatic tissue can be dissected off the underlying vessels by grasping the tissue and placing it under tension. The argon-beam coagulator is used to bluntly free the lymphatic tissue and apply coagulation when hemostasis is required. The lymphatic tissue may be retracted laterally (**a**) or medially (**b**) to provide the best orientation for lymph node removal. This will be dependent upon the location of the lymphatic tissue, as well as the orientation of the instruments.

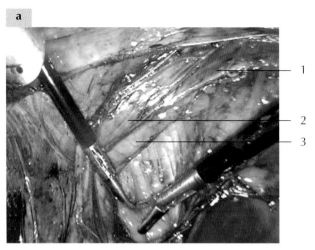

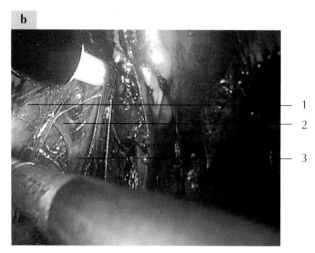

1 – Right deep circumflex iliac vein
2 – Right external iliac vein
3 – Right external iliac artery

1 – Left external iliac artery
2 – Left deep circumflex iliac vein
3 – Left external iliac vein

Figure 5.12. Distal limit of the external iliac dissection.
The distal extent of the external iliac dissection is the deep circumflex iliac vein. (**a**) Normally, the deep circumflex iliac vein passes over the external iliac artery, but in certain cases (**b**) the vein may pass beneath the artery. Removal of the nodal tissue surrounding the external iliac vessels should proceed with caution in this region as injury to these vessels may be difficult to control.

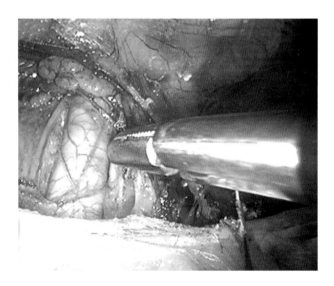

Figure 5.13. Identifying the external iliac vein.
After the nodal tissue from the external iliac artery has been removed, the external iliac vein should be identified. Once again, this can be done with careful blunt dissection using atraumatic forceps or the tip of the argon-beam coagulator. This photograph illustrates the identification of the left external iliac vein, just below the external iliac artery.

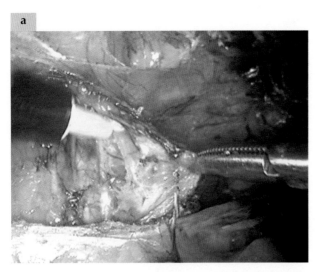
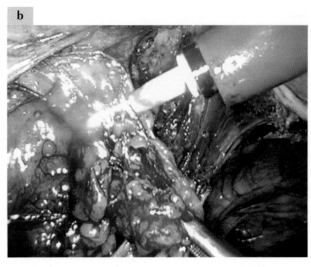

Figure 5.14. Removing nodal tissue from the external iliac vein.
(**a**) After identifying the external iliac vein, the surrounding nodal tissue can be grasped and dissected free using the argon-beam coagulator (ABC). Since the wall of the vein is pliable, it can easily be damaged if one is not careful during the dissection. Additionally, carbon dioxide gas that has been used to insufflate the peritoneum often compresses the vein. (**b**) Since the ABC will deliver a short stream of electrical current, care should also be taken to ensure that the energy is not misdirected into one of the vascular structures.

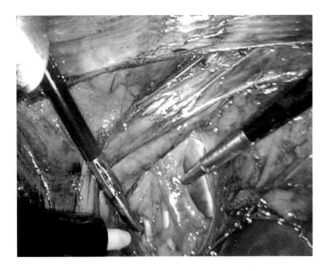

Figure 5.15. Exposing the obturator space.
After the external iliac vessels have been cleaned of the surrounding lymphatic tissue, they can be retracted medially to expose the obturator space. This must be done carefully, so as not to disrupt the network of veins that inhabit the obturator space. If the external vessels have been thoroughly cleaned from the bifurcation of the common iliac vessels down to the deep circumflex iliac vein, they will have sufficient mobility to permit adequate access to the obturator space.

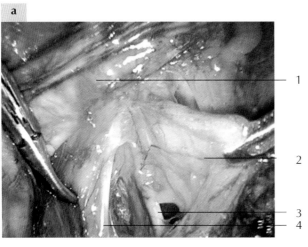

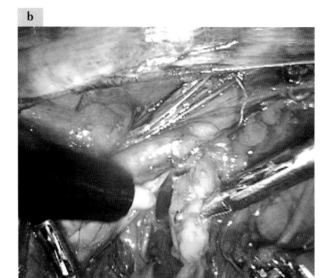

1 – Right external iliac artery
2 – Right obturator lymph nodes
3 – Right obturator nerve
4 – Right superior vesical artery

Figure 5.16. Identifying the obturator nerve.
After exposing the obturator space, the obturator nerve must be identified before attempting to remove any lymphatic tissue. The nerve can be identified with gentle blunt dissection of the lymphatic tissue in the obturator space. (**a**) Once the obturator nerve has been identified, the lymphatic tissue can be grasped and elevated away from it. (**b**) The argon-beam coagulator can now be used safely to free the nodal package from its attachments.

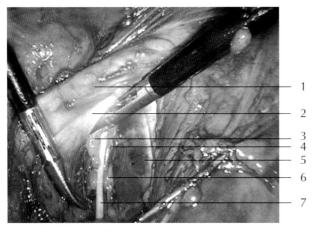

1 – Right external iliac artery
2 – Right external iliac vein
3 – Remaining obturator lymph nodes
4 – Right obturator vein
5 – Right obturator internus muscle
6 – Right obturator artery
7 – Right obturator nerve

Figure 5.17. Final dissection of the obturator space.
The last remaining nodal tissue can be easily removed from the obturator space once the obturator nerve and obturator internus muscle are visualized. The obturator artery and vein lie below the obturator nerve, so caution must be used when dissecting in this region.

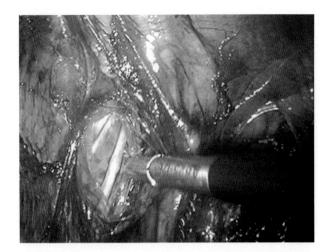

Figure 5.18. Medial approach to the obturator nodes.
An alternative approach to removing the obturator nodes is to expose the obturator space from the medial aspect. This is done by retracting the iliac vessels laterally and gently dissecting through the fatty lymphatic tissue to identify the obturator nerve. If the nerve is difficult to identify by one approach (medial or lateral) then the alternative approach may prove more fruitful.

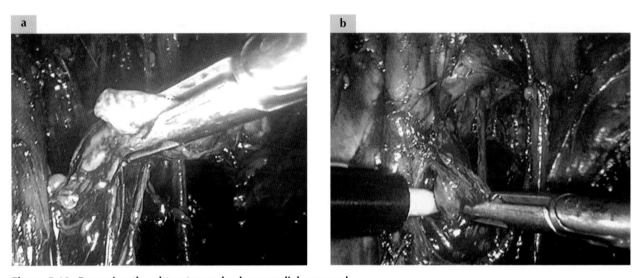

Figure 5.19. Removing the obturator nodes by a medial approach.
(a) The lymph nodes above the obturator nerve and below the external iliac vein can be grasped and dissected using a combination of blunt dissection and coagulation. (b) This should be done carefully, since the presence of an accessory obturator vein, also known as the anastomotic pelvic vein, may not be initially apparent.

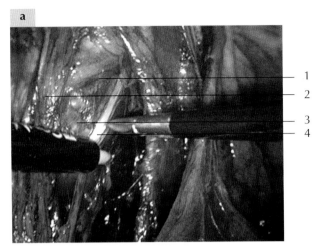

1 – Left accessory obturator vein
2 – Left external iliac vein
3 – Left obturator internus muscle
4 – Left obturator nerve

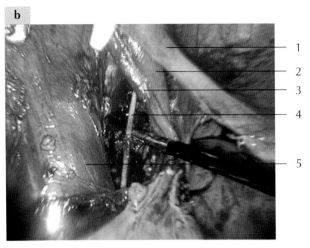

1 – Left round ligament
2 – Left external iliac vein
3 – Left external iliac artery
4 – Left obturator nerve
5 – Left psoas muscle

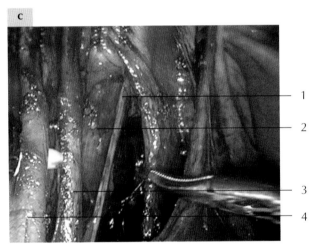

1 – Left obturator nerve
2 – Left obturator internus
3 – Left external iliac vein
4 – Left external iliac artery

Figure 5.20. Completed pelvic lymphadenectomy.
Once the pelvic lymphadenectomy is complete, no further lymph node tissue is visible. (**a**) The medial view of the obturator space dissection shows that all the nodal tissue has been removed and that the normal anatomic structures remain. (**b**) From the lateral approach, many of the same structures are visible; however, the most lateral aspect of the deep pelvic sidewall is not seen. (**c**) A view showing the external iliac dissection, as well as the obturator space dissection, demonstrates that after completely removing all lymphatic tissue, the external iliac artery and vein are completely separated from one another.

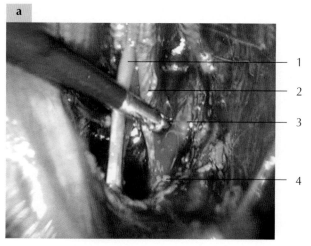

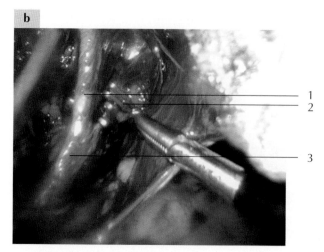

1 – Left obturator nerve
2 – Left superior vesical artery
3 – Left uterine artery
4 – Left hypogastric artery

1 – Left superior vesical artery
2 – Clips on left uterine artery
3 – Left hypogastric artery

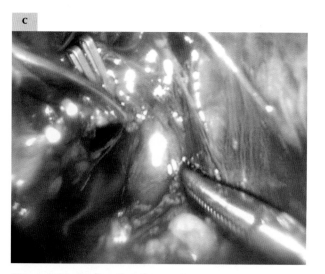

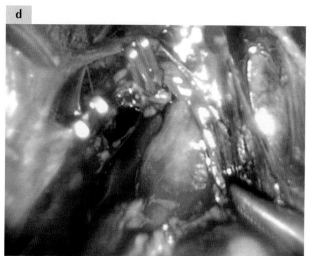

Figure 5.21. Transecting the uterine artery.
After completing the pelvic lymph node dissection, the uterine artery can be ligated at its origin. (**a**) This is done by dissecting it from the superior vesicle artery and applying hemostatic clips or staples. While not required to ligate the uterine artery at its origin during a staging procedure for endometrial or ovarian cancer, it can help to minimize bleeding during the hysterectomy portion of the procedure. (**b**) Typically, two clips are placed on either side of the point of transection. If the clips are placed securely across the entire vessel, (**c**) the artery can be transected with the endoscopic scissors (**d**) without significant bleeding.

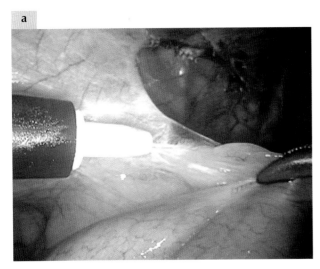
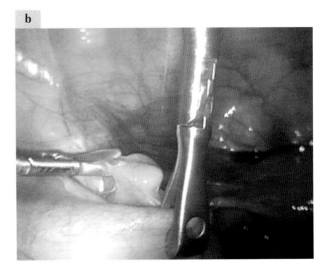

Figure 5.22. Freeing the sigmoid adhesions.
Before attempting the left-sided pelvic or paraaortic lymph node dissection, the sigmoid colon often needs to be mobilized to completely expose the left pelvic sidewall. (**a**) The argon-beam coagulator can be used to lyse any filmy attachments. Counter traction should be applied using atraumatic forceps on the sigmoid. (**b**) When lysing adhesions closer to the intestinal wall, it is often safer to employ sharp dissection with scissors.

Paraaortic lymphadenectomy

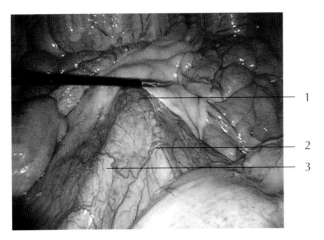

1 – Aortic bifurcation
2 – Left common iliac artery
3 – Right common iliac artery

Figure 5.23. Preparation for the paraaortic lymph node dissection.
Following the pelvic lymph node dissection, attention is turned to the paraaortic region. In preparation for the paraaortic lymph node dissection, the small bowel should be packed into the left upper quadrant to expose the aortic bifurcation. Meticulous packing of the bowel will facilitate the dissection.

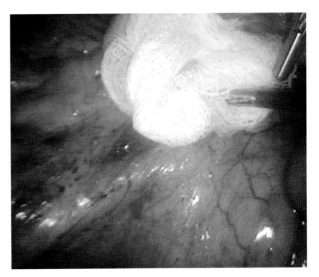

Figure 5.24. Insertion of a gauze sponge.
Prior to beginning the lymph node dissection, a radiopaque gauze sponge is inserted into the abdominal cavity. Unfolding the gauze completely will permit it to be placed through a 10-mm trocar. It can be used to blot the operative field or to tamponade any bleeding (in a similar fashion to that in which a laparotomy pad is used for open cases). It is important to keep close track of how many sponges have been placed intraperitoneally so that none inadvertently remain in the patient postoperatively.

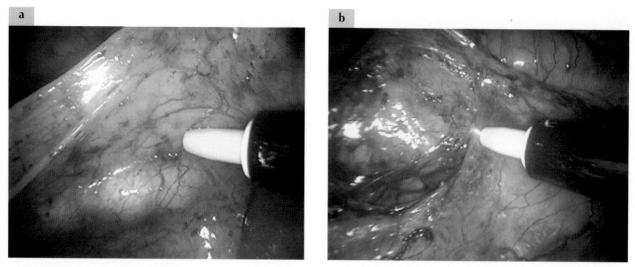

Figure 5.25. Opening the peritoneum.
The transperitoneal paraaortic lymph node dissection is begun by identifying the right common iliac artery. (**a**) The peritoneum over the artery is tented up with a grasper and is incised with the argon-beam coagulator or similar instrument. (**b**) Once the peritoneum has been incised, the incision is extended cephalad from the right common iliac artery to the bifurcation of the aorta. The pneumoperitoneum may help with the dissection – when gas enters the retroperitoneal space it helps elevate the posterior peritoneum off the underlying vessels.

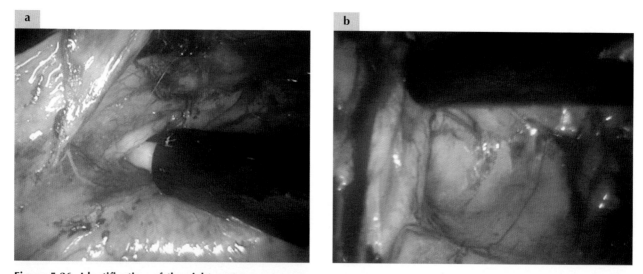

Figure 5.26. Identification of the right ureter.
Prior to beginning the right paraaortic dissection, the right ureter must be identified and retracted laterally. This entails elevating the posterior peritoneum while exploring, with blunt dissection, the retroperitoneal space lateral to the right common iliac artery. (**a**) Once the ureter is identified (**b**) it can be moved out of the operative field.

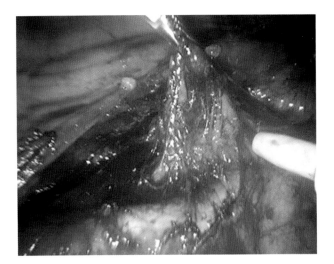

Figure 5.27. Beginning the right paraaortic dissection.
The nodal tissue overlying the vena cava is grasped and elevated. Using gentle blunt dissection this tissue is separated from the underlying vessel. The vena cava should be clearly identified before any attempt is made to remove the lymphatic tissue.

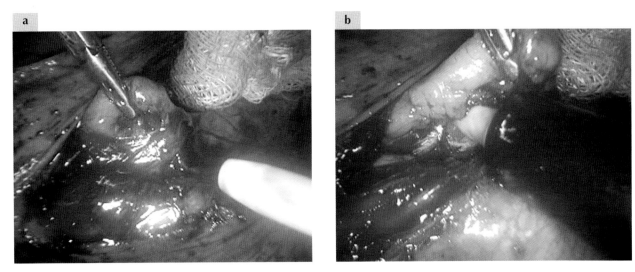

Figure 5.28. Removing the right paraaortic lymph nodes.
Once the vena cava has been identified, the process of removing the overlying lymphatic tissue can begin. This region has many perforating vessels from the vena cava to the lymphatic tissue. These small vessels should be coagulated prior to removing the nodal package. (**a**) The lymphatic tissue is elevated with a laparoscopic grasper; (**b**) pedicles are created with the argon-beam coagulator or another blunt-tipped instrument. The base of these nodal packets is then transected with cautery. The gauze placed into the peritoneum previously is seen in the background of these images.

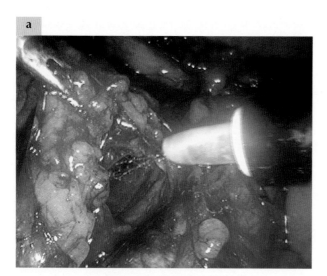
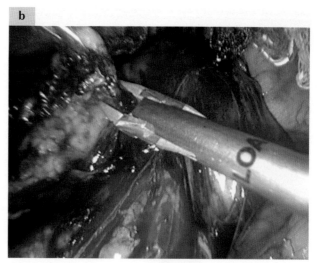

Figure 5.29. Identifying the 'fellow's vein'.
The precaval lymphatic package contains the 'fellow's vein'. Avulsing this vessel can lead to profuse bleeding that may be difficult to control laparoscopically. (**a**) As the nodal package is dissected from the vena cava, the surgeon must note the presence of this vessel. (**b**) Once the vessel is identified, it should be clipped, or coagulated and cut.

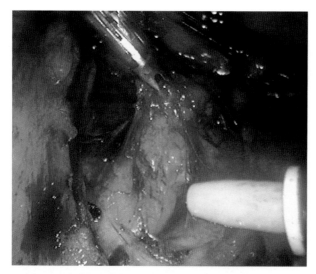

Figure 5.30. Removing the lateral caval nodes.
Lymph nodes lateral to the vena cava are removed in similar fashion. They are grasped and dissected off the vena cava using blunt dissection and coagulation with the argon-beam coagulator. Careful attention should be given to the location of the ureter and the underlying lumbar veins.

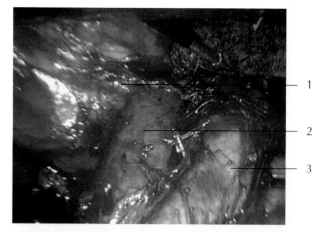

1 – Right ovarian vein
2 – Inferior vena cava
3 – Aorta

Figure 5.31. Identification of the right ovarian vein.
The precaval and lateral caval lymph nodes are removed to the level of the right ovarian vein. This is important given the drainage pattern of the right ovary. The lymphatic tissue typically runs in the same direction as venous drainage. The insertion of the ovarian veins is the prime landing zone for nodal metastases. If the dissection is not carried up to this level, important sites of metastatic disease may be overlooked.

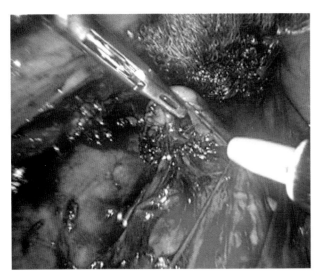

Figure 5.32. Removing interaortocaval lymph nodes.
The interaortocaval lymph nodes are removed in similar fashion. They are grasped and elevated off the aorta. The aorta is visualized, and the nodes are removed using a combination of blunt dissection and coagulation.

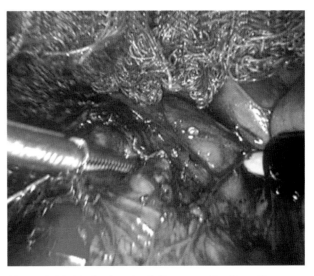

Figure 5.33. Beginning the left paraaortic dissection.
The left-sided dissection can be more challenging. This is in part due to the presence of the inferior mesenteric artery. Prior to beginning, the left ureter should be identified and pushed laterally.

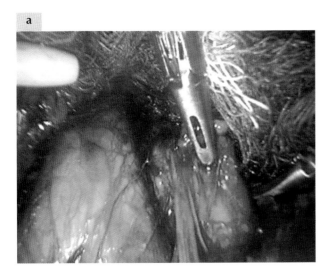

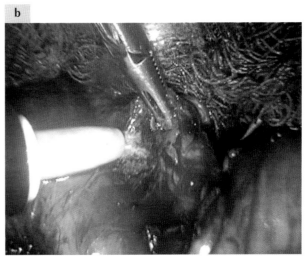

Figure 5.34. Removing the left paraaortic lymph nodes.
After retracting the ureter laterally, dissection of the left paraaortic nodes can be undertaken. (**a**) The nodal packages are elevated with laparoscopic grasping forceps as described previously. (**b**) The argon-beam coagulator, or other coagulating device, can be used to create pedicles that can then be detached from the aorta.

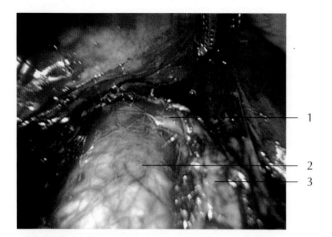

1 – Inferior mesenteric artery
2 – Aorta
3 – Lymph nodes surrounding the IMA

Figure 5.35. Superior aspect of the dissection.
The lymph nodes should be removed to the level of the
inferior mesenteric artery (IMA) for cases of endometrial
cancer. The IMA is usually surrounded by lymphatic
tissue and should be cleared to identify it unmistakably
to avoid injuring this vessel, and to ensure that the
dissection is carried out high enough. In cases of ovarian
cancer, the upper limit of the dissection is the left renal
vein.

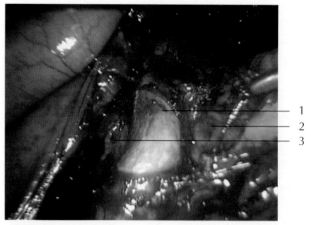

1 – Right common iliac artery
2 – Left common iliac vein
3 – Right common iliac vein

Figure 5.36. Removing the subaortic lymph nodes.
The subaortic lymph nodes can be removed using a
similar technique to that described previously. This nodal
package overlies the left common iliac vein. There may
be some vascular connections to the nodal package and
thus this area must be approached with caution. The
lymph nodes should be fully freed from the vein to
prevent tearing during nodal removal. The dissection
should be performed carefully so that the underlying
vascular structure is not punctured or lacerated. Not
being aware of this anatomic relationship can lead to
serious injury to the left common iliac vein, resulting in
a potential life-threatening hemorrhage.

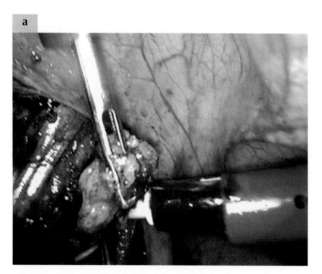

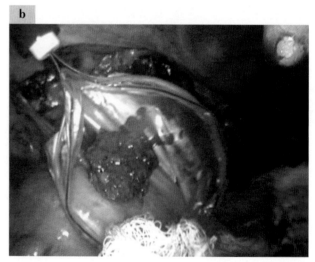

Figure 5.37. Removing the specimens.
(a) The harvested lymph nodes may be removed directly through the trocar using a strong, reliable grasper. (b) Larger
lymph node packets, or those suspicious for metastatic disease, may be removed in an endoscopic bag. The bag can
be removed through a large diameter trocar (10 or 12 mm) or, if a hysterectomy is to be performed as part of the
staging procedure, placed into the pouch of Douglas and removed at the time of vaginal colpotomy.

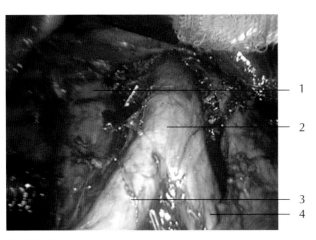

Figure 5.38. Completed inframesenteric dissection.
This figure illustrates the completed paraaortic dissection to the level of the inferior mesenteric artery (IMA). Note that left paraaortic lymph nodes will be found between the IMA and the aorta, as well as lateral to the IMA.

1 – Inferior vena cava
2 – Aorta
3 – Right common iliac artery
4 – Left common iliac artery

Laparoscopic omentectomy

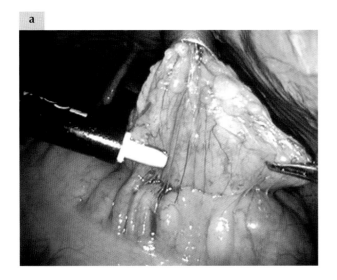

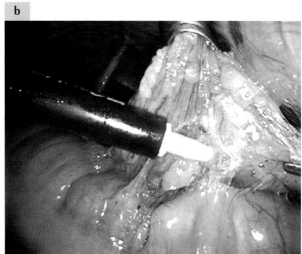

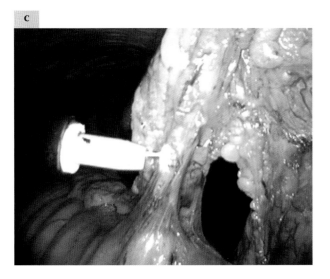

Figure 5.39. Freeing the transverse colon.
(**a**) The omentum is elevated and spread out to visualize the posterior leaf and the transverse colon. (**b**) The posterior leaf is incised to enter the lesser sac and to separate the omentum from the transverse colon. (**c**) The avascular portion of the omental attachment to the transverse colon is removed with the argon-beam coagulator (ABC) or a similar instrument. Other areas may be transected with cautery, but more energy will be required to adequately coagulate the small blood vessels that course through the omentum. The ABC should be activated a few millimeters away from the colon as some degree of thermal spread does occur.

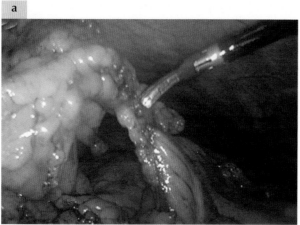

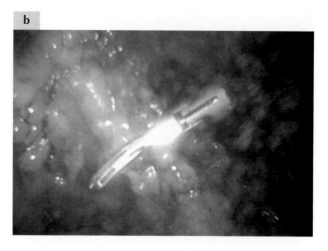

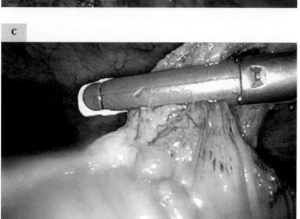

Figure 5.40. Transecting the gastrocolic ligament.
Once the omentum has been freed from the transverse colon, the gastrocolic ligament can be transected. This has a rich anastomosis of blood vessels and should be thoroughly cauterized. A number of different techniques may be employed to divide the gastrocolic ligament. (**a**) A harmonic scalpel uses ultrasonic energy, which can sequentially coagulate and cut across the gastrocolic ligament. (**b**) Ultrasound waves cause the tissue to be desiccated, which not only results in coagulation and cautery but also in the release of water as a byproduct. (**c**) Alternatively, a laparoscopic stapler with vascular loads may be used to transect the gastrocolic ligament, or to separate the omentum from the transverse colon.

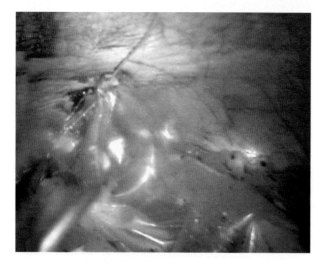

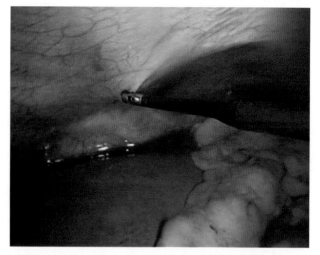

Figure 5.41. Specimen removal.
Once freed, the omentum can be placed into an endoscopic bag for removal. A very large omentum may need to be divided into parts to be removed, or a larger bag may need to be used. If a vaginal hysterectomy is to be performed as part of the staging procedure, the bag can be placed into the posterior cul-de-sac and removed at the time of vaginal colpotomy. Otherwise, one of the abdominal trocar sites should be extended slightly to remove the bag through the abdomen. The omentum is never removed by itself to prevent potential tumor contamination that may occur if it is brought through the abdominal wall without a bag.

Figure 5.42. Peritoneal biopsies.
Random peritoneal biopsies are obtained using biopsy forceps. Both diaphragms, the paracolic gutters, the pelvic sidewalls, the posterior cul-de-sac, and the bladder peritoneum are routinely sampled. If any suspicious nodules are found, these should be sampled or resected as well.

Laparoscopic portion of the hysterectomy

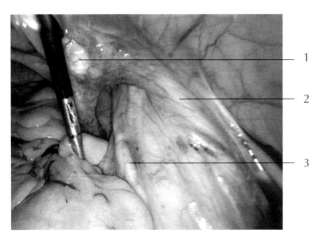

Figure 5.43. Identification of the ureter.
Prior to beginning the hysterectomy and bilateral salpingo-oophorectomy, it is important to visualize the course of the ureter. This can often be done transperitoneally by observing the ureter at the pelvic brim, where it crosses over the common iliac artery near its bifurcation, and tracing it down into the pelvis.

1 – Right ovary
2 – Right infundibulopelvic ligament
3 – Right ureter

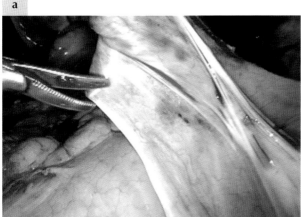

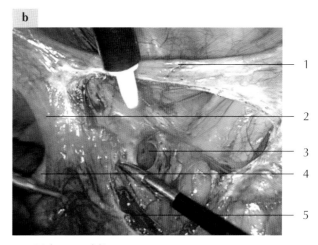

1 – Right round ligament
2 – Right fallopian tube
3 – Window in medial leaf of broad ligament
4 – Right ovary
5 – Right IP ligament

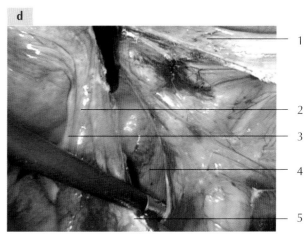

Figure 5.44. Isolating the infundibulopelvic (IP) ligament.
Since the broad ligament has been previously opened from the pelvic lymph node dissection, the IP ligament can be easily isolated. (**a** and **b**) Once the location of the ureter has been noted, a window is made in the medial leaf of the peritoneum with a grasper, scissors, or the argon-beam coagulator. (**c** and **d**) Creating countertraction with two instruments can easily extend this opening adequately to isolate the IP ligament.

1 – Right round ligament
2 – Right fallopian tube
3 – Right ovary
4 – Window in medial leaf of broad ligament
5 – Right IP ligament

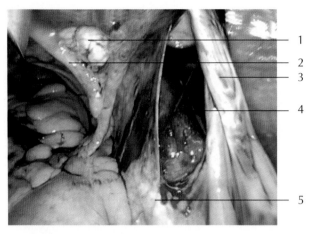

Figure 5.45. Rechecking the position of the ureter.
After creating the window in the medial leaf of the broad ligament the ureter is separated from the infundibulopelvic (IP) ligament. This should prevent it from being accidentally grasped when transecting the IP ligament. The figure illustrates the IP ligament after it has been isolated from the ureter.

1 – Right ovary
2 – Right fallopian tube
3 – Right infundibulopelvic ligament
4 – Window in medial leaf of broad ligament
5 – Right ureter

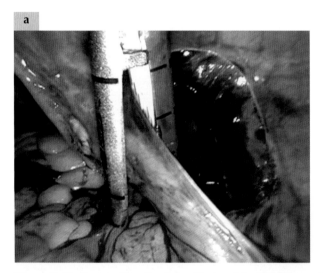
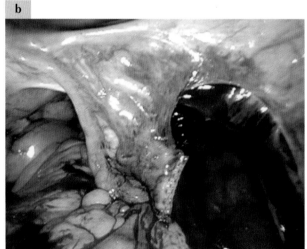

Figure 5.46. Transecting the infundibulopelvic (IP) ligament.
Once the IP ligament has been isolated from the ureter and surrounding structures, it can be safely transected. This can be accomplished with a stapling device (**a**), bipolar electrocautery (Kleppinger forceps, LigaSure, etc.), or endoscopic sutures. The tips of both jaws of the stapler should be visualized to ensure that the ureter is not inadvertently included in the jaws. (**b**) The entire ligament should be within the cut lines on the stapler to prevent bleeding when the tissue is released. It is also imperative that no ovarian tissue is captured in the stapling device as this can leave an ovarian remnant.

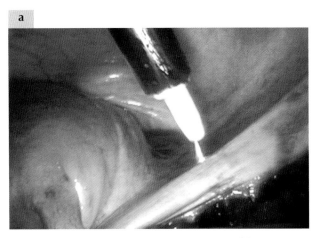
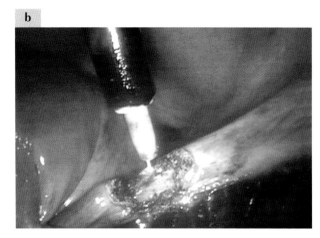

Figure 5.47 (a and b). Transecting the round ligament.
The development of a bladder flap begins with transecting the round ligament. The round ligament is placed under tension, and the argon-beam coagulator, or a similar device, is used to divide the ligament. If the ligament is transected without sufficient cautery, bleeding may occur from Samson's artery, which runs just beneath the round ligament proper.

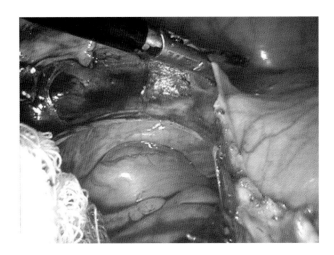

Figure 5.48. Creating the bladder flap.
The division of the round ligament provides access to the lateral border of the vesicouterine peritoneum. Using sharp dissection, the vesicouterine peritoneum can be incised to begin mobilizing the bladder.

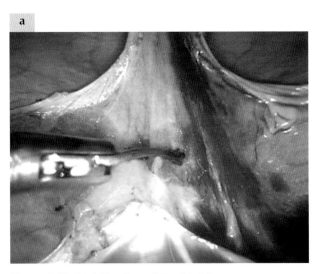
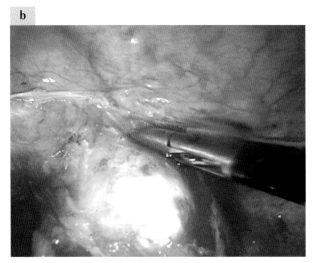

Figure 5.49. Mobilization of the bladder.
(a) The free edge of the bladder flap is elevated and the bladder is dissected from the underlying cervix using sharp dissection. Once the peritoneum has been transected, additional mobilization can be achieved by pushing the perivesical tissue caudad. (b) When the bladder has been fully mobilized off of the cervix the anterior intraperitoneal portion of the vagina will appear white and fibrous. This concludes the laparoscopic portion of the hysterectomy.

Vaginal portion of the hysterectomy

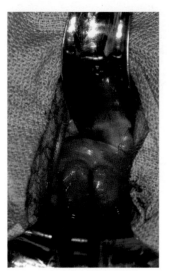

Figure 5.50. Beginning the vaginal hysterectomy. The vaginal portion of the procedure begins by inserting retractors into the vagina to expose the cervix. Typically, a weighted speculum is placed posteriorly and a Sims retractor or right-angled retractor is placed anteriorly. The cervix is grasped with two single-toothed tenacula or similar instruments.

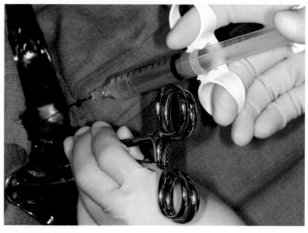

Figure 5.51. Injecting the cervix. The cervix is circumferentially injected at the cervico–vaginal junction with saline or a dilute solution of vasopressin (1 unit/ml). The vasopressin helps minimize bleeding when the vaginal cuff is incised and both solutions help to separate the planes of dissection.

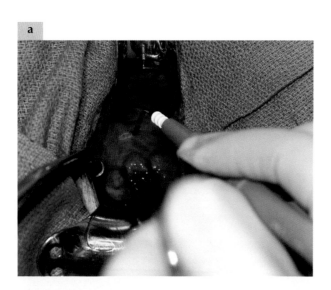

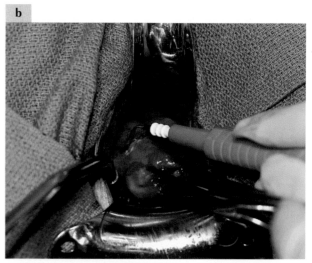

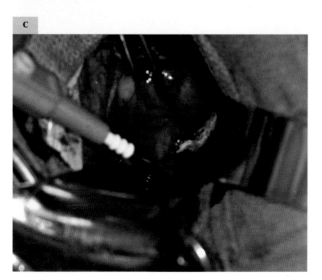

Figure 5.52. Circumscribing the vagina. (**a**) An initial incision is made anteriorly in the vaginal mucosa just below the level of the bladder. (**b**) The incision is extended laterally in both directions. This can either be performed with electrocautery (as illustrated) or a scalpel. (**c**) The incision is continued posteriorly until the anterior and posterior incisions meet. Once the initial incision is made, it is carried through the endopelvic fascia until a white and fibrous layer is reached. If the incision is not made deep enough, difficulty will be encountered while trying to enter the anterior or posterior cul-de-sac. To facilitate the dissection and achieve a natural separation of the tissue planes, strong traction is placed on the tenacula and the vaginal retractors to create countertraction.

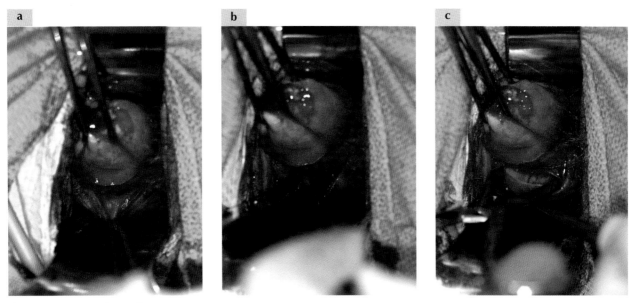

Figure 5.53. Posterior colpotomy.
(**a**) The cervix is pulled upward and the posterior vaginal mucosa is retracted inferiorly with forceps or the vaginal retractors. This allows the posterior peritoneum to be visualized and grasped. (**b**) The posterior cul-de-sac is entered by incising the posterior peritoneum with Mayo scissors. One broad cut with the scissors should be made to facilitate entry on the first attempt. If small cuts are made with the scissors, entry may not be achieved and the tissue planes will be disrupted making further dissection more difficult. (**c**) Once the pouch of Douglas has been entered the incision is enlarged bluntly with Mayo scissors. The posterior peritoneum is tagged with a suture and the weighted speculum is replaced with a Steiner retractor (long weighted speculum). This helps to keep the rectum out of the operative field during this portion of the procedure.

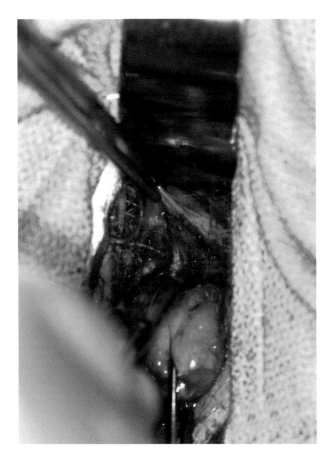

Figure 5.54. Dissecting the vesicouterine space.
The peritoneum overlying the anterior cul-de-sac is grasped with toothed forceps. The peritoneum is incised in a manner similar to that described for the posterior colpotomy. Once the peritoneum is entered, a narrow curved Deaver retractor is inserted beneath the bladder. The peritoneum should be entered in the midline to avoid injury to the bladder pillars. Concern for a cystotomy should be raised if urine begins to leak, or the catheter or balloon is seen.

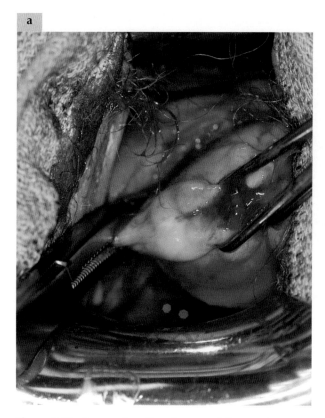

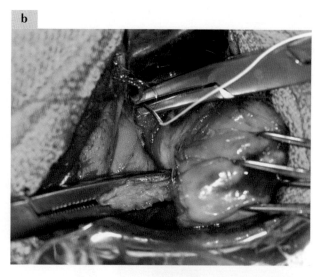

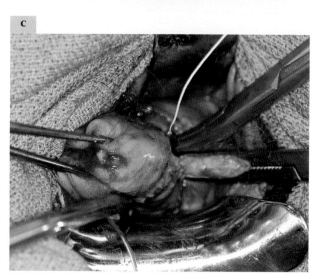

Figure 5.55. Transecting the uterosacral ligaments.
Once the posterior cul-de-sac has been entered, the uterosacral ligaments can be transected. (**a**) Traction is applied to the cervix to help expose the ligaments as a heavy clamp, such as a Heaney or Zeppelin, is placed. (**b**) The ligament is then transected with a Mayo scissors and suture ligated with a heavy delayed absorbable suture, such as 0-polyglactin. (**c**) The procedure is repeated on the contralateral side.

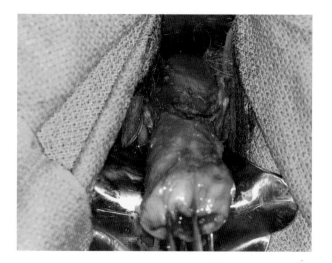

Figure 5.56. Cardinal ligaments.
Alternating side to side, the remainder of the cardinal ligaments and the lower portion of the broad ligaments are clamped, cut, and suture ligated. The uterine arteries are ligated during this step. The potential for bleeding is decreased if the uterine arteries have been previously ligated at their origin during the laparoscopic portion of the procedure. Once the lateral attachments have been released, the cervix and lower uterine segment appear free from the surrounding tissue.

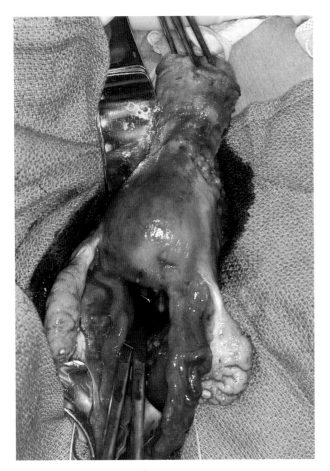

Figure 5.57. Delivering the uterus.
Once the uterine arteries have been secured and the
lateral attachments released, the uterine fundus can be
delivered through the posterior cul-de-sac. The adnexa
are then retrieved with the surgeon's finger, if they are
scheduled for removal. Usually, a small portion of the
broad ligament will remain and it should be clamped,
cut, and ligated. The specimen is then sent for routine
pathology.

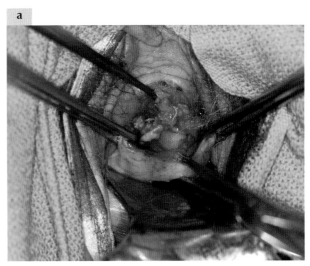

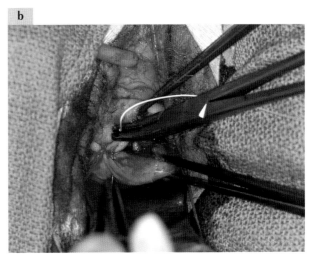

Figure 5.58. Closing the vaginal cuff.
(**a**) The vaginal cuff is grasped at the angles, anteriorly
and posteriorly. Delayed absorbable sutures are placed
and held at the vaginal angles. Classically, a Heaney-
type suture is placed in this position. The remainder of
the vaginal cuff is closed based upon surgeon preference.
(**b**) The vaginal cuff is then closed from anterior to
posterior using a continuous running-locked suture.

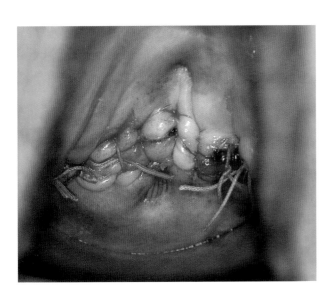

Figure 5.59. Closed vaginal cuff.
Once the vaginal cuff has been closed, the
pneumoperitoneum is re-established and the peritoneal
cavity is checked for adequate hemostasis. Copious
irrigation and suction are used to inspect all vascular
pedicles and lymph node basins. The fascia is closed for
all trocar sites ≥ 10 mm, and the skin is closed in the
usual fashion.

References

1. Dargent D, Salvat J. *L'Envahissement ganglionnaire pelvien.* (McGraw-Hill: Paris, 1989).

2. Querleu D, Leblanc E, Castelain B. Laparoscopic pelvic lymphadenectomy in the staging of early carcinoma of the cervix. *Am J Obstet Gynecol* 1991; **164**:579–81.

3. Childers JM, Surwit EA. Combined laparoscopic and vaginal surgery for the management of two cases of stage I endometrial cancer. *Gynecol Oncol* 1992; **45**:46–51.

4. Querleu D, LeBlanc E. Laparoscopic infrarenal paraaortic lymph node dissection for restaging of carcinoma of the ovary or fallopian tube. *Cancer* 1994; **73**:1467–71.

5. Scribner Jr DR, Mannel RS, Walker JL, Johnson GA. Cost analysis of laparoscopy versus laparotomy for early endometrial cancer. *Gynecol Oncol* 1999; **75**:460–3.

6. Lanvin D, Elhage A, Henry B et al. Accuracy and safety of laparoscopic lymphadenectomy: an experimental prospective randomized study. *Gynecol Oncol* 1997; **67**:83–7.

7. Gemignani ML, Curtin JP, Zelmanovich J et al. Laparoscopic-assisted vaginal hysterectomy for endometrial cancer: clinical outcomes and hospital charges. *Gynecol Oncol* 1999; **73**:5–11.

6 Laparoscopic radical hysterectomy

Douglas A Levine and Richard R Barakat

Laparoscopic radical hysterectomy is an alternative method to radical hysterectomy via laparotomy for the treatment of early invasive cervical cancer and, to a lesser extent, endometrial cancer. Patients with Stage IA2 or IB1 cervical cancers should be treated by radical hysterectomy and pelvic lymphadenectomy, with or without adjuvant radiation therapy, based upon pathologic findings.[1,2] Patients with Stage IA1 tumors and lymph–vascular space invasion (LVSI) should also undergo radical hysterectomy. The management of patients with Stage IB2 lesions is more controversial. Standard management had been either radical hysterectomy or radiation therapy, with the understanding that the two treatments were equally effective. With the recent discovery that chemoradiation is a superior treatment for patients with cervical cancer compared to radiation alone, there is a bias toward chemoradiation for Stage IB2 lesions instead of radical surgery.[3] Nonetheless, chemoradiation has never been directly compared to radical surgery for Stage IB2 tumors and definitive recommendations will have to await the results of randomized trials. Several recent studies have reported that radical hysterectomy for the treatment of Stage II endometrial cancer is associated with improved long-term survival.[4,5] Radical hysterectomy should be considered for endometrial cancer patients with preoperatively known cervical involvement.

The benefits of laparoscopic radical hysterectomy instead of traditional radical hysterectomy reflect the general benefits of laparoscopy. In particular, laparoscopic procedures for gynecologic malignancies result in decreased hospitalization, reduced blood loss, faster recovery, diminished overall hospital charges, and less postoperative pain.[6,7] The additional magnification of the laparoscope can be useful when performing complex parts of the procedure, such as ligating the uterine artery at its origin and dissecting the ureter from the parametrial tunnel. Nezhat et al first described the laparoscopic radical hysterectomy in 1992.[8] Since then many reports have appeared in the peer-reviewed literature regarding the outcomes of patients undergoing laparoscopic radical hysterectomy for early invasive cervical cancer. The largest series published to date was reported by Spirtos et al in 2002;[9] they evaluated 78 patients with Stage IA2 or IB cervical cancers who had negative paraaortic nodes, clinically normal pelvic nodes, and no evidence of extracervical disease. The operative time, estimated blood loss, and intraoperative complications compare very favorably to reports on radical hysterectomy via laparotomy. While the identical surgical procedure can be performed laparoscopically, there are no randomized data to prove the equivalence of laparoscopic and open radical hysterectomy. Future studies will need to determine if this procedure results in the similarly high cure rates seen when early-stage cervical cancer is treated by conventional radical surgery. The recurrence rates reported to date suggest that the two procedures have similar efficacy.

In this chapter, the technique of laparoscopic radical hysterectomy will be described in detail. One of the benefits for gynecologic oncologists wishing to learn these techniques is that the same procedure already performed via laparotomy is tailored to laparoscopic instrumentation. The laparoscopic procedure requires mastery of the standard radical hysterectomy followed by an adaptation to laparoscopic techniques in order to accomplish the required surgical objectives. There are variations in technique, and illustrated here is the use of the argon-beam coagulator (ABC) for dissection and hemostasis, along with the endoscopic stapler and hemostatic clips. The ABC is set at 70 W with a gas flow of 2–4 l/min. The endoscopic stapler is always used with vascular loads, and hemoclips can be placed with a 5- or 10-mm clip applier. As mentioned above, this procedure is intended for patients with early invasive cervical cancer (Stage IA1 with LVSI, and Stages IA2 and IB1). The treatment of Stage IB2 lesions is controversial and a full discussion outside of what has already been mentioned is beyond the scope of this text. Large lesions may be difficult to extract while following the strict principles of cancer surgery. Gross lesions < 2 cm in greatest dimension should be readily amenable to laparoscopic radical hysterectomy, but larger lesions should be carefully evaluated for resectability via the laparoscopic approach. An abdominal procedure may be more successful for patients with large lesions or lesions involving the upper vagina. The laparoscopic procedure may be contraindicated in patients with severe pulmonary disease or other comorbid conditions in which a steep Trendelenburg position, increased intra-abdominal pressure, or extended operative time would not be well tolerated. Other relative contra-indications to laparoscopy include multiple prior abdominal procedures, previous pelvic irradiation, abdominal wall defects, or bleeding diatheses. There are no weight restrictions for performing a laparoscopic radical hysterectomy, but many practitioners will not offer this approach to patients with a Quetelet index > 35.

The management of the ovaries at the time of radical hysterectomy has been the subject of many reports. The incidence of ovarian metastases is low enough that oophorectomy is not a standard part of the procedure.[10,11] The ovaries should be managed as they would be for any woman undergoing a hysterectomy for benign indications. If the ovaries are left in situ they may be transposed out of the pelvis in an attempt to reduce the exposure to postoperative radiation. However, only 40–50% of patients who undergo ovarian transposition and receive postoperative radiation therapy retain ovarian function.[12,13] Approximately 20% of patients with transposed ovaries will require additional surgery to manage symptomatic adnexal masses.[14,15] Furthermore, in those patients who underwent ovarian transposition and did not receive postoperative radiation therapy, the average age of menopause occurred 5 years earlier. Therefore, the decision to perform ovarian transposition should be carefully considered as it does not protect ovarian function after radiation in the majority of patients, can increase the risk for subsequent adnexal surgery, and can reduce overall endocrine function. Finally, it was once thought that pelvic drains should be placed at the time of radical hysterectomy. Multiple studies have established that pelvic drains do not alter the incidence of postoperative lymphocyst formation.[16,17] In fact, febrile morbidity may actually be increased in patients who have had pelvic drains placed. Standard practice does not include the placement of pelvic drains to reduce lymphocyst formation or febrile morbidity.

Cystoscopy

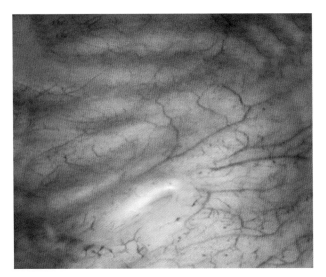

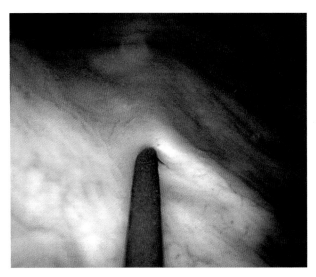

Figure 6.1. Cystoscopy.
The patient is placed in dorsal lithotomy position and draped for cystoscopy. The preparation for the laparoscopic radical hysterectomy and cystoscopy can be done at the same time with separate drapes for each procedure, or two preparations can be performed. Placing ureteral stents before the laparoscopic radical hysterectomy facilitates the ureteral dissection and may minimize injury to the ureters. This can usually be accomplished in 10–15 minutes and therefore adds little to the overall time under anesthesia. After introducing the cystoscope through the urethra, the ureteral orifice is identified. Shown here is the left ureteral orifice. If the ureteral orifice is difficult to locate, intravenous indigo carmine can be given to detect efflux through it.

Figure 6.2. Guidewire.
Ureteral catheters are usually placed preoperatively and removed at the end of the procedure. If the ureter is damaged or excessively manipulated during the procedure, the catheters can be changed over a wire, and stents may be left in for several days. Alternatively, double-J ureteral stents may be placed from the outset. Stents should be placed under fluoroscopy to ensure proper positioning, and a plain radiograph should be obtained at the conclusion of the procedure to ensure that operative manipulations have not resulted in stent migration. To place a ureteral stent, a guidewire is initially inserted through the ureteral orifice.

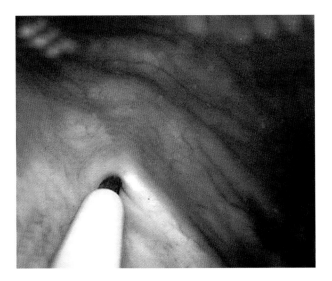

Figure 6.3. Ureteral stent.
The stent is placed over the guidewire and gently passed through the ureteral orifice. It is important to insert the stent slowly so that ureteral bleeding is not created, which will interfere with additional cystoscopy and increase postoperative hematuria. If available, fluoroscopy is used to confirm that the stent has reached the renal pelvis, prior to withdrawing the guidewire. A 20-cm stent is used for women ≤ 62 inches in height; a 30-cm stent is used for women ≥ 72 inches in height. For women taller than 62 inches but shorter than 72 inches, the following formula can be used as a guide to determine the proper length for the stent: height (inches) minus 42. If an odd number is returned, round up to the closest even number, as stents only come in even lengths.

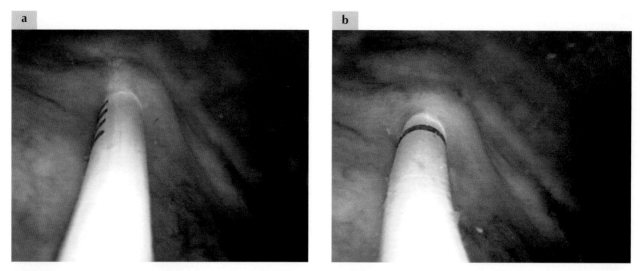

Figure 6.4. Advancing the stent.
A stent pusher (not shown) is used to advance the stent over the guidewire once it has entered the cystoscope. Usually, a 0.035-inch guidewire and a 6-French stent are used in adult women. The stents have markings every 5 cm to serve as a guide during placement. (**a**) The 20-cm marking is approaching the ureteral orifice. Each 5-cm marking has an additional band; therefore, the four bands seen in the figure confirm that the stent has been advanced 20 cm. The measurements do not include the pigtail portions of the catheter. (**b**) If the correct length stent has been chosen, a single circumferential band will reside at the ureteral orifice when the stent has been fully inserted into the ureter, which can be used later as a reference to determine if the stent has migrated. The procedure is repeated on the contralateral side.

Opening the spaces

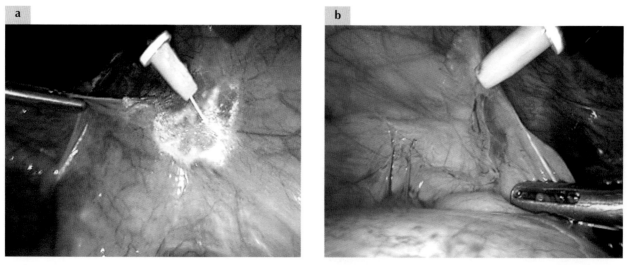

Figure 6.5. Entering the retroperitoneum.
Access is gained to the abdomen and pelvis in the usual manner for laparoscopy. A combination of 10- and 12-mm trocars is used, based upon operator preference. After completing a brief survey of the abdomen the retroperitoneum is opened. (**a**) The argon-beam coagulator is used for this step and throughout the procedure. The pelvic peritoneum is incised between the infundibulopelvic ligament and the external iliac vessels. This incision is extended from the round ligament to the pelvic brim. On the left side, the sigmoid is often adherent to the pelvic sidewall. (**b**) These adhesions need to be incised to gain access to the left pelvic retroperitoneum. The first step of the procedure is to define the paravesical and the pararectal spaces.

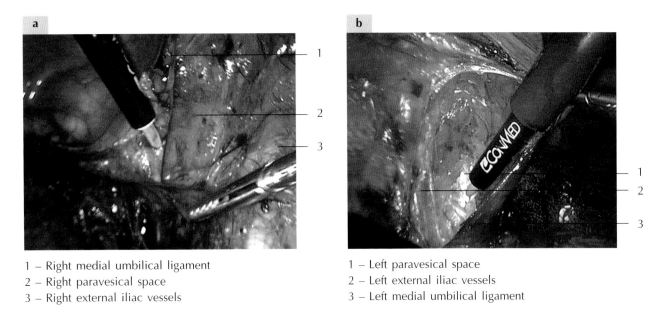

1 – Right medial umbilical ligament
2 – Right paravesical space
3 – Right external iliac vessels

1 – Left paravesical space
2 – Left external iliac vessels
3 – Left medial umbilical ligament

Figure 6.6. Paravesical space.
Incising the peritoneum parallel and lateral to the medial umbilical ligament opens the paravesical space. The medial boundary is the medial umbilical ligament and the lateral boundary the external iliac vessels. This avascular space can be bluntly dissected to mobilize the bladder from its lateral attachments. The right (**a**) and left (**b**) paravesical spaces have been partially opened and the relevant landmarks are demonstrated.

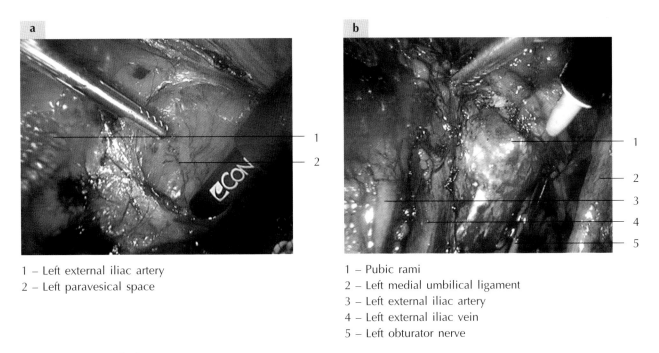

1 – Left external iliac artery
2 – Left paravesical space

1 – Pubic rami
2 – Left medial umbilical ligament
3 – Left external iliac artery
4 – Left external iliac vein
5 – Left obturator nerve

Figure 6.7. Paravesical space.
(**a**) Further dissection delineates the external iliac vessels and the areolar tissue that can be swept medially with the argon-beam coagulator. (**b**) After arriving at the base of the paravesical space, the pubic rami and distal aspect of the obturator nerve are seen. Completely opening the paravesical space facilitates the creation of the bladder flap and the lymph node dissection.

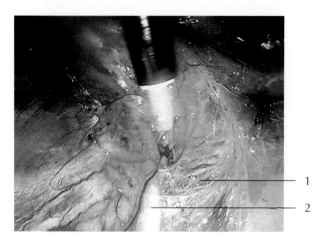

1 – Right pararectal space
2 – Right ureter

Figure 6.8. Pararectal space.
The pararectal space is opened by dissecting from the medial aspect of the infundibulopelvic ligament toward the obturator fossa. The areolar tissue is bluntly dissected with the argon-beam coagulator. The medial aspect of the pararectal space is the ureter and the lateral boundary the internal iliac vessels. Care should be taken not to injure the internal iliac vein, as this can be difficult to control laparoscopically. Once the paravesical and pararectal spaces are open, the parametrium is isolated between these two areas of dissection.

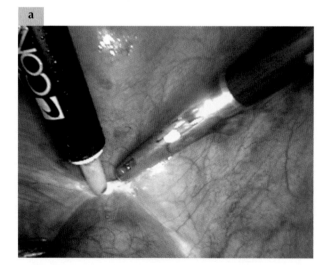
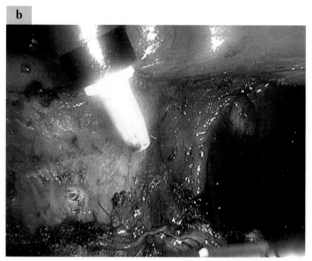

Figure 6.9. Vesicouterine peritoneum.
After opening the pelvic spaces, the next step in the procedure is to incise the vesicouterine peritoneum to ensure that the bladder has sufficient mobility. (**a**) The bladder peritoneum is grasped with an atraumatic forceps and elevated to delineate the junction of the bladder and the uterus; the peritoneum is incised just superior to this area. The vesicouterine incision will span the distance between the cut edges of the peritoneum. (**b**) After incising the peritoneum, the relatively avascular areolar tissue is dissected bluntly with the argon-beam coagulator or a similar instrument. Cautery is applied as needed for hemostasis. When the bladder has been completely mobilized, the pelvic surface of the vagina will appear white and uniform.

Pelvic lymphadenectomy

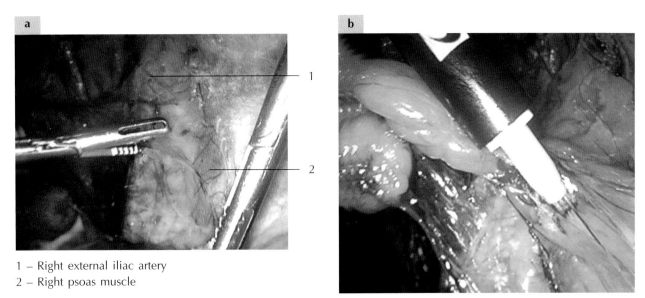

1 – Right external iliac artery
2 – Right psoas muscle

Figure 6.10. Identifying the external iliac vessels.
The external iliac lymph nodes are removed first to gain additional exposure and access to the pelvic sidewall. (**a**) After opening the retroperitoneum, the external iliac vessels still remain covered with a cohesive layer of areolar tissue. (**b**) Often, adipose tissues that may not contain lymph nodes need to be removed to adequately visualize the vessels. These tissues should all be sent for routine pathologic evaluation, as the difference between lymph-node-bearing tissue and adipose tissue can be difficult to discern with the naked eye.

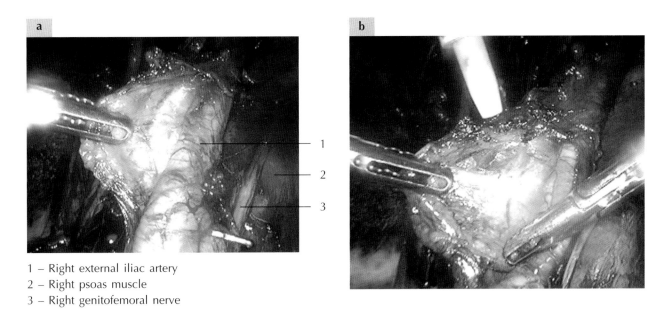

1 – Right external iliac artery
2 – Right psoas muscle
3 – Right genitofemoral nerve

Figure 6.11. Removing the lymph nodes.
The lymphatic tissue is adherent to the vessels as lymph node channels run parallel to arteries and veins; larger vessels will contain greater amounts of lymphatic tissue. (**a**) The lymph nodes are grasped with a toothed forceps and retracted away from the external iliac artery. (**b**) The argon-beam coagulator is then used to transect the pedicle from its attachment to the artery with both cautery and blunt dissection. Care is taken not to injure the genitofemoral nerve, which runs over the psoas muscle, parallel and lateral to the external iliac artery.

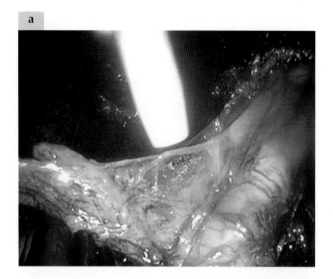

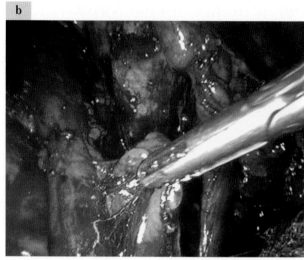

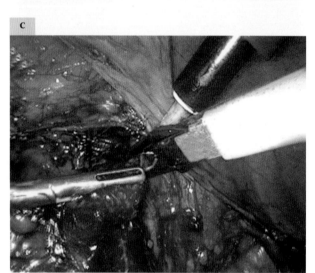

Figure 6.12. External iliac lymph nodes.
Additional nodes are removed along the external iliac artery and vein as described. (**a**) Nodal tissue being removed from the right external iliac artery; (**b**) lymphatic tissue being removed from the left external iliac artery. In contrast with adipose tissue, the nodal tissue is more 'sticky' and does not come away from the vessels as easily. Blunt dissection alone will lead to bleeding from small perforating vessels and result in unnecessary leakage of lymphatic fluid, which can result in postoperative lymphocyst formation. (**c**) Thus, coagulation or hemostatic clips should be used as part of the lymph node dissection to minimize bleeding and lymphatic leakage. Generally, coagulation is used for small perforators and clips are reserved for larger pedicles.

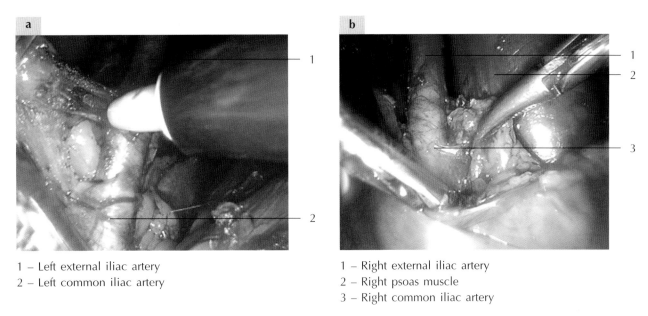

1 – Left external iliac artery
2 – Left common iliac artery

1 – Right external iliac artery
2 – Right psoas muscle
3 – Right common iliac artery

Figure 6.13 (a and b). Common iliac lymph nodes.
The proximal extent of the lymph node dissection is the common iliac lymph nodes that overlie the common iliac artery. In certain high-risk lesions (large primary tumor, unfavorable histology, etc.), paraaortic nodes are sampled as well. Care should be taken to avoid injury to the ureter, which crosses over the common iliac artery in proximity to the common iliac lymph nodes. Some practitioners send the common iliac lymph nodes for intraoperative pathologic evaluation prior to performing the radical hysterectomy. This may be warranted if it would result in either abandoning the procedure or altering the extent of the lymph node dissection. It is operator dependent and beyond the scope of this text. Nonetheless, the common iliac nodes should be sent separately from the rest of the pelvic lymph nodes.

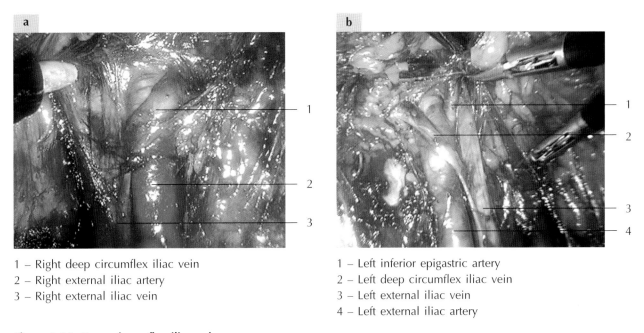

1 – Right deep circumflex iliac vein
2 – Right external iliac artery
3 – Right external iliac vein

1 – Left inferior epigastric artery
2 – Left deep circumflex iliac vein
3 – Left external iliac vein
4 – Left external iliac artery

Figure 6.14. Deep circumflex iliac vein.
The distal extent of the pelvic lymphadenectomy is the point where the deep circumflex iliac vein crosses over (or under, in certain cases) the external iliac artery. This vein should be carefully dissected to ensure that an adequate lymphadenectomy has been performed. (**a**) The right deep circumflex iliac vein is seen crossing over the right external iliac artery. (**b**) In addition to the left deep circumflex iliac vein, the origin of the left inferior epigastric artery is also clearly demonstrated.

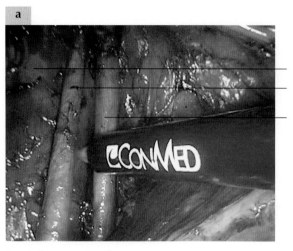

1 – Left psoas muscle
2 – Left external iliac artery
3 – Left external iliac vein

Figure 6.15. Completed external iliac lymphadenectomy.
It is important to dissect between the artery and vein to completely remove all lymphatic tissue. (a) The lymph node tissue between the artery and vein has been completely removed. (b) Nodal tissue will also be found lateral to the external iliac artery and should be completely removed as well. At the conclusion of the external iliac lymphadenectomy, both the artery and the vein should be freely mobile from the common iliac bifurcation to the deep circumflex iliac vein.

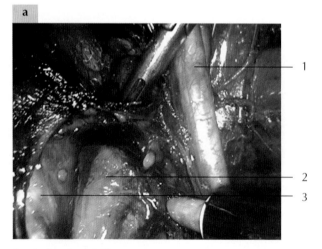

1 – Left external iliac artery
2 – Left obturator space
3 – Left pelvic sidewall

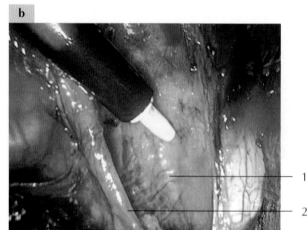

1 – Right obturator nerve
2 – Right ureter

Figure 6.16. Entering the obturator space.
The obturator space can be entered lateral or medial to the external iliac vessels. (a) The left external iliac vessels are retracted medially and the lymphatic tissue is seen in the left obturator space inferior to the psoas muscle. Perforating vessels and lymphatics, which travel between the external iliac vein and the psoas muscle, should be clipped or cauterized. (b) The right ureter is retracted medially, and right obturator lymph nodes are seen overlying the right obturator nerve, which has not yet been dissected.

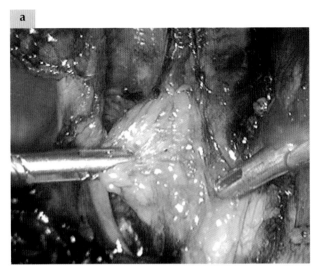

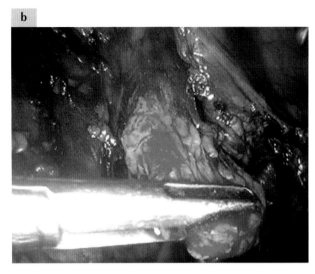

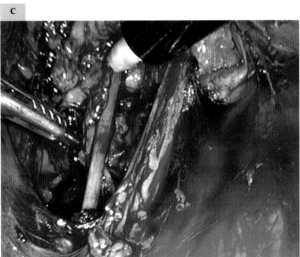

Figure 6.17. Obturator lymph nodes.
Obturator lymphatic tissue is grasped with a forceps and elevated. Blunt dissection is used initially until the obturator nerve is clearly identified. The nodes are not cauterized or transected until the nerve is readily apparent. (**a** and **b**) The nodal tissue is dissected bluntly since the nerve has not yet been seen. (**c**) The nerve has been visualized and cautery can be carefully used to transect the base of the nodal packet. Typically, the obturator fossa will yield a greater number of lymph nodes than the external iliac dissection.

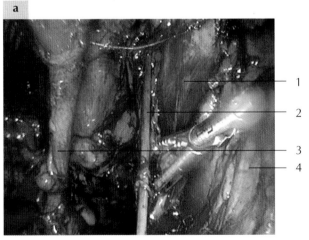

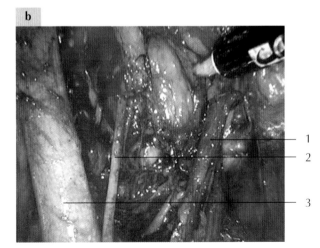

1 – Right obturator internus muscle
2 – Right obturator nerve
3 – Right ureter
4 – Right external iliac vein

1 – Left ureter
2 – Left obturator nerve
3 – Left external iliac vein

Figure 6.18. Obturator nerve.
The obturator nerve is plainly visible after the nodal tissue has been removed. It is customary to remove nodal tissue above and below the obturator nerve when performing a lymphadenectomy for cervical cancer, though some practitioners may only remove nodal tissue above the nerve. At the conclusion of the obturator lymphadenectomy, the area between the ureter and the obturator internus muscle should be devoid of nodal tissue. The right (**a**) and left (**b**) obturator fossae; (**a**) shows the small amount of remaining tissue being removed with the toothed forceps.

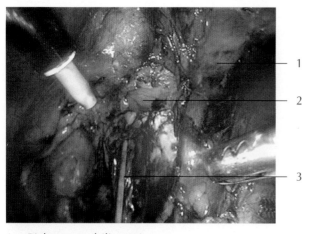

Figure 6.19. Pelvic vein.
The anastomotic pelvic vein, also referred to as the accessory obturator vein, has a variable course and may drain into the obturator vein or the underside of the external iliac vein. While not uniformly present, it should be kept in mind during the obturator lymphadenectomy as injury to this vein may result in troublesome bleeding. Here, the pelvic vein is seen crossing over the obturator internus fascia and draining into the external iliac vein.

1 – Right external iliac vein
2 – Right anastomotic pelvic vein
3 – Right obturator nerve

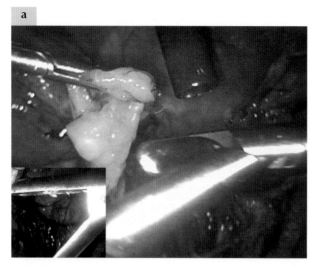

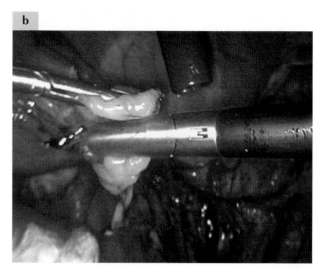

Figure 6.20. Retrieving the nodes.
Large packets of lymph nodes can be difficult to remove through the 10-mm trocars, so it is good practice to use a large, sturdy grasping device to remove the nodes from the patient. (**a**) A spoon grasping forceps, which has a wide opening and a concave center to hold and compress the nodal tissue; (**b**) when grasped firmly, large nodal packets are unlikely to be lost in the trocar during retrieval.

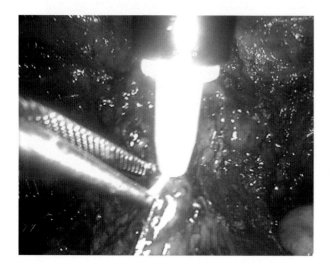

Figure 6.21. Argon-beam coagulator (ABC).
The ABC is used extensively during the procedure described. It has the ability to coagulate and cut simultaneously. Additionally, the tip permits blunt dissection without the need to change instruments. It is highly accurate and, when used properly, has minimal lateral thermal spread. Care should be taken not to use the ABC in close proximity to metal instruments. As shown in the figure, the beam can arc onto the tips of a metal instrument, leading to unintended thermal injury. Typical laparoscopic settings are 70 W with a gas flow of 2–4 l/min.

Uterine artery and adnexa

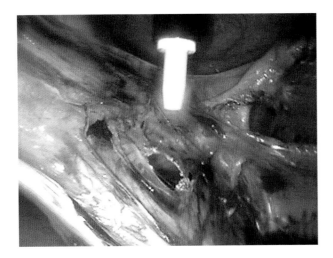

Figure 6.22. Infundibulopelvic (IP) ligament.
A window is created beneath the IP ligament, between it and the ureter. This can be accomplished bluntly, with coagulation, or with endoscopic scissors. The window is then extended in both directions (not shown). In a postmenopausal patient or a patient who does not wish to retain her ovaries, the IP ligament is transected proximally at the pelvic brim, taking care to avoid the ureter and iliac vessels. It is important to completely excise the entire ovary to prevent an ovarian remnant syndrome. In a patient who wishes to retain her ovaries, the utero-ovarian ligament is transected close to the uterine body so that the IP ligament and ovary remain intact.

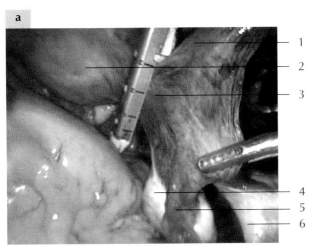

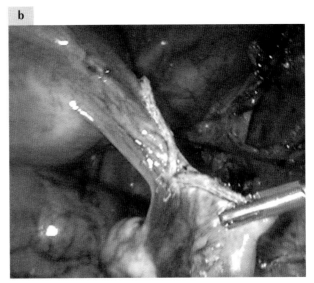

1 – Right round ligament
2 – Uterus
3 – Right utero-ovarian ligament
4 – Right ovary
5 – Right fallopian tube
6 – Right infundibulopelvic ligament

Figure 6.23. Utero-ovarian ligament.
In this patient, the ovaries were not scheduled for removal; therefore, the endoscopic stapler with vascular loads is placed across the utero-ovarian ligament. (**a**) Care is taken to ensure that all tissue is within the cut line so that the entire ligament will be transected when the stapler is fired. (**b**) If this is not possible, two fires may be used to accomplish complete transection of the ligament.

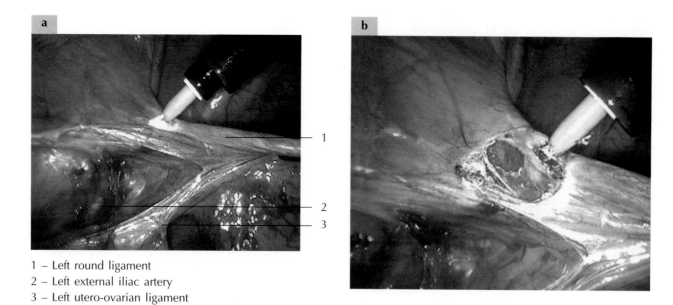

1 – Left round ligament
2 – Left external iliac artery
3 – Left utero-ovarian ligament

Figure 6.24 (a and b). Round ligament.
The round ligament is transected after completion of the pelvic lymphadenectomy. If need be, it may be transected earlier in the procedure, but the round ligament can provide useful traction during the lymph node dissection. Unlike a simple hysterectomy, during a radical hysterectomy the round ligament is intentionally transected as close to the pelvic sidewall as possible. This can be accomplished with the argon-beam coagulator, as shown in these images, or with monopolar cautery, bipolar cautery, hemostatic clips, the harmonic scalpel, or an endoscopic stapler.

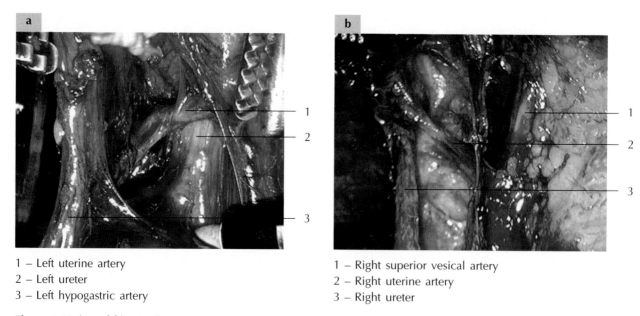

1 – Left uterine artery
2 – Left ureter
3 – Left hypogastric artery

1 – Right superior vesical artery
2 – Right uterine artery
3 – Right ureter

Figure 6.25 (a and b). Uterine artery.
The uterine artery is carefully dissected at its origin from the hypogastric artery. In a radical hysterectomy the uterine artery is taken at its origin, whereas in a modified radical hysterectomy the uterine artery is transected at the point where it crosses the ureter. The right and left uterine arteries are shown, originating from the hypogastric arteries and crossing over the ureter. The uterine artery may be transected after completing the pelvic lymphadenectomy or during the pelvic lymphadenectomy depending on exposure and operator preference.

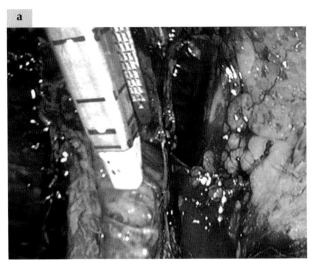
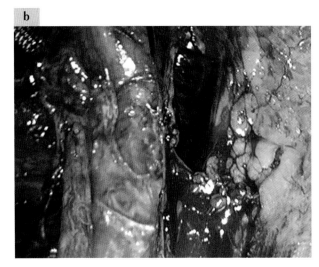

Figure 6.26. Transecting the uterine artery.
The uterine artery may be transected using the endoscopic stapler, the harmonic scalpel, or hemostatic clips. (**a**) The endoscopic stapler is placed across the uterine artery and vein, which have been dissected free from their surrounding attachments. (**b**) Staples are seen on the proximal and distal aspects of the transected artery and vein.

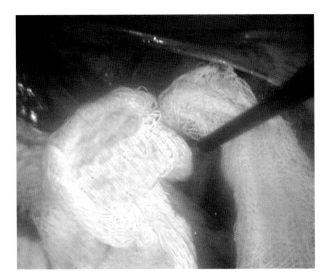

Figure 6.27. Gauze.
A 4 × 4 inch radiopaque gauze is inserted through a 10-mm trocar; a 4 × 8 inch gauze can also be used. This is very effective in cleaning the operative field and helps to obtain hemostasis. The gauze may be applied to small blood vessels in a manner similar to an open technique. Pressure is applied with one of the laparoscopic instruments. Maintaining meticulous hemostasis is a crucial component of advanced laparoscopy for optimal visualization. Irrigation during the procedure should be avoided as it is difficult to completely suction all infused fluid and this too will compromise visualization.

Uterosacral ligament

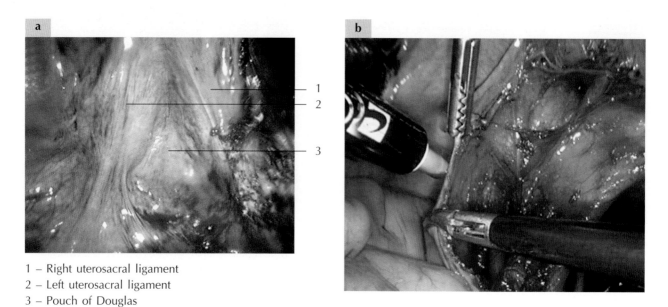

1 – Right uterosacral ligament
2 – Left uterosacral ligament
3 – Pouch of Douglas

Figure 6.28. Defining the uterosacral ligaments.
(**a**) The uterus is anteverted while the rectum is retracted out of the pelvis. This defines the uterosacral ligaments and the pouch of Douglas. (**b**) The peritoneal reflection beneath the transected infundibulopelvic ligament is incised to the level of the uterosacral ligament. The uterosacral ligament is a fibrous band that extends from the lateral rectal pillars to the posterior inferior aspect of the uterus. It is less well defined than other pelvic structures, and normal anatomic relationships can help guide the dissection. Small vessels coursing through the uterosacral ligament require some form of hemostasis to be employed when transecting the ligaments.

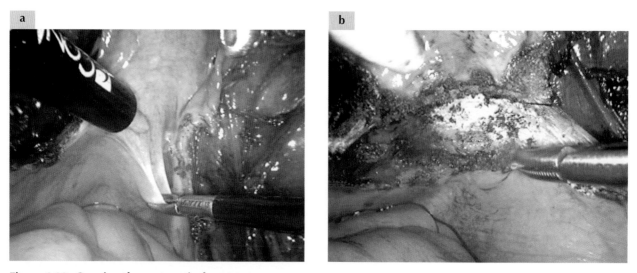

Figure 6.29. Opening the rectovaginal septum.
The rectovaginal septum is entered prior to transecting the uterosacral ligaments. (**a**) To gain access to this area, the peritoneum above the rectum is first tented outward. It is then incised from each cut edge of the peritoneum. (**b**) Blunt or sharp dissection may also be used further to separate the upper and lower aspects of the peritoneal edges.

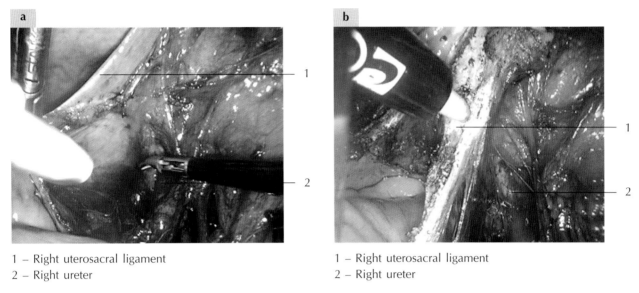

1 – Right uterosacral ligament
2 – Right ureter

1 – Right uterosacral ligament
2 – Right ureter

Figure 6.30. Mobilizing the ureter.
The ureter is reflected laterally to free it from the uterosacral ligament. (**a**) Careful manipulation with a closed grasping forceps can accomplish lateral mobilization. (**b**) The uterosacral ligament may be partially or completely transected with cautery, taking care to ensure that the ureter is out of the operative field. Although the argon-beam coagulator is shown here, monopolar and bipolar cautery are also effective methods to transect fibrous tissue.

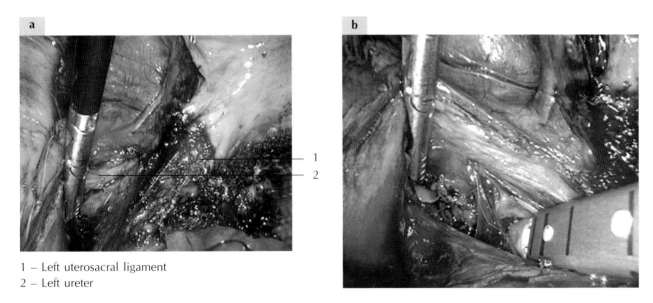

1 – Left uterosacral ligament
2 – Left ureter

Figure 6.31. Transecting the uterosacral ligament.
(**a**) The ureter is retracted laterally before transecting the uterosacral ligament. Once the ureter has been sufficiently mobilized, the uterosacral ligament can be transected with cautery (as shown in the previous figure), the harmonic scalpel or the endoscopic stapler. (**b**) The ureter is completely freed prior to placing any device across the uterosacral ligament.

Parametrial dissection

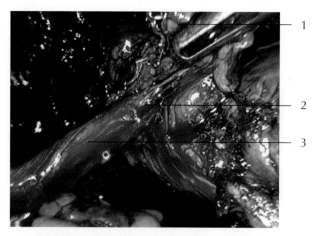

1 – Left uterine artery and lateral parametrial tissues on traction
2 – Left ureter entering the parametrial tunnel
3 – Left ureter

Figure 6.32. Parametrial tunnel.
At this point in the procedure, the ureter is already partially freed from its surrounding attachments. It has been carefully identified at several points during the procedure thus far: prior to transecting the infundibulopelvic ligament, during the isolation of the uterosacral ligaments, during the pelvic lymph-adenectomy, and when ligating the uterine artery. The next step is to release the ureter from the parametrial tunnel and by doing so bringing the lateral parametrial tissue over the ureter and toward the uterus. This is the most technically complex portion of the procedure. The ligated uterine artery is elevated with a grasping forceps and the ureter is seen heading directly into the parametrium.

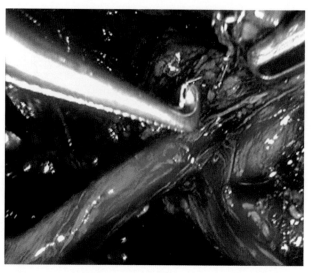

Figure 6.33. Instrumentation.
A laparoscopic right angle clamp (laparoscopic Mixter) is used to dissect the ureter out of the parametrial tunnel, while retracting the lateral parametrial tissue medially over the ureter and toward the uterus. The fine tips of the laparoscopic right angle clamp are useful during the meticulous dissection that is required during this portion of the procedure.

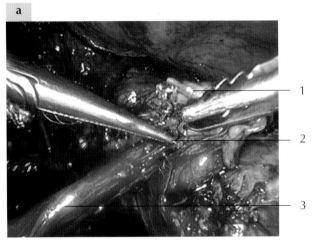

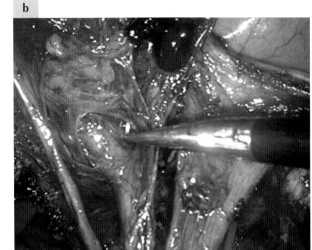

1 – Left uterine artery and lateral parametrium
2 – Laparoscopic right angle clamp in the ureteral tunnel
3 – Left ureter

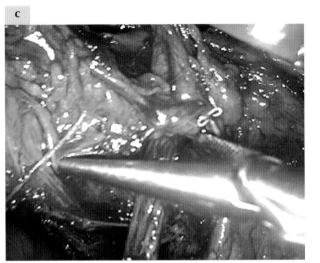

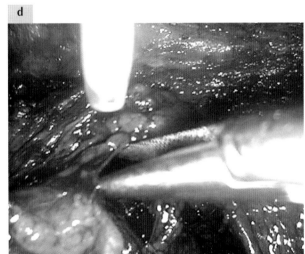

Figure 6.34. Ureteral dissection.
The tip of the laparoscopic right angle clamp will slide easily on top of the left (**a**) or right (**b**) ureter. (**c**) Opening the tips of the instrument when it is overlying the ureter permits dissection of the parametrial tissues. A variety of instruments can be used to transect the parametrial tissue. Maintaining medial traction is important during this part of the procedure in order to resect as much parametrium as possible. (**d**) The argon-beam coagulator can be activated to transect the parametrial tissue. Other commonly used instruments include the harmonic scalpel, hemostatic clip or the endoscopic scissors without cautery. The advantage of the argon-beam coagulator and the harmonic scalpel is that thermal spread is minimal, which decreases the likelihood of ureteral injury during this challenging part of the procedure.

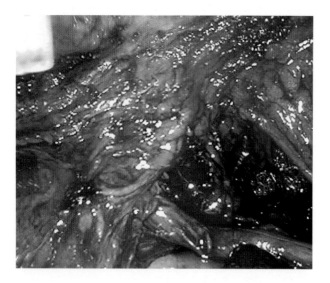

Figure 6.35. Ureteral insertion.
After completely extirpating the ureter from the parametrial tunnel it will insert directly into the urinary bladder. The ureteral dissection can result in devascularization, subsequent complications, such as ureteral stricture or fistula formation, thermal damage, inadvertent ligation, compression, or other unrecognized injury. While the ureter must be freed from the parametrial tunnel as part of the radical hysterectomy, it is not necessary to completely skeletonize the ureter since the vascular supply runs longitudinally along its length. Leaving a bit of areolar tissue on the ureter is advantageous.

Specimen removal

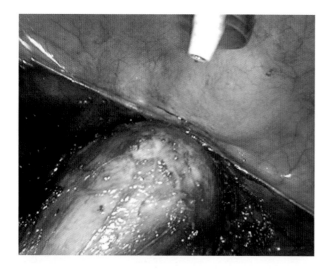

Figure 6.36. Preparing the vagina.
Once the bladder has been fully mobilized and the ureters are directly entering the bladder, the vagina is ready to be incised. A rectal probe or similar device (i.e. sponge stick) is placed into the vagina to provide traction and distend the vaginal tube. The anterior wall of the vagina is displaced ventrally with the vaginal/rectal probe in preparation for the vaginal incision.

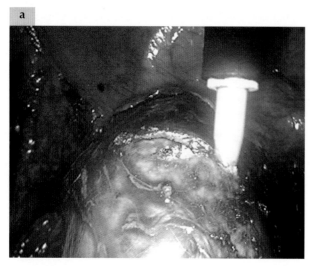

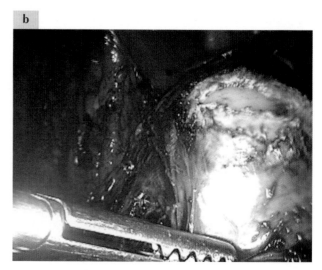

Figure 6.37. Opening the vagina.
(**a**) The anterior vagina is incised with the argon-beam coagulator. This part of the procedure produces considerable smoke and therefore the trocars should be fully vented. (**b**) After traversing the full thickness of the vagina, the vaginal/rectal probe appears through the incision.

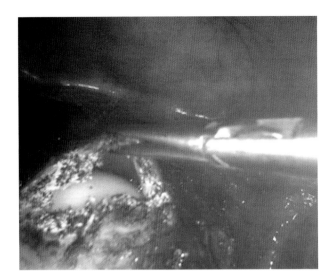

Figure 6.38. Traction.
After extending the incision, a strong clamp should be placed on the anterior vaginal wall to provide traction while the remainder of the vagina is opened. This figure shows that a laparoscopic tenaculum has been placed on the anterior vaginal wall and the vaginal/rectal probe is still in the vagina. Traction is important to maintain tissue tension while the lower vagina is separated from the specimen.

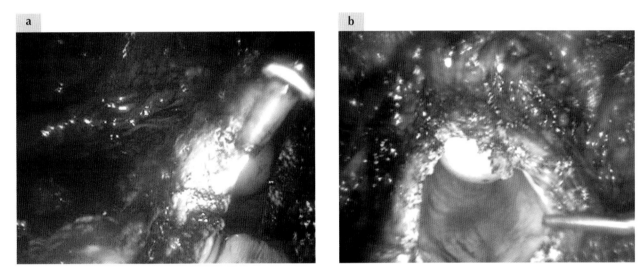

Figure 6.39 (a and b). Circumscribing the vagina.
The vaginal incision is continued in both directions. The lateral aspects of the vagina are incised before continuing to the posterior side, which is the most difficult area to transect safely. Part of the intricacy stems from the fact that more carbon dioxide escapes as the vagina is opened further. To prevent the escape of carbon dioxide, the rectal/vaginal probe is removed and the second assistant places a moist laparotomy pad into the vagina. This is usually effective in maintaining pneumoperitoneum. Additionally, two carbon dioxide insufflators are used throughout the procedure to preserve stable intraabdominal pressures.

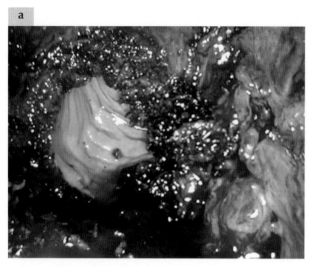

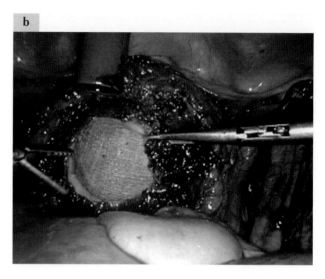

Figure 6.40. Vaginal cuff.

(a) Once the vagina has been completely circumscribed, the specimen is free and the lumen of the vagina can be seen through the pelvis. (b) At this point, if not sooner, the pneumoperitoneum will be lost and the vagina is closed off with a laparotomy pad or large sponge to prevent the egress of carbon dioxide. A laparoscopic grasper is used for traction on the vaginal cuff to maintain patency while the specimen is removed transvaginally.

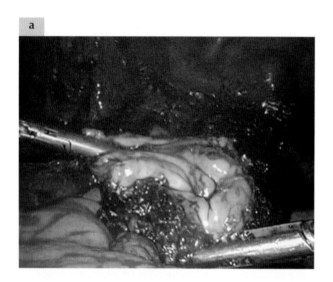

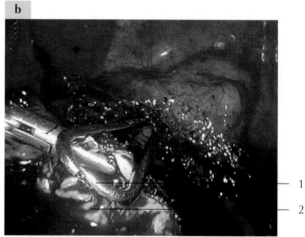

1 – Single-tooth tenaculum coming through vaginal cuff
2 – Cervical os

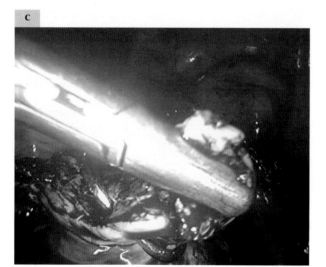

Figure 6.41. Specimen removal.

The specimen is grasped by the cervix or lower uterine segment with a laparoscopic forceps. (a) The cervical os is seen rotated toward the laparoscope. (b) The second assistant, who stands between the patient's legs, places a single-tooth tenaculum through the vagina. (c) The specimen is then grasped at or near the cervix and drawn through the vagina. Once removed, the specimen is sent for routine pathologic analysis. Frozen section is not necessary unless there is concern for a close vaginal margin, and an additional portion of the upper vagina could be resected if need be.

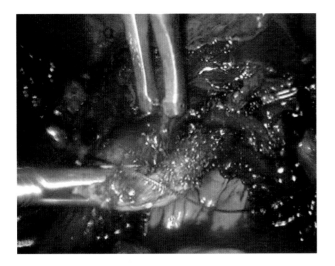

Figure 6.42. Closing the vaginal cuff.
An endoscopic suture device (EndoStitch, US Surgical Corp., Norwalk, CT) is used to close the vaginal cuff. This device features a suture attached to the midportion of a needle that is sharp at both ends. The vaginal cuff is grasped with forceps and the EndoStitch, in the closed position, is inserted through the suprapubic trocar. A slipknot is tied on the end of the suture and is inserted into the pelvis along with the instrument. It is the authors' practice to close the vaginal cuff from anterior to posterior, although other practitioners may close the cuff from side to side.

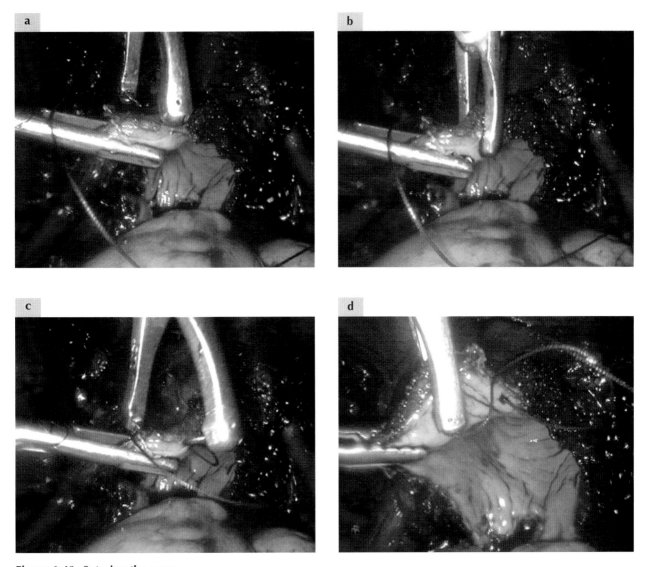

Figure 6.43. Suturing the apex.
(**a**) The EndoStitch is opened and (**b**) the needle is placed through the top of the vagina from outside to inside. (**c**) The needle is transferred to the opposite jaw of the EndoStitch and brought out the other side of the vagina. (**d**) The needle is then placed directly back through the vaginal cuff from inside to outside at a position a few millimeters away from where it was brought through.

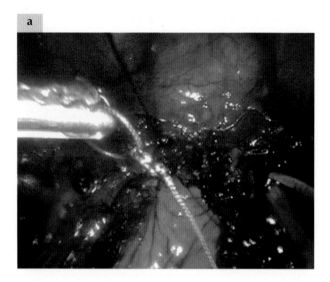

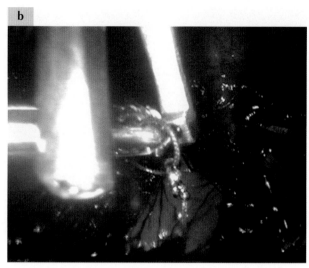

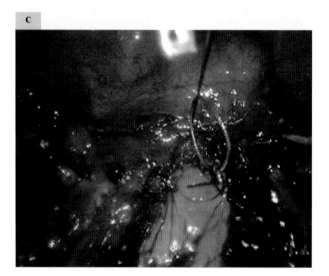

Figure 6.44. Tying the first knot.
Passing the suture through the slipknot that was made
extracorporally creates the first knot. (**a**) The slipknot is
grasped with a forceps and (**b**) the needle is placed
through the loop in the suture. (**c**) After being brought
through the loop, it is cinched down by pulling on the
free end of the suture.

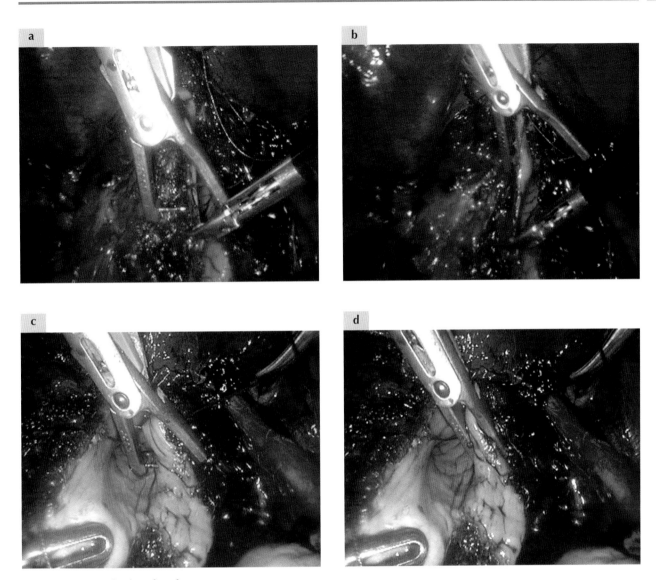

Figure 6.45. Continuing the closure.
Traction is maintained with the previously placed sutures. Passing the suture from side to side with the EndoStitch closes the midportion of the vaginal cuff. (**a**) The needle is passed from the peritoneal side of the vagina (**b**) into the luminal side of the vagina. (**c**) The needle is then transferred back to the opposite jaw to be ready for placement through the other side of the vagina. (**d**) It is placed into the contralateral vaginal wall and brought out the other side by toggling it between the two jaws.

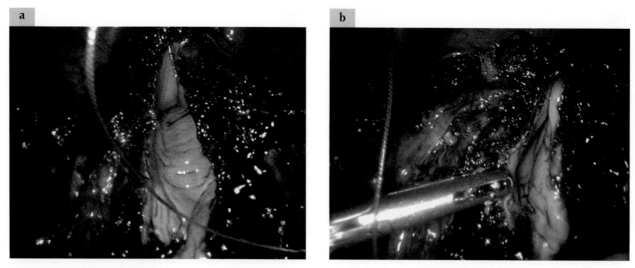

Figure 6.46. Progressive closure.
Using the technique described in the previous figures, the vaginal cuff is progressively closed from anterior to posterior. Contrast (**a**) and (**b**) to appreciate the sequential closure of the vaginal cuff.

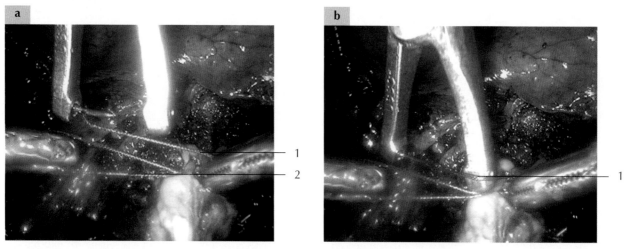

1 – Suture that has been passed through the vaginal cuff
2 – Suture being held to create a loop

1 – Suture that has been rotated over the empty jaw of the EndoStitch

Figure 6.47. Tying the last knot.
(**a**) The knot at the posterior aspect of the vaginal cuff is created by initially having the first assistant grasp the suture before pulling it completely through the vagina to create a loop. (**b**) The EndoStitch is then rotated so that the suture crosses over the empty jaw of the instrument.

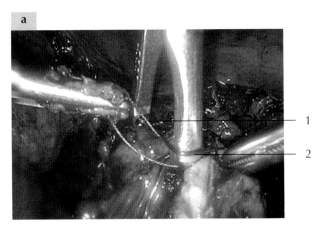

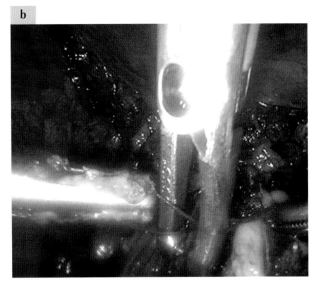

1 – Suture loop being placed between the jaws of the EndoStitch

2 – Suture wrapped around empty jaw of instrument, beneath which suture loop is placed

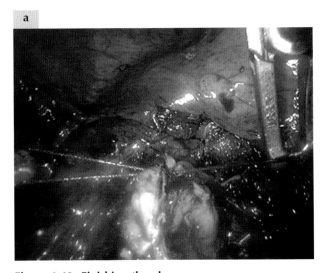

Figure 6.48. Passing the suture.
(**a** and **b**) The loop is then brought in between the jaws of the instrument and the needle is passed beneath the suture loop. (**c**) The needle is then withdrawn on the other side and brought out through an internal loop, which creates a flat knot.

1 – Suture loop that is now within newly created knot

2 – Suture that is over the empty jaw is also wrapped over the suture loop to create the new knot

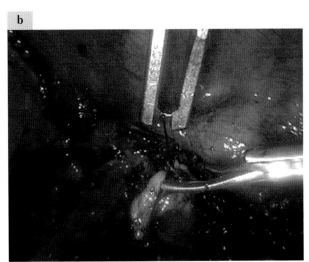

Figure 6.49. Finishing the closure.
(**a**) After completing the knot, the ends of the suture are pulled in opposite directions to cinch it down. (**b**) Once three to four intracorporeal knots have been placed, the suture is cut with the endoscopic scissors and the EndoStitch is removed.

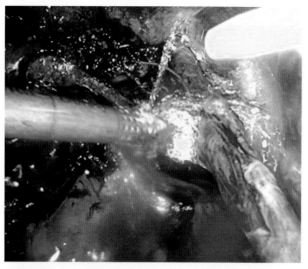

Figure 6.50. Irrigation.
At the completion of the procedure, the pelvis is copiously irrigated and suctioned to assess hemostasis. All vascular pedicles are closely examined and hemostasis may be achieved with a combination of coagulation, hemostatic clips, and sutures as necessary.

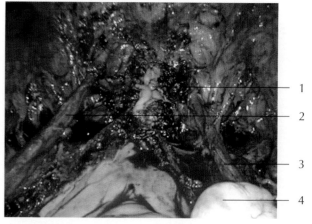

1 – Vaginal cuff
2 – Left ureter
3 – Right ureter
4 – Right ovary

Figure 6.51. Completed procedure.
Both ureters can be seen directly entering the urinary bladder, and the vaginal cuff has been closed laparoscopically. If the ovaries have not been removed, they are restored to their normal anatomic location and may be sutured to the pelvic peritoneum at the discretion of the operator. Some practitioners will transpose the ovaries out of the pelvis in a premenopausal patient, but this decision should be individualized as discussed previously.

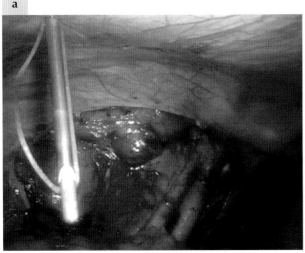

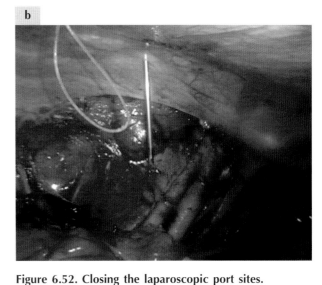

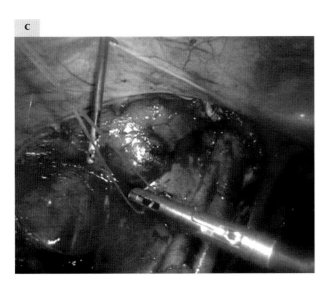

Figure 6.52. Closing the laparoscopic port sites.
The fascia is closed for all the port sites since 10- and 12-mm trocars were used. They can be closed traditionally from above or laparoscopically using an endoscopic needle. (**a**) A delayed absorbable suture is placed into the groove at the tip of the needle and introduced lateral to the port site, through the fascia and peritoneum, but not through the skin or subcutaneous tissue. (**b**) The suture is released and remains inside the peritoneal cavity as the needle is removed. (**c**) The needle is reintroduced on the opposite side of the port site to grasp and remove the suture, which can be accomplished with or without a second grasper to manipulate the suture. The pneumoperitoneum is let down and the suture is tied. The port site is interrogated with the surgeon's finger, and if any defect is noted an additional suture is placed. This technique can be used for all port sites except the last one, since the laparoscope is required to view the closure.

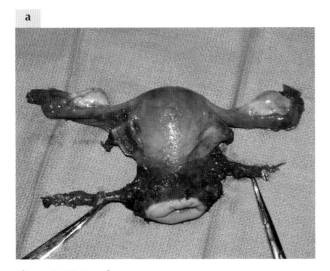

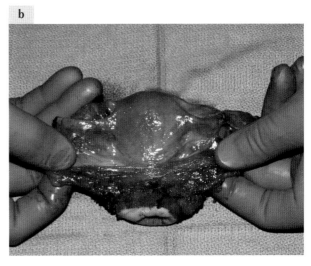

Figure 6.53. Specimen.
This is the laparoscopic radical hysterectomy specimen. It was performed on an older patient and therefore the ovaries were removed along with the main specimen. Contrasting (**a**) and (**b**) illustrates the ordinary appearance of the parametrium, which without stretch is very unimpressive. Substantial effort is made in a radical hysterectomy to resect as much of the parametrium as possible. When placed under tension the resected parametrial tissues become readily apparent.

References

1. Sedlis A, Bundy BN, Rotman MZ et al. A randomized trial of pelvic radiation therapy versus no further therapy in selected patients with stage IB carcinoma of the cervix after radical hysterectomy and pelvic lymphadenectomy: a Gynecologic Oncology Group Study. *Gynecol Oncol* 1999; **73**:177–83.

2. Peters 3rd WA, Liu PY, Barrett 2nd RJ et al. Concurrent chemotherapy and pelvic radiation therapy compared with pelvic radiation therapy alone as adjuvant therapy after radical surgery in high-risk early-stage cancer of the cervix. *J Clin Oncol* 2000; **18**:1606–13.

3. Keys HM, Bundy BN, Stehman FB et al. Cisplatin, radiation, and adjuvant hysterectomy compared with radiation and adjuvant hysterectomy for bulky stage IB cervical carcinoma. *N Engl J Med* 1999; **340**:1154–61.

4. Mariani A, Webb MJ, Keeney GL et al. Role of wide/radical hysterectomy and pelvic lymph node dissection in endometrial cancer with cervical involvement. *Gynecol Oncol* 2001; **83**:72–80.

5. Sartori E, Gadducci A, Landoni F et al. Clinical behavior of 203 stage II endometrial cancer cases: the impact of primary surgical approach and of adjuvant radiation therapy. *Int J Gynecol Cancer* 2001; **11**:430–7.

6. Gemignani ML, Curtin JP, Zelmanovich J et al. Laparoscopic-assisted vaginal hysterectomy for endometrial cancer: clinical outcomes and hospital charges. *Gynecol Oncol* 1999; **73**:5–11.

7. Malur S, Possover M, Michels W, Schneider A. Laparoscopic-assisted vaginal versus abdominal surgery in patients with endometrial cancer – a prospective randomized trial. *Gynecol Oncol* 2001; **80**:239–44.

8. Nezhat CR, Burrell MO, Nezhat FR et al. Laparoscopic radical hysterectomy with paraaortic and pelvic node dissection. *Am J Obstet Gynecol* 1992; **166**:864–5.

9. Spirtos NM, Eisenkop SM, Schlaerth JB, Ballon SC. Laparoscopic radical hysterectomy (type III) with aortic and pelvic lymphadenectomy in patients with stage I cervical cancer: surgical morbidity and intermediate follow-up. *Am J Obstet Gynecol* 2002; **187**:340–8.

10. Sutton GP, Bundy BN, Delgado G et al. Ovarian metastases in stage IB carcinoma of the cervix: a Gynecologic Oncology Group study. *Am J Obstet Gynecol* 1992; **166**:50–3.

11. Natsume N, Aoki Y, Kase H et al. Ovarian metastasis in stage IB and II cervical adenocarcinoma. *Gynecol Oncol* 1999; **74**:255–8.

12. Feeney DD, Moore DH, Look KY et al. The fate of the ovaries after radical hysterectomy and ovarian transposition. *Gynecol Oncol* 1995; **56**:3–7.

13. Buekers TE, Anderson B, Sorosky JI, Buller RE. Ovarian function after surgical treatment for cervical cancer. *Gynecol Oncol* 2001; **80**:85–8.

14. Chambers SK, Chambers JT, Holm C et al. Sequelae of lateral ovarian transposition in unirradiated cervical cancer patients. *Gynecol Oncol* 1990; **39**:155–9.

15. Anderson B, LaPolla J, Turner D et al. Ovarian transposition in cervical cancer. *Gynecol Oncol* 1993; **49**:206–14.

16. Jensen JK, Lucci 3rd JA, DiSaia PJ et al. To drain or not to drain: a retrospective study of closed-suction drainage following radical hysterectomy with pelvic lymphadenectomy. *Gynecol Oncol* 1993; **51**:46–9.

17. Lopes AD, Hall JR, Monaghan JM. Drainage following radical hysterectomy and pelvic lymphadenectomy: dogma or need? *Obstet Gynecol* 1995; **86**:960–3.

7 Second-look laparoscopy with intraperitoneal catheter placement

Christopher S Awtrey and Nadeem R Abu-Rustum

A common approach to the patient with advanced epithelial ovarian cancer involves initial staging and attempted optimal cytoreduction followed by platinum-based chemotherapy. For most patients with advanced-stage epithelial ovarian cancer this approach leads to a period of clinical remission or, for a minority, complete cure of disease. Physicians monitor patients for disease recurrence by clinical examination, imaging studies, and tumor markers. Even in combination, these are not always highly sensitive for disease persistence or recurrence. The ability to detect tumor deposits < 1 cm with currently utilized techniques, such as computed tomography (CT), sonography, and magnetic resonance imaging (MRI), are limited.[1] Furthermore, tumor markers that are initially elevated and normalize after primary therapy do not always guarantee a biopsy-proven remission. In patients with no clinical evidence of tumor after primary surgery and adjuvant chemotherapy, persistent disease is noted in 60% of surgically evaluated patients.[2] A secondary surgical evaluation is the most accurate method for assessing the status of disease.

A second-look laparotomy is defined as a comprehensive diagnostic surgical evaluation performed in patients with a history of epithelial ovarian cancer who are deemed clinically free of disease by physical examination, imaging studies and tumor markers. The procedure consists of a thorough evaluation of the peritoneal cavity and obtaining biopsies of any suspicious nodules or adhesions. In the absence of gross disease, biopsies and washings of normal-appearing surfaces are taken in a systematic manner to be evaluated for microscopic involvement. The procedure also permits resection of any gross disease and the placement of an

intraperitoneal catheter to infuse chemotherapy as consolidation treatment in patients who have no evidence or microscopic evidence of disease. Hoskins et al reported that complete resection of visible disease at the time of second-look laparotomy was associated with an improved survival.[3] Laparoscopy appears to be an acceptable alternative to laparotomy and is associated with less morbidity, shorter operating time, shorter hospital stay, and lower hospital charges.[4] With current technology, laparoscopy should not be associated with a decreased sensitivity of the procedure.[4,5]

The second-look procedure can be divided into three separate components. As with the initial surgical evaluation, the first step is abdominal entry, restoration of normal anatomy, and evaluation of the peritoneal cavity. Unlike primary evaluation, adhesions often markedly hinder this process. Indeed, in some cases the adhesions can be so dense that incidental enterotomy may occur upon attempted abdominal entry. Adhesions can be due either to postoperative changes or to microscopic tumor deposits. Biopsies should be taken from the adhesions and sent for pathologic evaluation. Upon abdominal entry, washings are also taken to be assessed for microscopic cytologic evidence of disease.

Evaluation of the abdominal cavity involves visualizing and palpating the bowel and its mesentery, the liver edge and diaphragmatic surfaces, as well as the pelvic peritoneal surfaces. If there is no evidence of disease, the second portion of the procedure is to obtain multiple random biopsies from these peritoneal surfaces. The paracolic gutters, diaphragmatic surfaces, entire abdominopelvic peritoneum and remaining omentum are all biopsied. The third portion of the procedure is to evaluate the nodal basins. Again, this is done by palpation and biopsy from the pelvic and paraaortic regions. In general, patients who had advanced disease and did not undergo lymph node sampling at the time of initial cytoreductive surgery are candidates for lymph node sampling at the time of second-look laparoscopy.

The substitution of video laparoscopy for laparotomy clearly benefits the patient with respect to postoperative recovery; however, it does present the surgical team with a unique set of challenges. Due to the high frequency of intestinal adhesions to the previous midline abdominal incision, blind introduction of a Veress needle in the periumbilical area is dangerous. The preferred method of abdominal entry is an open laparoscopic technique, away from the prior incision site. This reduces, but does not eliminate, the risk of bowel injury upon entry. A shortcoming with the application of minimally invasive techniques to this procedure is the limited tactile sensation available to palpate the peritoneal and diaphragmatic surfaces and nodal basins. To a certain extent, this can be overcome by close visual inspection with the laparoscope and use of a straight, blunt probe. For the patient needing nodal sampling, this is performed in the same manner as in an open procedure. Laparoscopic lymph node sampling is described elsewhere in this text.

Since approximately half of the patients found to be disease free at second-look evaluation go on to develop recurrent disease, several consolidation strategies have been designed to improve survival. Intraperitoneal (IP) chemotherapy offers many theoretical advantages over intravenously administered agents, including the ability to deliver extremely high concentrations of drug to the IP compartment. Barakat et al recently described the long-term follow-up of patients treated at Memorial Hospital with IP chemotherapy.[6] Patients treated with IP therapy after a negative second-look evaluation had a median survival of 8.7 years, and in those with microscopic disease the median survival was 4.8 years. Although never studied in a prospective randomized manner, the use of IP chemotherapy as a consolidation technique appears promising. Placement of the IP catheter at the time of second-look laparoscopy is simple and safe. The criteria for placing an IP port at the time of second look include a lack of significant adhesions, so as not to interfere with IP drug distribution, and disease of no greater than 5 mm in any dimension. The use of laparoscopy in second-look procedures is likely to expand as gynecologic oncologists become more familiar and comfortable with these techniques. Moreover, minimally invasive technology continues to advance, and operative gynecologic oncology will benefit from these developments.

Survey and biopsies

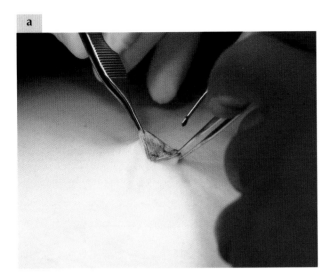

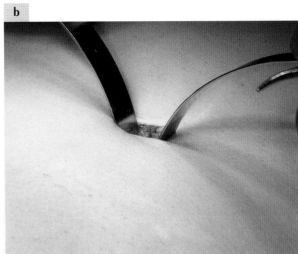

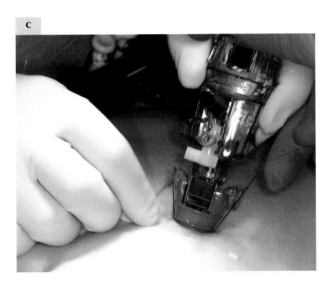

Figure 7.1. Open laparoscopy.
The procedure begins by placing a Hassan canula via the open technique. Abdominal access is typically obtained though a periumbilical incision; however, an alternative location is chosen if it is distant from the previous abdominal scar. (**a** and **b**) After the incision in the skin is made, dissection is carried down to the level of the fascia with narrow curved retractors. Once the fascia is identified, it is grasped and incised. The peritoneum is then entered under direct vision. (**c**) After the intra-abdominal location is confirmed with the laparoscope, two stay sutures are placed through the fascia and secured to the canula.

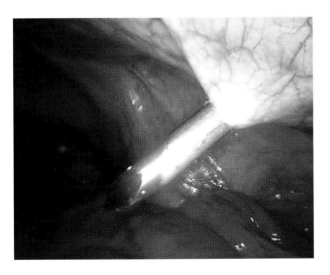

Figure 7.2. Placement of additional trocars.
Once pneumoperitoneum has been obtained, additional trocars are inserted through the lower quadrants. Under direct visualization, the lower quadrant trocars are introduced with care to avoid the inferior epigastric vessels. They are placed 1–2 cm medial and superior to the anterior superior iliac crests. Extensive adhesions, when present, should be taken down prior to inserting the lower quadrant trocars. If this is not possible (i.e. bilateral or extremely dense adhesions), the trocars are placed in alternative sites where direct entry can be observed with the laparoscope.

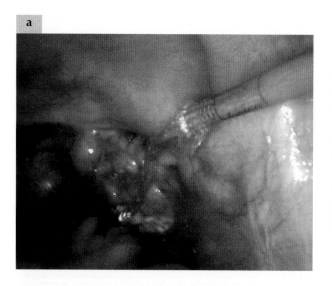

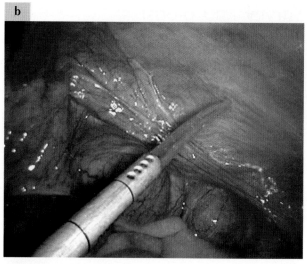

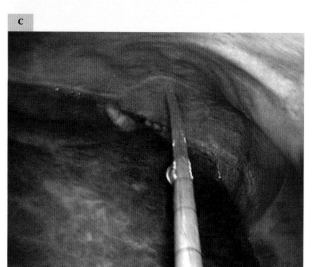

Figure 7.3. Washings.
With the patient in steep Trendelenburg position, the bowel is mobilized out of the pelvis. Copious irrigation is used in a systematic fashion starting from the pelvis and working clockwise along the peritoneal surfaces. Important areas to include are the (**a**) pelvis, (**b**) bilateral paracolic gutters and (**c**) bilateral diaphragmatic surfaces. Washings may be sampled separately from each of these surfaces or combined together, as long as all sites have been included. The washings are collected into a trap attached to the suction tubing.

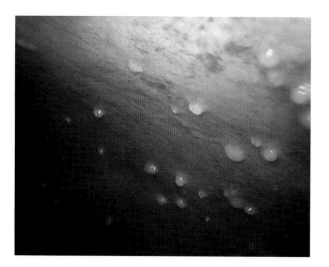

Figure 7.4. Peritoneal nodules.
Although patients undergoing a second-look laparoscopy have no clinical evidence of disease, tumor is often discovered intraoperatively. Isolated small tumor nodules, carcinomatosis, or substantial masses may be found. Shown here is peritoneal carcinomatosis discovered at the time of a second-look laparoscopy. Frozen-section biopsies should be obtained from any suspicious areas. If a positive biopsy is returned, the diagnostic portion of the procedure is complete. A careful survey should continue to determine the extent of disease and the need for resection.

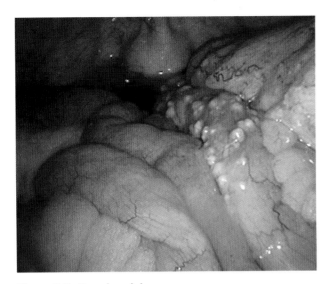

Figure 7.5. Bowel nodules.
Tumor nodules can be diffuse or localized. In this patient, tumor nodules were found in a segmental manner along the small bowel serosa. This underscores the need for systematic evaluation of the entire small bowel to search for unanticipated disease.

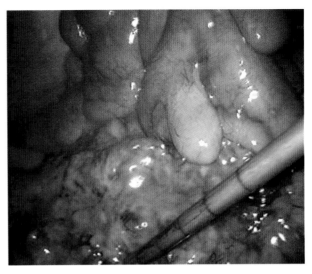

Figure 7.6. Large tumor mass.
Occasionally, a large tumor mass will be found at the time of a second-look laparoscopy. Care should be taken to evaluate the mass and the rest of the peritoneal cavity. Isolated sites of disease should be considered for resectability. Patients who have complete gross resection of tumor at the time of the second look have a better overall prognosis. Laparotomy or hand-assisted laparoscopy are considerations for tumor resection at the time of the second-look procedure.

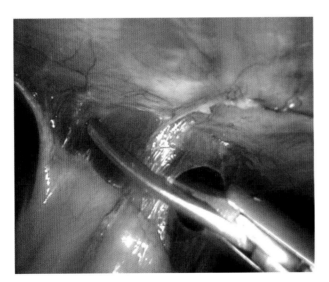

Figure 7.7. Adhesions.
Adhesions are frequently noted at the time of re-exploration. The adhesions should be lysed and biopsied, as tumor deposits are often discovered microscopically at the site of adhesions. Filmy adhesion can easily be released by cutting through the clear, avascular portion with the endoscopic scissors. Use of monopolar cautery should be limited as thermal injuries may occur. Patients suffering unrecognized bowel injuries may present several days later with signs of intestinal perforation.

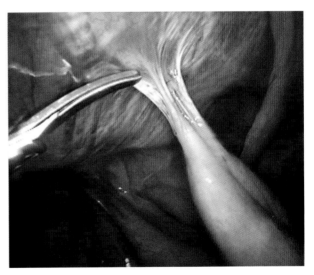

Figure 7.8. Dense adhesions.
Dense intestinal adhesions can present a challenging problem. The adhesions should be transected close to the anterior abdominal wall in order to minimize the risk of enterotomy. However, if too much anterior abdominal wall is incised, the dissection may track into the retroperitoneum. Care should be taken to identify the occasional patient who has herniated tissue through the previous laparotomy scar.

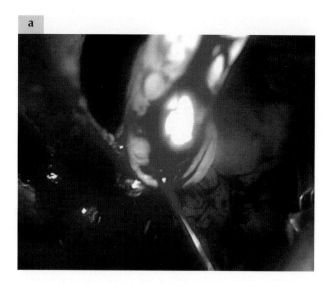

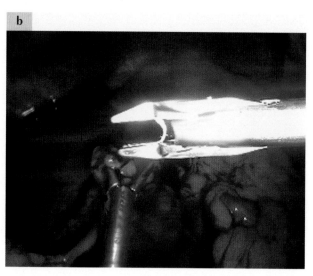

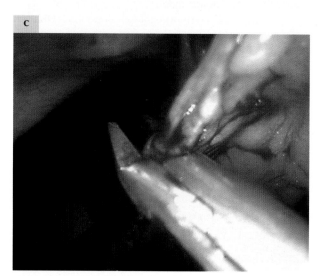

Figure 7.9. Hemostasis.
Dense adhesions may contain moderate-sized blood vessels. If bleeding is encountered, several techniques can be used to obtain hemostasis, including coagulation, sutures, or clips. (**a**) Bleeding is seen coming from the site of a dense omental adhesion. (**b**) The bleeding vessel is grasped with a forceps and the clip applier is introduced through a 5-mm trocar. (**c**) The clip is then applied to control the bleeding. Suction and irrigation are used as needed to clear the surfaces of blood and to look for additional sites of bleeding.

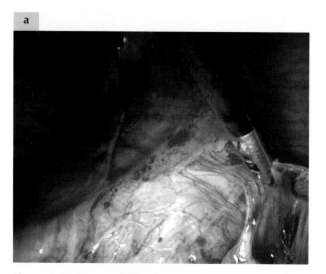

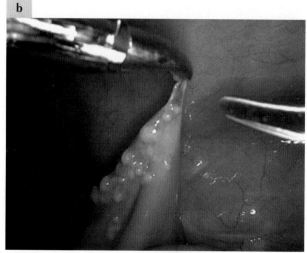

Figure 7.10. Targeted biopsies.
Biopsies are taken from all suspicious areas, adhesions, and normal surfaces. (**a**) In this case, a biopsy forceps is used to take a biopsy through the thin, avascular portion of an adhesion. Once the biopsy is taken, the adhesion should be inspected for hemostasis. Small perforating vessels may bleed once tension is released. (**b**) Excisional biopsies of suspected tumor nodules may be taken with the scissors after placing the specimen on traction to define a clear, avascular plane.

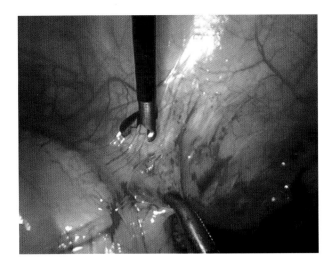

Figure 7.11. Random biopsies.
Random biopsies are taken from the pelvic peritoneum, left and right paracolic gutters, the diaphragmatic surfaces, and anterior peritoneal surfaces. This is in addition to any suspicious sites and areas of adhesions, which should be sampled as well. If a positive biopsy is found on frozen section, additional random biopsies are unnecessary.

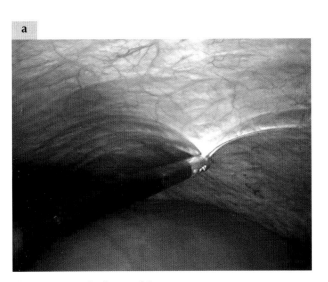

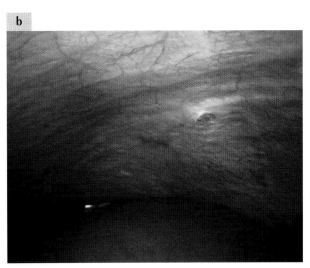

Figure 7.12. Diaphragm biopsy.
The biopsy forceps is used for most of the random biopsies. (**a**) The peritoneum is pulled inferiorly to obtain the biopsy. The biopsy is obtained by using a short jerking motion to remove the tissue while the jaws of the instrument remain closed. This instrument has a sharp cutting edge that facilitates specimen retrieval. If bleeding is encountered, electrocautery is used to achieve hemostasis. (**b**) While a generous biopsy specimen is desired, overzealous sampling could lead to inadvertent perforation of the diaphragm. The diaphragm is seen here before and after biopsy.

Intraperitoneal catheter placement

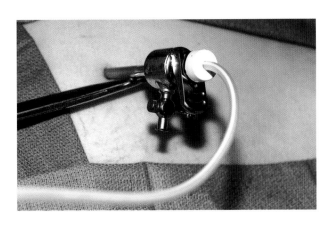

Figure 7.13. Introducing the catheter.
Once the examination, washings, and biopsies have all been completed, the intraperitoneal (IP) catheter is placed. All operative sites should be re-examined for hemostasis. The IP catheter is inserted through the 5-mm left lower quadrant trocar. IP catheters are placed in patients who are found to have no gross residual disease or only small-volume disease, making them candidates to receive IP chemotherapy.

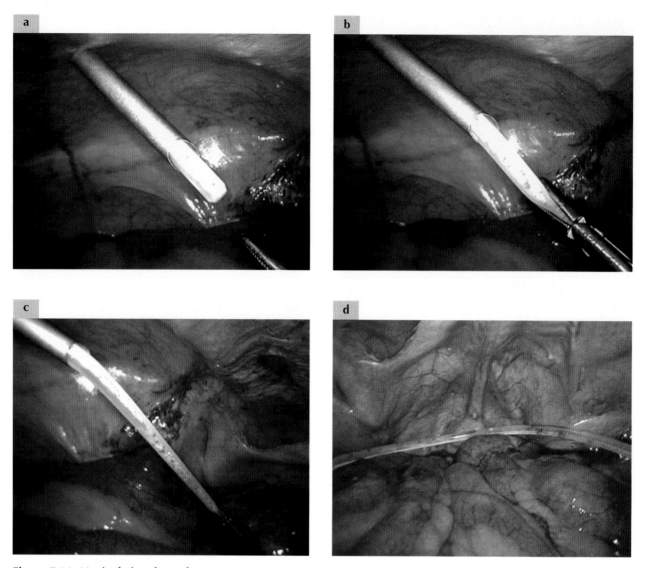

Figure 7.14. Manipulating the catheter.
(**a**) Once introduced through the trocar, further manipulation of the catheter is accomplished under direct visualization with the assistance of an atraumatic grasper. (**b** and **c**) The intraperitoneal (IP) catheter is guided into the pelvis using the grasper. (**d**) The catheter should curve through the base of the pelvis and the tip should reside on the contralateral side, still within the true pelvis. It extends from the left lower quadrant port site down into the pelvis and ends in the right lower quadrant to allow for dispersion of the infused agents across all of these areas. The trocar through which the catheter was inserted is now removed.

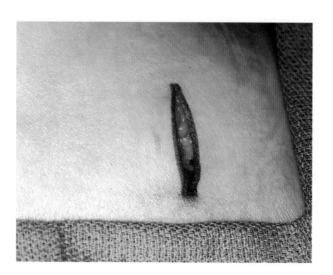

Figure 7.15. Port site location.
The port is placed in the midclavicular line over the second lowest ipsilateral rib. A small horizontal incision is made to accommodate the diameter of the port, which is approximately 4 cm. The incision is carried down to, but not through, the level of the fascia. If the port is not placed over the ribs, it may invert, rendering the reservoir inaccessible.

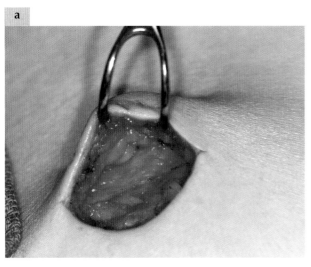

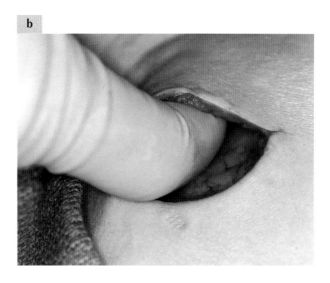

Figure 7.16. Developing the pocket.
(**a**) The inferior edge of the incision is elevated and undermined with electrocautery. (**b**) Blunt dissection is also used to mobilize the subcutaneous tissues and create a pocket for the intraperitoneal (IP) port. The reservoir is inserted to assess the size of the pocket. The reservoir should have limited mobility when placed into the pocket so that it rests firmly on the chest wall, providing the necessary support to facilitate access. Once the pocket is the correct size, hemostasis should be achieved, as it can be difficult to obtain once the port is in situ.

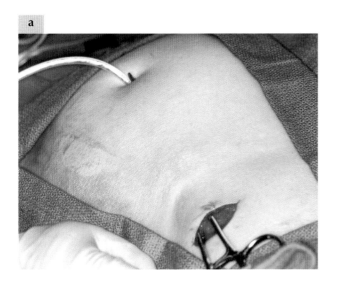

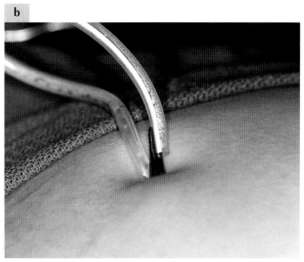

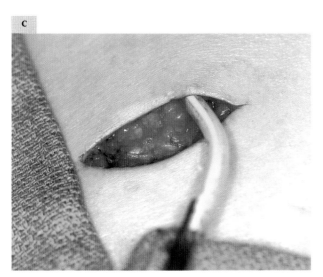

Figure 7.17. Subcutaneous tunneling.
(**a**) A long fine-tipped clamp is advanced from the pocket inferiorly through the subcutaneous tissues to the lower quadrant port site. The tip of the clamp should be oriented superiorly to assist in grasping the catheter. If a suitable clamp is not available, a laparoscopic grasper may be used as an alternative. (**b**) Once the lower quadrant port site is reached with the tip of the clamp, the end of the catheter is securely grasped. (**c**) The catheter is then pulled through the subcutaneous tunnel.

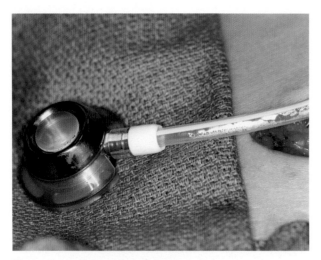

Figure 7.18. Connecting the reservoir.
The catheter tubing is connected to the port and the catheter lock is applied; the clear end of the lock is placed against the hub. Once attached, heparinized saline is infused through the catheter. The attachment between the tubing and the port must be secure to prevent inadvertent infusion of chemotherapeutic agents into the subcutaneous tissues.

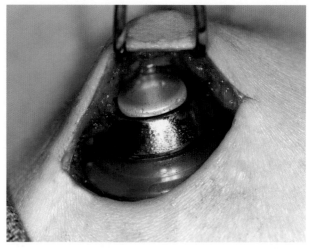

Figure 7.19. Inserting the port.
The port is then advanced into the pocket to ensure that it will fit correctly. Adjustments can be made at this point if the pocket is not the correct size.

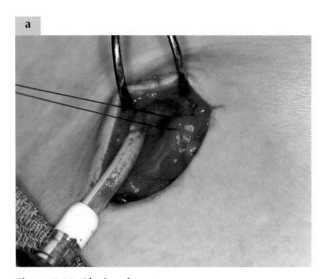

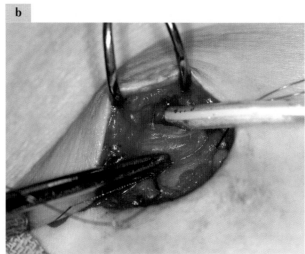

Figure 7.20. Placing the sutures.
3–0 Polypropylene sutures are used to anchor the port in place. Three sutures are placed to prevent rotation of the reservoir. (**a**) All the sutures are inserted through the fascia before placing any of them through the port. (**b**) Care is taken to ensure that the catheter is not damaged during placement of the sutures. An inadvertent needle stick through the catheter can cause leakage of chemotherapeutic agents.

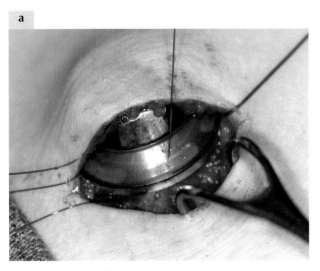
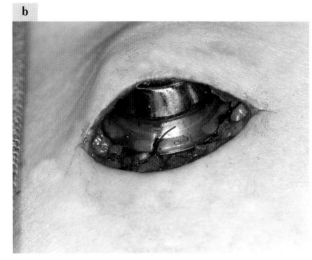

Figure 7.21. Suturing the port.
(**a**) After all the sutures have been placed through the fascia, they are then placed through the port; the sutures are inserted through openings provided at the port edges. Once all sutures have been placed, the port is tied down, starting first with the most distal suture. (**b**) When all the sutures have been tied, the port should be correctly oriented within the pocket, with the infusion site close to the skin surface.

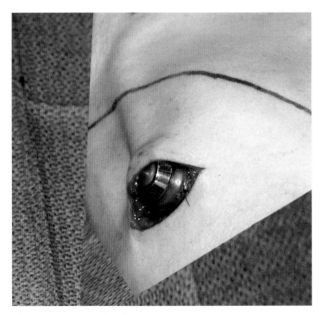

Figure 7.22. Port in situ.
In this particularly thin patient, the course of the catheter can be seen as it passes from the reservoir to the left lower quadrant port site. The outlined costal margin demonstrates the proper placement of the port in relation to the lower ribs.

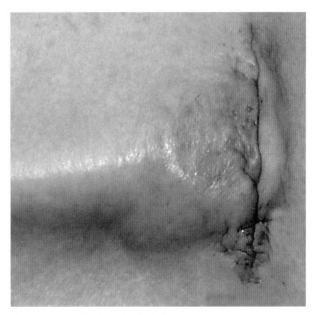

Figure 7.23. Closing the incision.
The skin incision is closed in two layers. Interrupted delayed absorbable sutures are used to approximate the subcutaneous tissue and to take tension off the skin sutures. The skin is closed in a running subcuticular fashion with 4–0 poliglecaprone sutures.

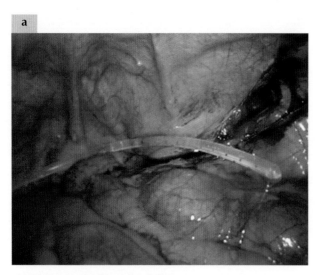 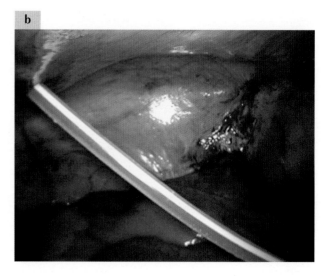

Figure 7.24. Flushing the catheter.
The peritoneum is re-examined laparoscopically for hemostasis and to assess placement of the catheter. (**a**) The catheter is repositioned as needed and then flushed transcutaneously with heparinized saline to ensure patency. (**b**) The course of the catheter through the subcutaneous tunnel is examined, and any slack is removed laparoscopically by gently tugging on the catheter. The remaining trocars are removed under direct visualization, and the port sites are closed in the standard fashion.

References

1. Ozols RF, Rubin SC, Thomas G, Robboy S. Epithelial ovarian cancer. In: (Hoskins WJ, Perez CA, Young RC, eds) *Principles and Practice of Gynecologic Oncology*, 3rd edn. (Lippincott-Raven: Philadelphia, 2000) 1025.

2. Rubin SC, Hoskins WJ, Hakes TB et al. Serum CA 125 levels and surgical findings in patients undergoing secondary operations for epithelial ovarian cancer. *Am J Obstet Gynecol* 1989; **160**:667–71.

3. Hoskins WJ, Rubin SC, Dulaney E et al. Influence of cytoreductive surgery at the time of second look laparotomy on survival of patients with epithelial ovarian cancer. *Gynecol Oncol* 1989; **34**:365–71.

4. Abu-Rustum NR, Barakat RR, Siegel PL et al. Second-look operation for epithelial ovarian cancer: laparoscopy or laparotomy? *Obstet Gynecol* 1996; **88**:549–53.

5. Hussain A, Chi DS, Prasad M et al. The role of laparoscopy in second-look evaluations for ovarian cancer. *Gynecol Oncol* 2001; **80**:44–7.

6. Barakat RR, Sabbatini P, Bhaskaran D et al. Intraperitoneal chemotherapy for ovarian carcinoma: results of long-term follow-up. *J Clin Oncol* 2002; **20**:694–8.

8 Extraperitoneal lymph node dissection

Yukio Sonoda, Denis Querleu and Eric Leblanc

The laparoscopic extraperitoneal approach for surgically staging patients with advanced cervical cancer is a new procedure that combines the benefits of laparoscopy with those of an extraperitoneal dissection. Given the inability of modern radiological modalities to accurately detect subclinical paraaortic lymphatic spread, surgical sampling remains the gold standard. Patients with metastasis to this region are candidates for extended-field radiation therapy. Traditional transperitoneal paraaortic lymph node sampling via laparotomy has been associated with increased radiation-induced gastrointestinal toxicity secondary to resulting bowel adhesions. An extraperitoneal approach has been shown to decrease toxicity due to the decreased incidence of bowel adhesions. Transperitoneal laparoscopy has also been employed to sample the paraaortic nodes with much success. Benefits of the laparoscopic extraperitoneal approach compared to a laparoscopic transperitoneal approach include operative feasibility (in spite of previous abdominal surgery), decreased risk of direct bowel injury, and decreased bowel adhesion formation. Benefits over an extraperitoneal laparotomy include decreased wound complications and possibly decreased hospital stay and treatment delays.

This procedure is used in the management of patients with advanced cervical cancer who are about to undergo radiation therapy. The incidence of paraaortic lymph node metastases increases with advancing tumor stage. Given that the status of the paraaortic lymph nodes may alter the radiation fields, this procedure is intended to sample these nodes while minimizing morbidity. The authors routinely perform this procedure on all patients with FIGO Stages IB2–IVA with no clinical or radiological evidence of distant spread.

Laparoscopic anatomy of the retroperitoneum via a left-sided extraperitoneal view may initially be difficult to interpret; however, knowledge of such a view is crucial for this procedure as the dissection takes place around major vascular structures. Additionally, surgeons working in this region should be comfortable managing possible vascular injuries either by laparoscopy or by laparotomy.

Prior to undertaking the procedure, the surgeon should obtain a radiological study (i.e. a computed tomography (CT) scan) to evaluate the retroperitoneal structures and to rule out any vascular abnormalities. Careful identification of the major landmarks is crucial for the success of this dissection. The remainder of this chapter illustrates the technical steps for this procedure.

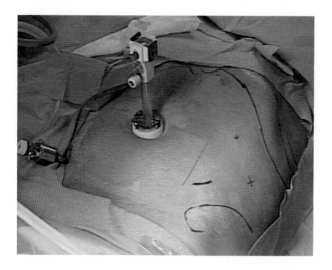

Figure 8.1. Diagnostic laparoscopy and trocar placement.
Diagnostic laparoscopy is performed prior to the extraperitoneal dissection to inspect the peritoneal cavity and to rule out carcinomatosis. This is carried out using an umbilical port and a right lower quadrant port and, if needed, a suprapubic port. During this step, the pelvis can be inspected for bulky lymphadenopathy. Trocar placement for the extraperitoneal dissection is illustrated in this photograph. A 15-mm incision for the finger dissection is made 3–4 cm medial to the left iliac spine. Two accessory trocars are used: a 10-mm trocar is placed in the left mid-axillary line and a 5-mm trocar is placed in the anterior axillary line approximately 5 cm below the rib cage.

a

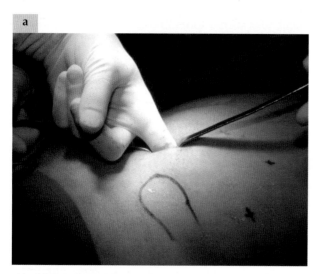

b

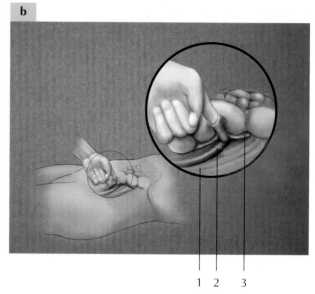

1   2   3

1 – Psoas muscle
2 – Left common iliac artery
3 – Ureter

Figure 8.2. Finger dissection.
The opening of the extraperitoneal space begins with a finger dissection. (**a**) Using the incision medial to the iliac spine, the surgeon introduces an index finger through the abdominal fascia and muscles, being careful not to perforate the peritoneum. (**b**) The dissection begins by first identifying the psoas muscle followed by the left common iliac artery. After identifying these two landmarks, the peritoneum is freed in the cephalic direction off the abdominal wall muscles. The finger dissection can be done under laparoscopic guidance using the umbilical port or blindly after carefully dissecting through the various layers of the abdominal wall to identify the preperitoneal space.

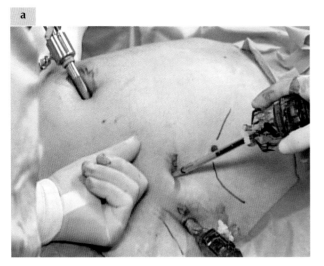

Figure 8.3. Additional trocar.
(**a**) After the separation of the peritoneal sac from the abdominal wall, accessory trocars can be placed; placement of these trocars is accomplished under finger guidance. The surgeon must be sure to have separated the peritoneum off the abdominal wall at the points where the accessory ports are to be placed. (**b**) The operator should ensure that the trocar does not accidentally pierce the peritoneal reflection, which would make insufflation of the retroperitoneal space difficult. This photograph illustrates how the accessory trocar is introduced into the extraperitoneal space at a point where the peritoneal sac has been separated from the abdominal wall.

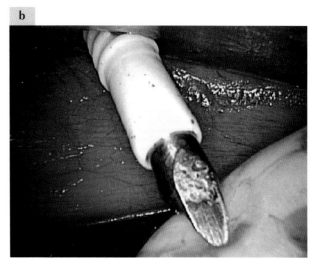

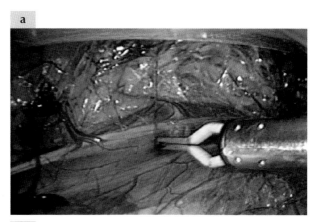

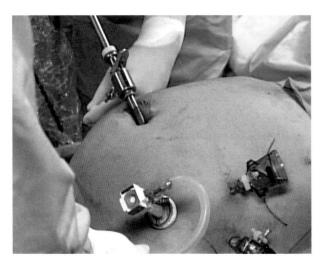

Figure 8.4. Final port placement.
Once the additional two trocars have been placed, the surgeon's index finger is removed and a balloon trocar is placed into the extraperitoneal space under laparoscopic guidance – this balloon trocar ensures pneumostasis. The laparoscope is placed through the balloon trocar. This photograph illustrates the three ports that are required for this procedure.

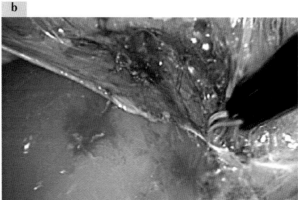

Figure 8.5. Psoas muscle.
(**a**) The psoas muscle is the first landmark that is identified. The peritoneal sac has been partially released off the psoas muscle with the finger dissection; however, occasionally this must be completed under visual guidance using the laparoscopic instruments. (**b**) Using both blunt and sharp dissection, the psoas can be released from the overlying tissue. The psoas is released up to the fascia of the kidney; the kidney may need to be elevated off the psoas to provide adequate room to operate. Additionally, this creation of space allows for the pooling of both blood and irrigation fluid away from the operative field.

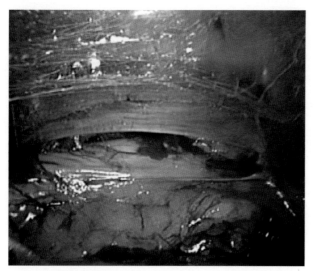

Figure 8.6. Identifying the left common iliac artery.
Once the peritoneal sac has been freed off the psoas, attention is turned to identifying the left common iliac artery, which is done by careful blunt dissection. The left ureter and ovarian vessels are attached to the peritoneal sac and elevated off the psoas and common iliac artery. This photograph illustrates the appearance of the left common iliac artery as it is first identified.

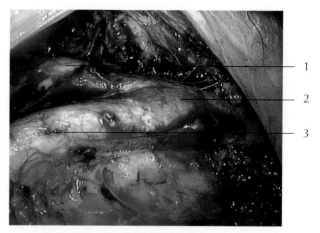

1 – Right common iliac artery
2 – Aorta
3 – Left common iliac artery

Figure 8.7. Aortic bifurcation.
Once the left common iliac artery is identified, it can be traced to the aortic bifurcation and the right common iliac artery. This is done using both blunt and sharp dissection to open the areolar tissue and elevate the peritoneal sac.

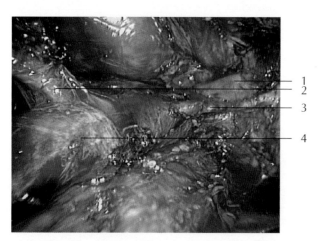

1 – Left renal vein
2 – Inferior mesenteric artery
3 – Left renal artery
4 – Aorta

Figure 8.8. Inferior mesenteric artery and left renal vein.
The inferior mesenteric artery is the next structure that should be identified; this can be done by tracing the aorta cranially. Postganglionic sympathetic fibers usually converge in this region and may give the surgeon clues as to its whereabouts. The next structure to be identified is the left renal vein. This can be found by continuing up the aorta cranially to the crossing of the left renal vein.

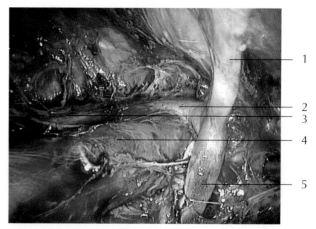

1 – Left ovarian vein
2 – Left renal vein
3 – Inferior vena cava
4 – Aorta
5 – Azygos vein

Figure 8.9. Left renal vein.
An alternative approach is to identify the left ovarian vein and trace it to the left renal vein. Dissection of the left renal vein and removal of the lymph nodes in this region must be done with caution so as not to injure the azygos vein. One of the reasons the authors prefer a left-sided approach is the complexity of the left infrarenal dissection.

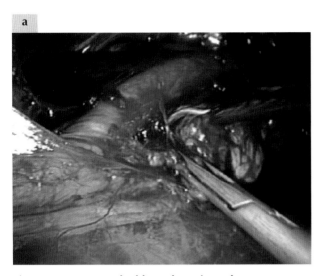 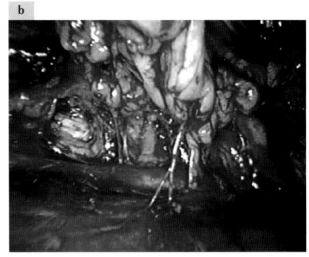

Figure 8.10. Removal of lateral aortic nodes.
(a) The lateral aortic nodes and the left common iliac nodes can be easily detached from the large vessels using sharp and blunt dissection. Cephalad to the inferior mesenteric artery is the origin of the left ovarian artery. This artery is not easily seen and can be avulsed, which may result in excessive bleeding. (b) Posteriorly, the lateral aortic nodes should be removed above the sympathetic chain. Below this level lie the lumbar vessels that can cause significant bleeding if injured. The postganglionic fibers can be cut at their origin.

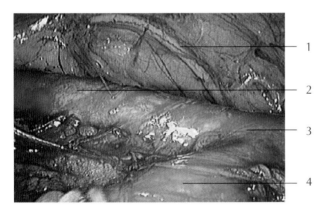

1 – Right ureter
2 – Right common iliac artery
3 – Aorta
4 – Left common iliac artery

Figure 8.11. Right common iliac artery.
Prior to removing the lymph nodes from the right common iliac artery, the right ureter should be visualized. As it is still attached to the peritoneum, it can be swept laterally and away from the dissection.

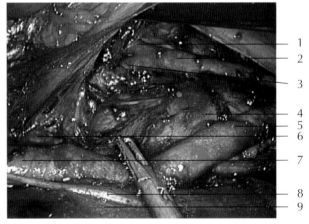

1 – Right external iliac artery
2 – Right common iliac artery
3 – Right internal iliac artery
4 – Left common iliac vein
5 – Left common iliac artery
6 – Left internal iliac artery
7 – Left external iliac artery
8 – Left genitofemoral nerve
9 – Left psoas muscle

Figure 8.12. Subaortic and right common iliac artery.
The left common iliac vein and both of the common iliac arteries are illustrated in this photograph. The lymph nodes can be removed from the common iliac arteries to the level of the iliac bifurcation. The subaortic lymph nodes have been removed, but the surgeon must be aware of the middle sacral vein.

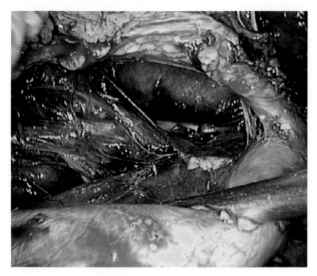

Figure 8.13. Precaval lymph nodes.
Precaval and lateral caval lymph nodes can be removed using a left-sided approach. The nodes must be grasped firmly and dissected from the vena cava. Small perforating vessels from the vena cava to the nodal package should be identified and coagulated. Avulsing these vessels may cause severe hemorrhage.

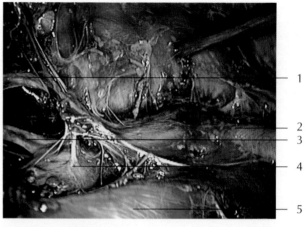

1 – Right ovarian artery
2 – Left renal vein
3 – Right ovarian vein
4 – Inferior vena cava
5 – Aorta

Figure 8.14. Right ovarian vessels.
The high pre-aortic and interaortocaval nodes are removed with careful attention to the right ovarian artery, which may be difficult to identify. This should be coagulated and cut prior to removing the nodal package. The duodenum should be freed from the left renal vein to access this area.

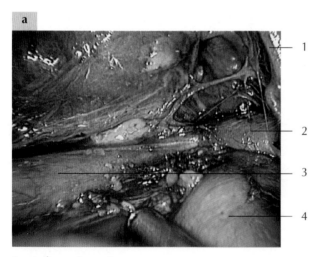

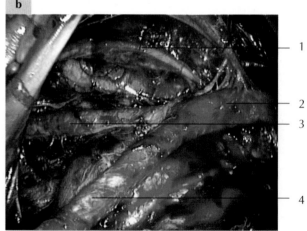

1 – Left ovarian vein
2 – Left renal vein
3 – Inferior vena cava
4 – Aorta

1 – Right ureter
2 – Aorta
3 – Right common iliac artery
4 – Left common iliac artery

Figure 8.15. Extent of the dissection.
(a) The superior limit of the dissection is the left renal vein as it inserts into the vena cava. The interaortocaval and high precaval nodes have been removed. This area is rich in lymphatics and these channels should be thoroughly coagulated. (b) This photograph demonstrates the finished dissection below the inferior mesenteric artery. The common iliac, subaortic, precaval, and paraaortic nodes have been removed.

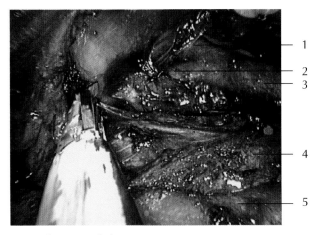

1 – Right external iliac artery
2 – Right internal iliac artery
3 – Right common iliac artery
4 – Left common iliac vein
5 – Left common iliac artery

Figure 8.16. Marking lower limits.
The inferior limits of the dissection are marked with clips at the level of the bifurcation of the common iliac artery. This allows the radiation oncologist to accurately design the radiation fields.

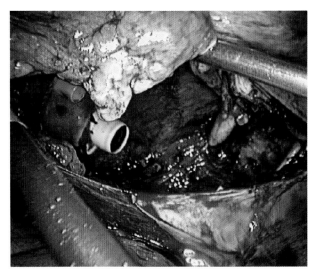

Figure 8.17. Marsupialization.
Symptomatic lymphoceles comprised the majority of postoperative complications in the authors' early experience. Thus, it became routine to marsupialize the peritoneum in the left paracolic gutter using the initial transperitoneal approach initiated for the diagnostic step, and no further symptomatic lymphoceles have been witnessed.

9 Surgery for carcinoma of the vulva

Mary L Gemignani

Vulvar cancer is relatively rare among the female genital tract cancers. In 2003, it is estimated that only 4000 cases of cancer of the vulva will be diagnosed in the USA.[1] The surgical procedures performed for this cancer have changed drastically over the past several decades. Initially, the surgical treatment was an en-bloc removal of the vulva to include bilateral inguino-femoral lymphadenectomy. The morbidity associated with this radical approach included wound complications and lymphedema in almost all patients.

Currently, less radical approaches and improvements in perioperative techniques have resulted in fewer complications, without a compromise in outcome. The en-bloc removal of the vulva and inguino-femoral nodes has been replaced by lymphadenectomy, performed through separate incisions from those of the radical vulvectomy. Depending on tumor location and size, often this can be accomplished by a partial radical vulvectomy and ipsilateral inguino-femoral lymphadenectomy. A midline lesion is treated with bilateral inguino-femoral lymphadenectomy.

The majority of the complications still associated with treatment of this disease are a direct consequence of the lymphadenectomy. Investigative work into the use of sentinel node procedure holds promise in this area. The sentinel node concept has been validated in melanoma and breast cancer.[2,3] The sentinel node is predictive of the status of the regional lymphatic basin.[4] In breast cancer and melanoma, if the sentinel node is examined and does not demonstrate metastatic disease, a regional lymphadenectomy is not routinely performed. The sentinel node procedure holds promise in the treatment of vulvar carcinoma by reducing the need for complete lymphadenectomy in all patients.[5] This could be accomplished without compromising adequate staging and allowing for lymphadenectomy in only those patients with positive nodes.

In this chapter, the anatomical and surgical techniques of radical vulvectomy, skinning vulvectomy, inguino-femoral lymphadenectomy, and sentinel node biopsy will be demonstrated.

Radical vulvectomy

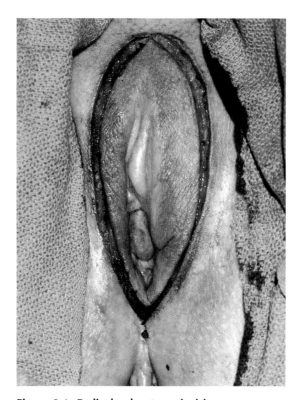

Figure 9.1. Radical vulvectomy incision.
The radical vulvectomy incisions are placed according to the location and size of the primary tumor. The surgeon should attempt to obtain a 2-cm margin of normal tissue around the tumor in all directions. However, a 1-cm margin is reasonable around the urethral meatus, clitoris, and anus: in these areas, this is necessary to preserve the structures and their function.

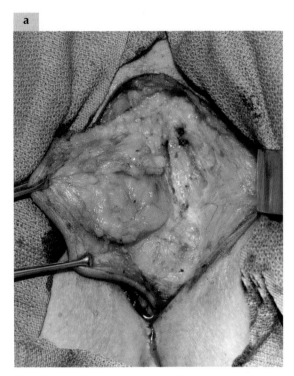

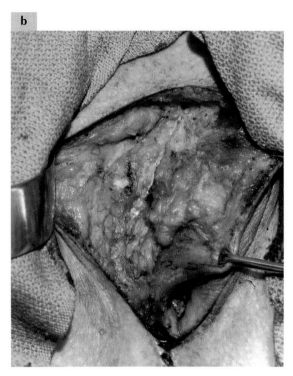

Figure 9.2 (a and b). Deep fascia of the urogenital diaphragm.
The labiocrural incisions are carried through the fatty tissue bilaterally; extension through the tissue is necessary to the level of the deep fascia of the urogenital diaphragm bilaterally, and this is usually performed with electrocautery. Care should be taken to identify the internal pudendal vessels at about the 4 o'clock and 8 o'clock positions during this part of the dissection; these can be individually clamped, transected, and ligated. Inferiorly, the perineal body and posterior vulvar tissue are dissected away from the anus.

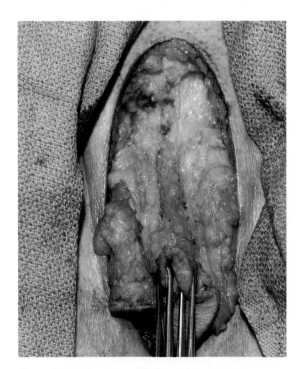

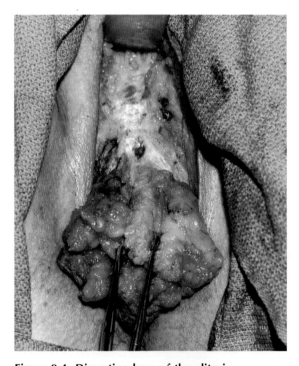

Figure 9.3. Dissection off the pubic periosteum.
Superiorly, the specimen is dissected off the pubic periosteum and adductor fascia; the dissection is continued in this manner inferiorly. The lateral portions of this part of the procedure are also taken deeply until the adductor fascia is encountered.

Figure 9.4. Dissection base of the clitoris.
The dissection of the superior portion of the vulva continues medially and laterally to expose the pubic periosteum and adductor fascia (bilaterally). The base of the clitoris is identified, clamped, transected, and ligated at this point. The dissection is completed and joined medially by making a transvestibular mucosal incision above the urethra.

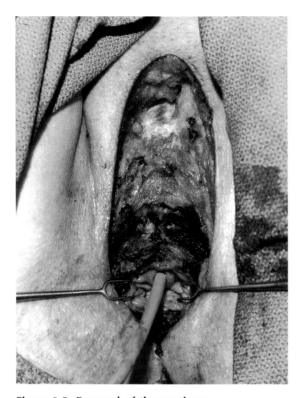

Figure 9.5. Removal of the specimen.
Inferiorly, the portions of the vulvar tissue along the perineum are dissected upward to the vagina; care should be taken to avoid injury to the rectum. The vascular vestibular tissue along the vagina is clamped and transected; the specimen is now free both superiorly and inferiorly, and removal of the vulva is complete. A Foley catheter is placed in the urethral meatus, and the vaginal opening is noted. The wound is irrigated and hemostasis is obtained.

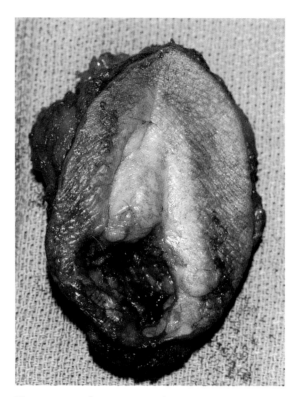

Figure 9.6. Vulvectomy specimen.

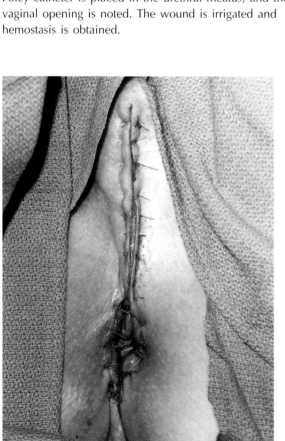

Figure 9.7. Closure of the radical vulvectomy wound.
Closure of the wound needs to be performed without tension to minimize wound breakdown. Any ischemic-appearing skin should be excised prior to closure. The edges of the wound and the perineum are closed with vertical mattress sutures. The urethra should be secured on a straight course without tension; a hood of skin above the urethra should be avoided because this can obstruct the urinary stream. The vaginal edges should be everted over the perineum and anus. It is important to avoid suturing the edges laterally over the perineum.

In some instances, such as when a large defect is present or the patient has had prior radiation, a primary tension-free closure is not possible. Incorporation of reconstructive techniques, including utilization of a myocutaneous flap, may be necessary to provide healthy tissue with adequate blood supply.

Skinning vulvectomy

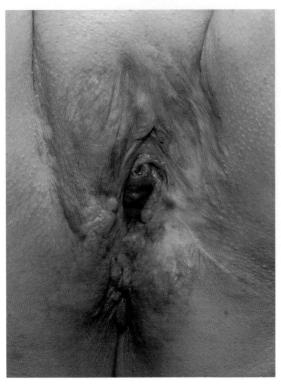

Figure 9.8. Skinning vulvectomy.
In select patients with extensive disease such as Paget's disease or vulval intraepithelial neoplasia (VIN), a vulvectomy incorporating all the skin/superficial tissue of the vulva may be indicated. In elderly patients with marked atrophy of the vulva, the demarcation of the labia minora and majora is unclear.

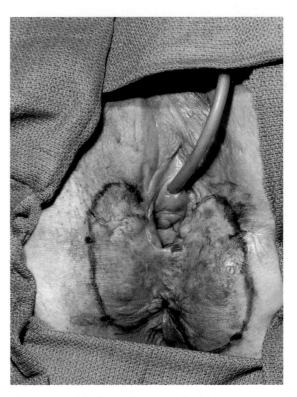

Figure 9.9. Skinning vulvectomy incision.
The incision lines are marked on the vulva. Incision is made to allow for adequate margins around the lesion(s).

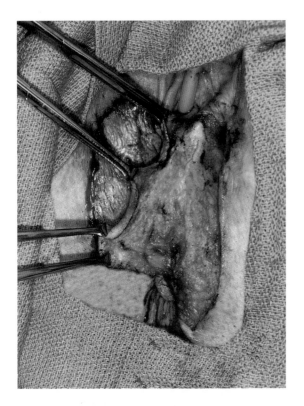

Figure 9.10. Superficial dissection.
The skin incision is made with a knife and remains a superficial dissection – it does not extend down to the deep fascia or the muscles of the urogenital diaphragm. Dissection can be accomplished with electrocautery or sharp instrumentation. Although it is unnecessary to remove the bulbocavernosus and ischiocavernous muscles, it may be difficult not to do so in patients with an atrophic vulva. The incision can be carried almost to the anal orifice. Care should be taken around the anus to avoid damage to the external anal sphincter.

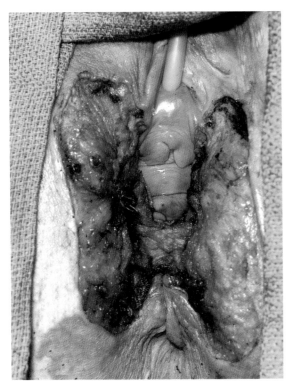

Figure 9.11. Removal of the specimen.
After removal of the specimen, it is evident that some of the mucosa along the anus has been dissected off the external anal sphincter anteriorly, and removed to allow for adequate tumor-free margins. The wound is irrigated and checked for hemostasis.

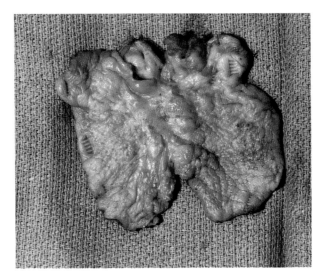

Figure 9.12. The skinning vulvectomy specimen.

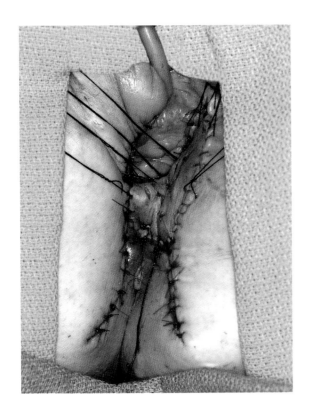

Figure 9.13. Wound closure.
The wound is closed primarily with delayed absorbable sutures. Closure of the perineal defect above the anal orifice requires everting the vaginal epithelium in this area. Lateral closure of skin edges across the posterior fourchette should be avoided. The wound is closed with interrupted sutures. A Foley catheter is left in the urinary bladder.

In cases where a primary tension-free closure is not possible, reconstructive options, such as utilization of a skin graft, are appropriate.

Inguinofemoral lymphadenectomy

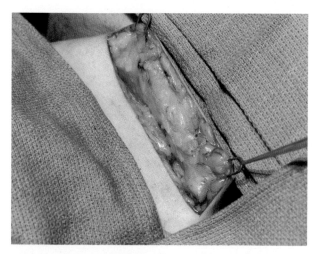

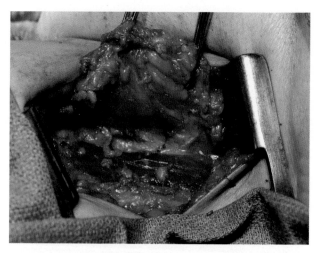

Figure 9.14. Skin incision.
The patient is placed in dorsolithotomy position, with minimal flexion at the hip to allow the groin area to be as flat as possible. The skin incision is 8–10 cm long, is made parallel to the inguinal ligament, and is carried down to Camper's fascia. This is not a true fascia and can be easily transected if not carefully identified. Skin hooks are used to elevate the skin and facilitate the creation of flaps, which separates the fat pad containing lymph nodes from the skin subcutaneous tissue. It is important not to make the skin flaps too thin, as doing so may lead to necrosis of the flaps. Either a knife or electrocautery is used during this part of the dissection.

Figure 9.15. Identification of the boundaries of the dissection.
It is important to identify the boundaries of the dissection. The adductor longus muscle is palpated medially and the incision is carried down to, but not through, the fascia of this muscle. Laterally, the sartorius muscle, shown in this figure, is identified. The upper dissection border consists of the mons pubis and pubic tubercle medially, and the external oblique aponeurosis overlying the inguinal canal superiorly.

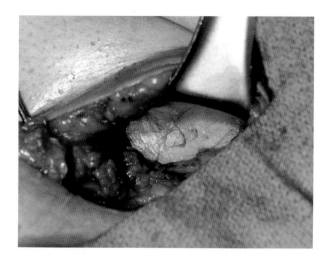

Figure 9.16. Clearing the external oblique aponeurosis.
Beginning superiorly, the fat pad is elevated from the external oblique aponeurosis. The fat pad is mobilized down to the inferior margin of the inguinal ligament. Medially, the external inguinal ring and the diverticular process containing the round ligament are identified. Branches of the superficial external pudendal and the superficial circumflex iliac vessels traverse over the inguinal ligament at the medial and lateral limits of the upper flap, respectively. This part of the dissection is carried superficial to the fascia lata; thus, the femoral vessels and nerve are not encountered.

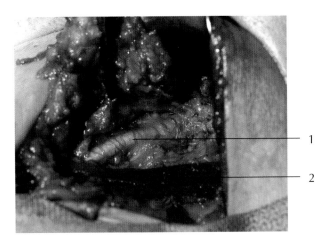

1 – Left femoral artery
2 – Sartorius muscle

Figure 9.17. Opening the cribriform fascia.
The dissection is carried deeper in the direction of the femoral triangle. Feeling for the pulsation of the femoral artery is helpful, and the femoral artery is identified by opening the cribriform fascia. The cribriform fascia should be opened along the anterior aspect of the femoral artery. The content of the fossa ovalis are noted. The dissection performed over the top of the artery is continued over the anterior surface of the vein, mobilizing the specimen to the medial aspect of the femoral vein. There is no need to dissect under the artery or between the femoral artery and vein.

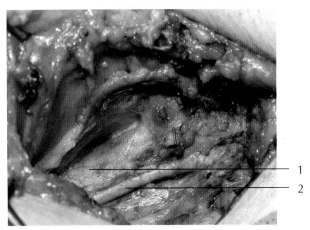

1 – Left femoral vein
2 – Left femoral artery

Figure 9.18. The common femoral vein.
Small tributaries of the saphenous vein are ligated as they are encountered during the medial part of the dissection. Dissection and clearing of the nodal tissue continues over the anterior surface of the common femoral vein with a combination of blunt and sharp dissection, using electrocautery and hemoclips as needed. Removal of the fat pad from the femoral triangle begins laterally and continues medially; the structures encountered laterally to medially are nerve, artery, vein, and lymphatics. The femoral nerve is best identified close to the inguinal ligament because it begins to branch more distally.

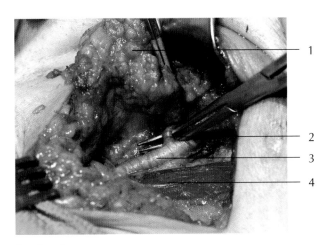

1 – Specimen
2 – Left superficial external pudendal artery
3 – Left femoral artery
4 – Sartorius muscle

Figure 9.19. External pudendal artery.
While clearing the femoral artery proximally, the most proximal branches are the superficial external pudendal artery, the superficial epigastric artery, and the superficial circumflex iliac artery. The superficial external pudendal artery, shown here, is the most medial proximal branch of the femoral artery. This small branch should be identified, isolated, and ligated.

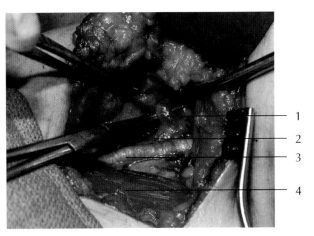

1 – Great saphenous vein
2 – Left femoral vein
3 – Left femoral artery
4 – Sartorius muscle

Figure 9.20. Saphenous vein identified at the saphenofemoral junction.
The great saphenous vein enters the common femoral vein cephalad at the point at which the external pudendal artery crosses the common femoral vein. The proximal 1–2 cm of the saphenous vein is isolated and ligated with permanent sutures at the level of the common femoral vein wall, and transected. It is important not to compromise the lumen of the femoral vein while ligating the saphenous vein.

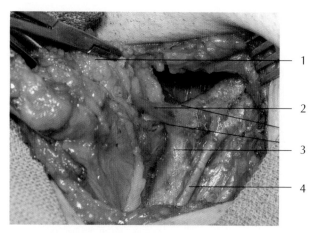

1 – Specimen
2 – Great saphenous vein
3 – Left femoral vein
4 – Left femoral artery

Figure 9.21. Saphenous vein.
The specimen side of the saphenous vein should also be ligated to avoid backbleeding.

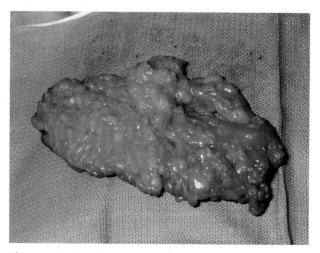

Figure 9.23. Specimen containing the inguino-femoral lymph nodes.

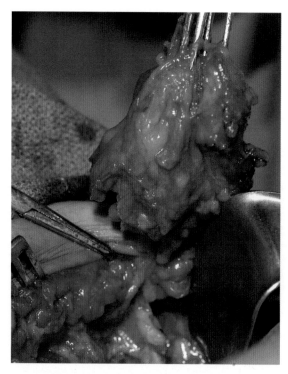

Figure 9.22. Removal of the specimen.
The bridge of tissue over the femoral vessels between the lateral and medial dissection is now ligated and divided. The specimen is freed from any remaining attachments and removed.

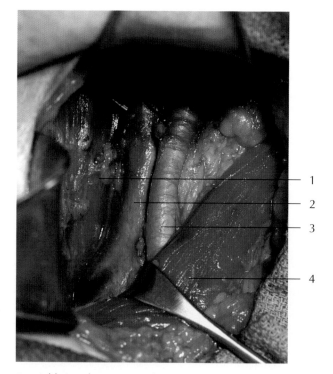

1 – Adductor longus muscle
2 – Left femoral vein
3 – Left femoral artery
4 – Sartorius muscle

Figure 9.24. Femoral triangle.
The anatomy of the femoral triangle is shown after removal of the specimen. At this point, the wound is checked for hemostasis. The sartorius can be transposed by transecting it with electrocautery at its tendinous attachment to the anterior superior iliac spine. It is then used to cover the vessels by suturing it to the inguinal ligament and pectineal fascia with interrupted delayed absorbable sutures.

Sentinel node biopsy

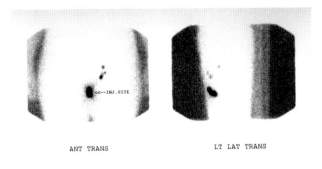

ANT TRANS   LT LAT TRANS

Figure 9.25. Lymphoscintigram.
In patients undergoing sentinel node biopsy, both radioisotope and blue dye are used to help in accurate localization of the sentinel node. In the Nuclear Medicine Department, an injection with filtered technetium-99m sulfur colloid is performed. Injection of 0.1–0.5 mci of the radiolabeled colloid is given at the leading edge of the vulvar lesion. A preoperative lymphoscintigram is shown: the scan demonstrates the localization of the sentinel 'hot' nodes to the ipsilateral groin. There can be one or more sentinel nodes. The radioisotope concentrates in the sentinel nodes and remains there for at least 2–6 hours after injection.

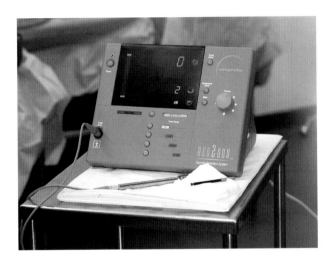

Figure 9.26. Gamma probe.
Shown here is the neo2000™ intraoperative gamma probe (Neoprobe Corporation, Dublin, OH). The probe identifies the sentinel lymph nodes by localizing the radioisotope signal that has concentrated in the nodes.

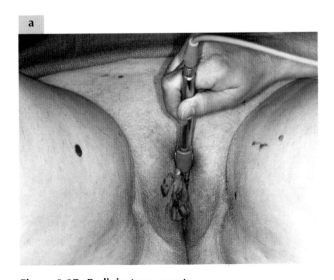
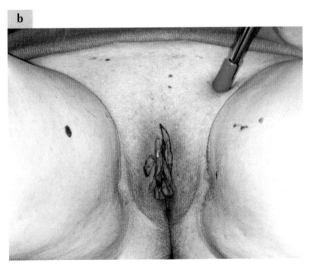

Figure 9.27. Radioisotope counts.
(**a**) Radioisotope counts are obtained over the injection site (primary lesion) and (**b**) the site of the sentinel lymph node (groin) as seen on the lymphoscintigram. These are recorded for later use.

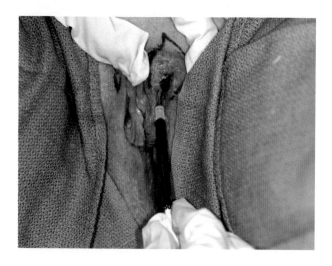

Figure 9.28. Isosulfan blue dye.
After the patient is anesthetized, 4 ml of isosulfan blue dye is circumferentially injected around the lesion. Injection is at the normal skin interface around the lesion, and not directly into the lesion. The injection is mostly intradermal; however, intraparenchymal injection is also effective, particularly in larger lesions. Injection should be performed at least 10 minutes before the groin incision is made. The sentinel lymph node biopsy is performed before excision of the primary vulvar lesion.

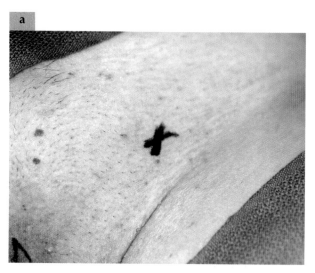
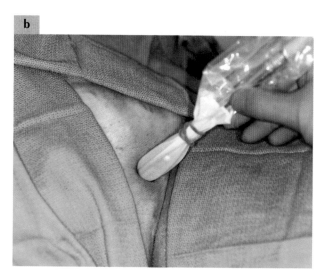

Figure 9.29. Marking the skin for groin incision.
(a) A small incision will be made in the groin directly over the point of maximum radioactivity, so the area with the highest radioisotope counts is initially marked. (b) The area is then prepped and draped in the usual sterile fashion, and the counts obtained again under sterile conditions.

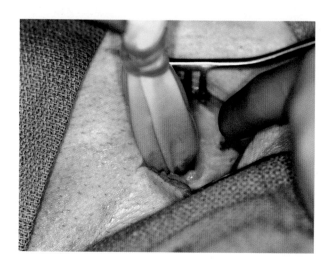

Figure 9.30. Intraoperative lymphatic mapping.
The gamma probe is used to help identify the 'hot' nodes, guiding the surgeon to the sentinel nodes. An incision is made parallel to the inguinal ligament. In cases where an inguino-femoral lymphadenectomy is planned, the incision can be extended after the sentinel node procedure is completed. The fatty tissue is carefully dissected through this area for identification of blue channels.

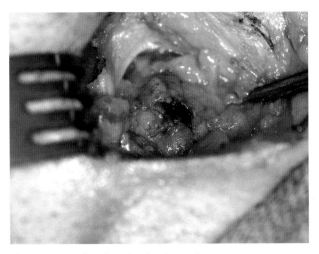

Figure 9.31. Blue lymphatic channels.
Blue lymphatics are noted leading to the sentinel node. The use of both isosulfan blue dye and a radioisotope help steepen the learning curve, and increase the success in identification of the sentinel node.

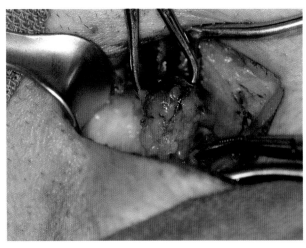

Figure 9.32. Sentinel node.
An Adair clamp is used to grasp the node – blue lymphatics are seen. The lymphatic tissue around the node is dissected with a hemostat and electrocautery.

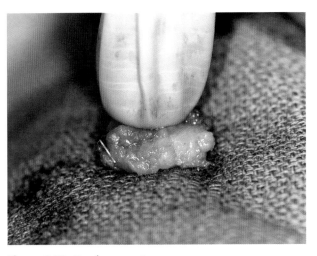

Figure 9.33. Ex vivo counts.
The node is removed and checked for radioactivity: counts are recorded for each node that is removed. Data sheets are available to record whether the nodes are blue and/or 'hot'.

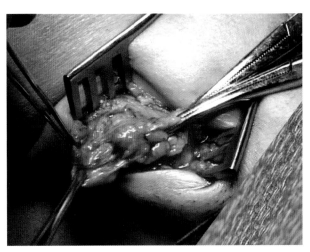

Figure 9.34. Sentinel node identification.
Any node that exhibits radioactivity or blue dye is removed.

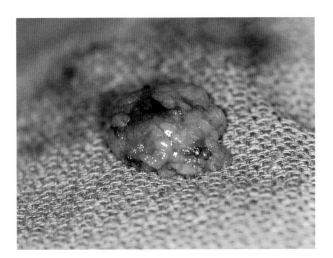

Figure 9.35. Specimen showing a blue sentinel node.

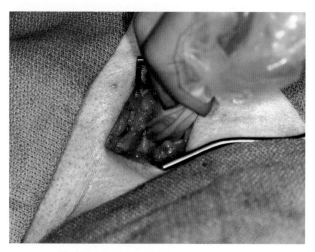

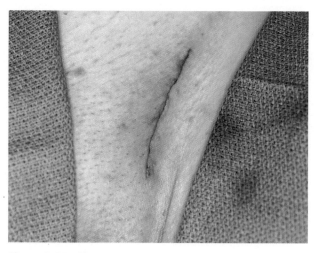

Figure 9.36. Postexcision counts.
The lymphatic basin is checked for residual radioactivity after removal of the sentinel node, and any discrete residual radioactivity is pursued. The counts should be minimal, with a more than 4- to 10-fold reduction over the maximum counts obtained at that site at the outset of the procedure. If significant counts remain, it is important to search the basin carefully for the possible presence of another sentinel node.

Figure 9.37. Closure.
The incision can be closed primarily with a rapidly dissolving suture in a subcuticular fashion. If an inguino-femoral lymphadenectomy is to follow, the incision can be extended, and the procedure completed as described previously.

References

1. Jemal A, Thomas A, Murray T, Thun M. Cancer statistics, 2002. *CA Cancer J Clin* 2002; **52**:23–47.
2. Albertini JJ, Lyman GH, Cox C et al. Lymphatic mapping and sentinel lymph node biopsy in the patient with breast cancer. *JAMA* 1996; **276**:1812–22.
3. Thompson JF, McCarthy WH, Bosch CM et al. Sentinel lymph node status as an indicator of the presence of metastatic melanoma in regional lymph nodes. *Melanoma Res* 1995; **5**:255–60.
4. Cody HS III, Borgen PI. State-of-the-art approaches to sentinel node biopsy for breast cancer: study design, patient selection, technique, and quality control at Memorial Sloan-Kettering Cancer Center. *Surg Oncol* 1999; **8**:85–91.
5. Levenback C, Coleman RL, Burke TW et al. Intraoperative lymphatic mapping and sentinel node identification with blue dye in patients with vulvar cancer. *Gynecol Oncol* 2001; **83**:276–81.

10 Laparoscopically assisted vaginal radical hysterectomy

Michel Roy, Marie Plante and Marie-Claude Renaud

The vaginal radical hysterectomy was first described by Schauta[1] at the turn of the twentieth century. It had the advantage of a significantly lower mortality rate than the abdominal radical hysterectomy championed by Wertheim; however, a few years later, Wertheim[2] reported a better survival rate with his abdominal approach. Thus, the vaginal route fell into disfavor. In the 1940s, pelvic lymphadenectomy became part of the standard of care in the surgical treatment of cervical cancer. Obviously, the vaginal approach alone could not accommodate that new standard. This changed when Mitra[3] proposed the use of bilateral flank incisions to perform a retroperitoneal lymph node dissection, followed by the vaginal radical hysterectomy. However, the technique was more complicated than the abdominal approach alone and was not esthetically appealing; therefore, it did not gain popularity in North America. With the subsequent development of laparoscopic techniques to perform a complete pelvic and paraaortic lymph node dissection,[4] and the experience of vaginal surgery specialists, particularly Professor Daniel Dargent in France, the Schauta operation suddenly enjoys a renewed interest in the gynecologic oncology community, and has regained acceptance as an attractive and efficient alternative to the standard abdominal approach.

Advantages of the laparoscopically assisted vaginal radical hysterectomy (LAVRH) include the absence of an abdominal incision, shorter hospital stay, and lower morbidity.[5] Studies have shown that the specimen removed after an LAVRH is satisfactory. Furthermore, if positive lymph nodes are identified at laparoscopy, one has the option of offering patients combined chemotherapy and radiation therapy without having submitted them to a major laparotomy. Lastly, and perhaps more importantly, since there is a definite learning curve before one becomes comfortable with vaginal radical surgery,[6] the skills gained in LAVRH help the surgeon to offer selected young patients the more conservative fertility-preserving vaginal radical trachelectomy,[7,8] which is a modification of the Schauta–Amreich procedure (see Chapter 11). In this chapter, the technique for LAVRH will be reviewed.

Vaginal radical surgery requires the surgeon to master laparoscopic surgery in order to conduct a complete laparoscopic lymph node dissection. At the completion of the lymphadenectomy, the paravesical and pararectal spaces are defined laparoscopically. This dissection facilitates the transection of the uterine artery, after clipping or cauterization, at its origin from the internal iliac artery. The distal parametrial tissue, potentially bearing lymph nodes, is also removed laparoscopically to reduce the extent of the parametrectomy required vaginally.

Although investigational at this point, the technique for localization and retrieval of the sentinel node (SN) will be described. The concept of the SN is that the first lymph node in a regional lymphatic basin to receive drainage from a tumor accurately reflects the status of the nodes in that regional basin. Theoretically, if the SN is negative, the other lymph nodes are also likely to be negative. If this concept proves to be true in cervical cancer, one may potentially be able to avoid complete lymph node dissection in the future.[9] This would substantially reduce surgical time and potential complications; however, additional data from properly designed studies are needed before this procedure gains wide acceptance.

Laparoscopic portion – sentinel lymph node localization

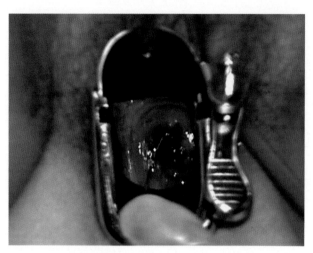

Figure 10.1. Injection of the cervix with colorant for sentinel lymph node identification.

Two techniques are currently used to identify the sentinel lymph node – visual localization by coloration of the node and lymphoscintigraphy with technetium-99m (Tc-99m labeled antimony sulfide). After examination under anesthesia and just prior to the initiation of surgery, 1 ml of Patent Blue or Lymphazurin solution is injected into each cervical quadrant. A 27-gauge needle is used and the injection is made superficially under the mucosa about 5 mm lateral to the external os, slowly and with constant pressure in order to minimize spillage. When needed, a small hook can be used to stabilize the cervix during the injection. A needle extender or spinal needle can also be used to facilitate the injection. If lymphoscintigraphy is used, the Tc-99m is injected in the same way 2–5 hours before surgery in order to allow time for the colloid to migrate to the lymph nodes.

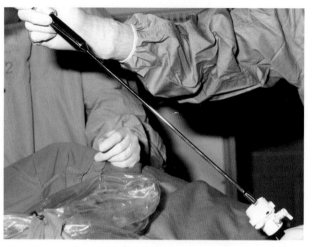

Figure 10.2. Laparoscopic probe for lymphoscintigraphy.
A laparoscopic probe is used to detect areas of high radioisotope activity. It is introduced through a 10 mm suprapubic trocar. Shown here is the Navigator GPS abdominal probe from US Surgical (Norwalk, CT).

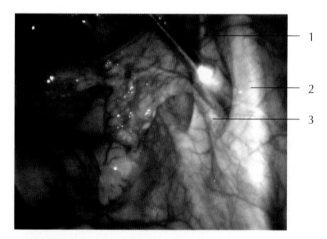

1 – Right obliterated umbilical artery
2 – Right external iliac vessels
3 – Right ovarian vessels

Figure 10.3. Laparoscopic localization of sentinel lymph node with lymphoscintigraphy.
The laparoscopic probe is swept along the pelvic sidewalls in search of the lymph nodes with greatest radioactivity. Areas of interest include the external iliac vessels, the hypogastric region, and the obturator fossa. Shown here is an evaluation of the right external iliac nodes.

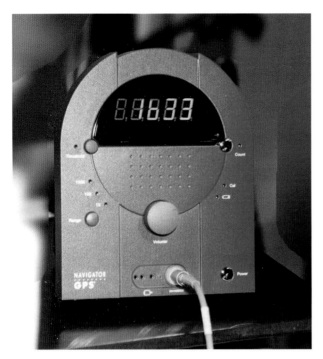

Figure 10.4. Measurement of radioactivity.
The radioactive counts are measured using the Navigator γ Position System or GPS (US Surgical, Norwalk, CT). These counts are recorded and used for comparison if additional hot spots are noted: nodes with activity > 10% of the sentinel node are excised.

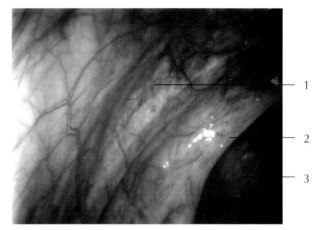

1 – Blue lymphatic channels
2 – Left uterosacral ligament
3 – Posterior cul-de-sac

Figure 10.5. Laparoscopic localization of the sentinel lymph node by Lymphazurin.
The injected blue dye is picked up by microlymphatics surrounding the tumor site; it then travels up through larger lymphatic channels. These can frequently be seen through the peritoneum and will, ultimately, lead to the sentinel lymph node, which appears blue.

Figure 10.6. Laparoscopic identification of lymphatic channels.
In order to localize the blue sentinel lymph node, after opening the peritoneum, the laparoscopist must search for the blue channels that, in 90% of cases, cross over the internal iliac artery. After removal of the sentinel lymph node, a detailed pathological evaluation is performed using serial sectioning and immunohistochemistry for the detection of micrometastasis.

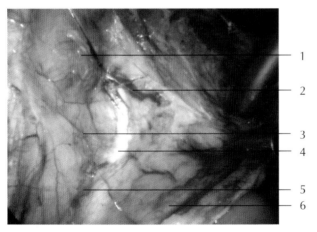

1 – Sentinel lymph node
2 – Blue lymphatic channel
3 – Left external iliac vein
4 – Left external iliac artery
5 – Secondary lymphatic channel
6 – Ureter retracted inferiorly

Laparoscopic preparation

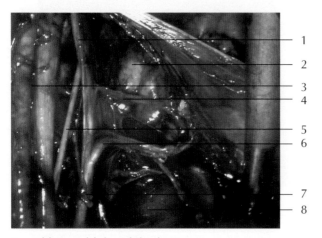

1 – Obliterated left umbilical artery
2 – Left paravesical space
3 – Left external iliac vessels
4 – Left superior vesical artery
5 – Left obturator nerve
6 – Left uterine artery
7 – Left internal iliac artery
8 – Left pararectal space

Figure 10.7. Laparoscopic preparation of the spaces.
After a complete pelvic lymphadenectomy, the pararectal and the paravesical spaces are opened laparoscopically. Shown here are the pelvic spaces in relation to the normal anatomical pelvic structures. The paravesical space is opened between the obliterated umbilical artery and the pelvic sidewall. Blunt dissection can then be used to gain access more medially. The pararectal space is opened between the ureter and the hypogastric artery.

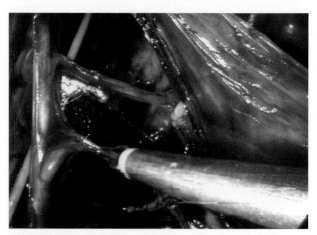

Figure 10.8. Laparoscopic ligation of the uterine artery.
The uterine artery is transected at its origin from the internal iliac artery. This can be performed with bipolar electrocautery (as shown in the figure), hemoclips, staplers, or suture ligatures.

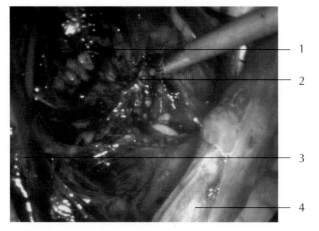

1 – Left obturator nerve
2 – Parametrium
3 – Left external iliac vein
4 – Left internal iliac artery, retracted medially

Figure 10.9. Laparoscopic parametrectomy.
The connective tissue of the parametrium, potentially containing lymph nodes, is gently dissected and removed using mostly blunt dissection with electrocautery as needed.

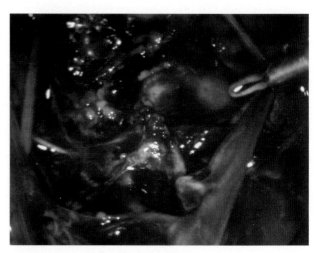

Figure 10.10. Left pelvic sidewall.
Once the parametrium is removed, only vessels and nerves are left between the pelvic sidewall and the proximal parametrium.

Vaginal portion – anatomical relationships

1 – Bladder
2 – Uterus
3 – Parametrium
4 – Ureter
5 – Uterine artery

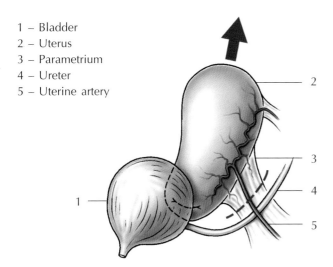

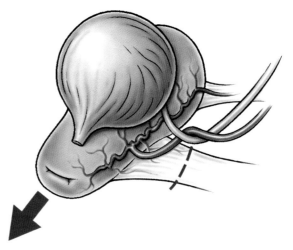

Figure 10.11. Abdominal radical hysterectomy: anatomical relationships.
When a radical hysterectomy is performed abdominally, the uterus is pulled upwards, taking with it the parametrium and the uterine vessels, while the bladder base is mobilized downwards. Therefore, the uterine vessels lie above the concavity of the ureters as the ureters course into the parametrial tunnel to enter the bladder base. Thus, after mobilization, the ureters are brought lateral and below the parametrium before it is divided. (From Plante and Roy[10] with permission.)

Figure 10.12. Vaginal radical hysterectomy: anatomical relationships.
Conversely, when the radical hysterectomy is done vaginally, the relationship between the structures is completely opposite to that when performed abdominally. The uterus is pulled downwards and the bladder base, along with the ureters, is mobilized upwards. As such, the uterine vessels end up below the concavity, or the 'knee', of the ureter. After mobilization, the ureters course above the parametrium when it is clamped. The radical vaginal surgical approach requires the surgeon to understand clearly the relationship between the ureter, the uterine artery, and the cardinal ligament (parametrium), as well as the relationship between the bladder base and the lower uterine segment. (From Plante and Roy[10] with permission.)

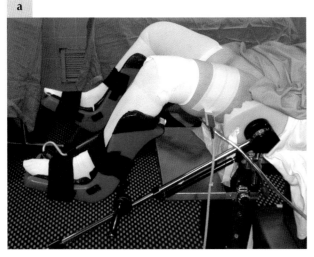

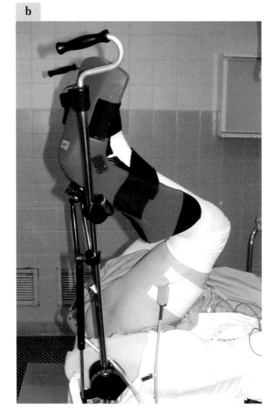

Figure 10.13. Positioning of the patient.
In order to facilitate the vaginal approach, the patient's legs are slightly extended, but the thighs are hyperflexed onto the abdomen. To avoid having to redrape after the laparoscopic lymphadenectomy and parametrectomy, hydraulic leg holders are very useful. (**a**) The legs are down for laparoscopy and (**b**) are moved up in order to attain a vertical line between the feet and the buttocks for the vaginal surgery.

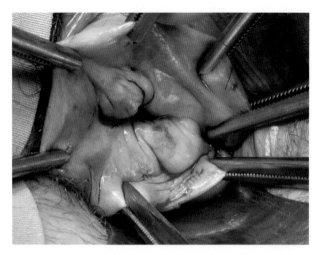

Figure 10.14. Defining the vaginal cuff.
The size and location of the cervical tumor are considered when determining the amount of vaginal tissue to be removed. Usually, 1–2 cm of vaginal cuff is scheduled for removal. The vaginal mucosa around the cervix is grasped circumferentially with six or seven Kocher clamps.

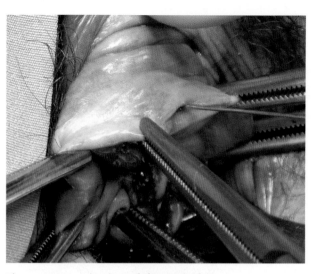

Figure 10.15. Injection of the vaginal mucosa.
A 10–20 ml solution of 1% lidocaine mixed with epinephrine 1:100,000 is injected between each Kocher clamp. This separates the mucosa from the underlying tissue and causes vasoconstriction, which will reduce bleeding.

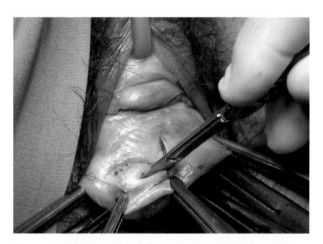

Figure 10.16. Incision of the vaginal mucosa – marking the midline.
A small vertical incision is made to mark the midline and another incision is made with the scalpel just above the Kocher clamps. It is carried through the vaginal mucosa anteriorly and posteriorly, but only superficially laterally. The mark in the midline helps to maintain orientation throughout the procedure.

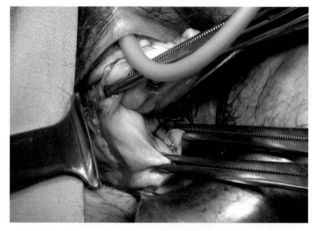

Figure 10.17. Incision of the vaginal mucosa – lateral incision.
The incision is made only superficially through the lateral vaginal mucosa so as not to enter the underlying tissues. A sidewall retractor toed in laterally is useful to retract the vaginal mucosa as it is incised.

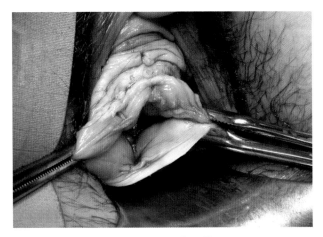

Figure 10.18. Closing the vaginal cuff.
Chrobak clamps (Lépine, France) applied side by side, are used to close the vaginal cuff in front of the cervix. This maintains important anatomic relationships, as well as assisting with the en-bloc removal of the specimen.

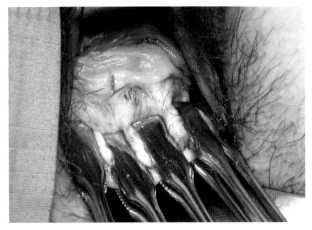

Figure 10.19. Uterine traction.
When all clamps are applied, the vaginal cuff is closed over the cervix. This provides an organized fulcrum that is strong enough to give a good traction on the uterus throughout the procedure.

Pelvic spaces

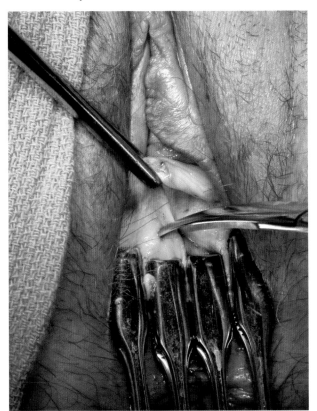

Figure 10.20. Dissection of the vesicouterine space – area of incision.
The specimen is pulled downward and the anterior vaginal mucosa is held upwards. This allows stretching of the connective tissue, which is incised with scissors held perpendicular to the cervix.

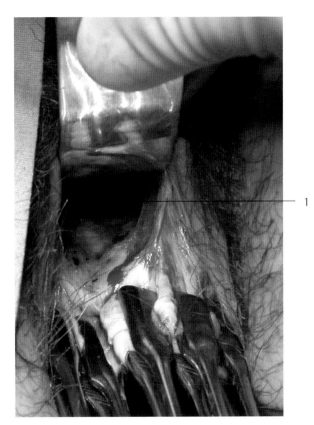

1 – Vesicouterine space

Figure 10.21. Dissection of the vesicouterine space – base of the bladder.
The index finger is also used to push the tissue until the anterior peritoneum is felt, or visualized. It is important to stay in the midline to avoid bleeding and injury to the ureter and the base of the bladder. Once the vesicouterine space is dissected, the bladder is retracted anteriorly, defining the bladder pillars on each side of the cervix.

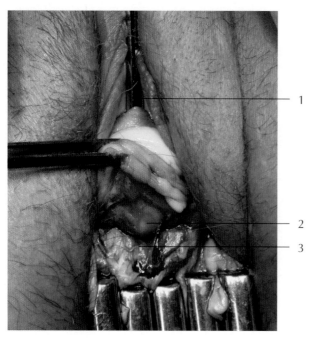

1 – Metal catheter
2 – Base of bladder pushed by metal catheter
3 – Vesicouterine space

Figure 10.22. Dissection of the vesicouterine space – identification the bladder base.
When dissection of the bladder is difficult, a metal catheter can be introduced through the urethra to localize the base of the bladder. This can help to identify the anatomic relationships that may be distorted due to prior surgery or other factors.

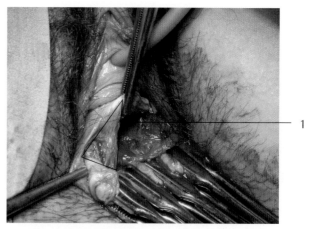

1 – Vesicouterine space
Triangle – Area of entry

Figure 10.23. Right paravesical space.
Using clamps, the anterior vaginal mucosa is grasped at 9 o'clock and 11 o'clock, and stretched. This forms a triangle where the space should be entered.

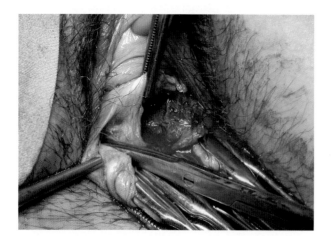

Figure 10.24. Opening the right paravesical space.
With the scissors directed upwards and outwards, the connective tissue of the triangle is blindly separated, making possible the junction with the same space already dissected laparoscopically. A rotating movement toward the midline, under the pubic bone, then enlarges the space.

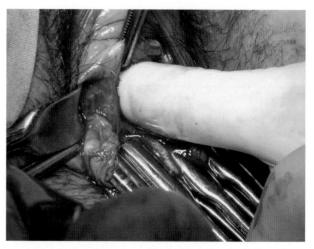

Figure 10.25. Palpation of the right ureter.
A Breisky retractor is introduced into the right paravesical space. The location of the ureter is verified by palpating the tissue between the surgeon's right index finger which is introduced in the vesicouterine space and the retractor in the paravesical space. The typical feeling and sound of the ureter indicates if the ureter is high or low in the septum between these spaces.

Dissection of the right ureter

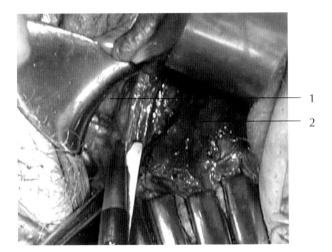

1 – Right paravesical space
2 – Vesicouterine space

Figure 10.26. Dissection of the bladder pillars.
The bladder pillars are identified between the
vesicouterine space and the right paravesical space. To
visually identify the ureter, the bladder pillars are
transected midway between the base of the bladder and
the cervix. Before cutting, the surgeon should always
palpate the tissue to confirm that the ureter is still above
the site of incision.

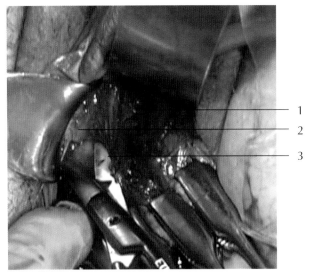

1 – Vesicouterine space
2 – Right ureter
3 – Bladder pillars

Figure 10.27. Visualization of the ureter.
After cutting the anterior bladder pillars, the ureter is
visualized medially and superiorly to the paravesical
space.

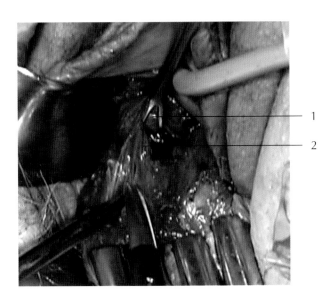

1 – Right ureter
2 – Posterior bladder pillars

Figure 10.28. Mobilization of the ureter.
Mobilization upwards of the ureter is accomplished by
grabbing the base of the bladder and the distal portion of
the ureter with a Babcock clamp. Placing this connective
tissue on tension exposes the posterior bladder pillars.
Without releasing these attachments further, mobility of
the ureter is limited.

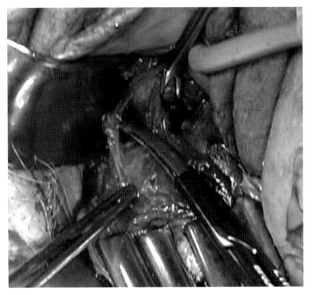

Figure 10.29. Posterior bladder pillars.
The remaining posterior and anterior attachments are
transected, enabling the surgeon to elevate the ureter
outside the parametrium. Medial and superior dissection
of the ureter should be avoided because of the risk of
injury to the bladder base.

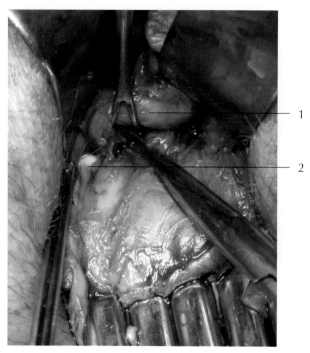

1 – Right ureter
2 – Right uterine artery

Figure 10.30. Identification of the uterine artery.
After the posterior fibers are fully transected, the uterine artery can be visualized beneath the knee of the ureter.

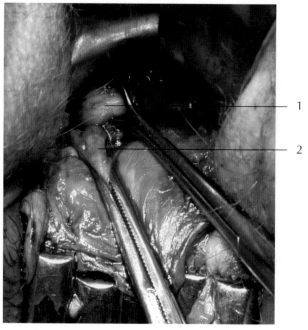

1 – Right ureter
2 – Right uterine artery

Figure 10.31. Manipulation of the uterine artery.
Gentle traction can be placed on the uterine artery with a small clamp or other instrument in order to gain additional mobility. This will help to ultimately transect the uterine artery as close to its origin as possible. Often, remaining fibers between the ureter and the parametrium can be identified and transected.

Figure 10.32. Retrieval of the uterine artery.
The entire uterine artery is removed from its origin at the hypogastric artery. The ligation of the uterine artery has been previously performed laparoscopically. The proximal portion of the vessel is identified by the clip or cautery burn that had been placed laparoscopically. An identical procedure is performed on the contralateral side.

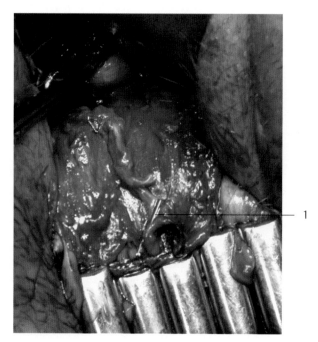

1 – Clip on right uterine artery

Parametrium

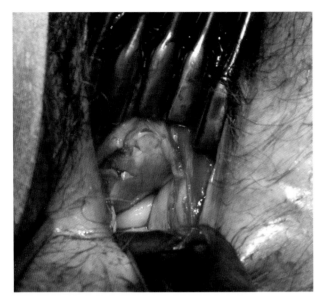

Figure 10.33. Opening the pouch of Douglas.
After both ureters have been dissected and pushed up, the peritoneum is entered by opening the posterior cul-de-sac with scissors while the uterus is pulled upwards.

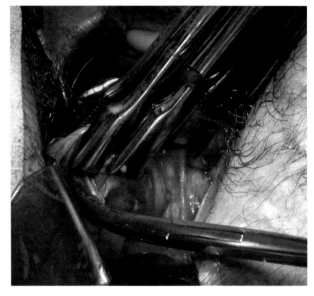

Figure 10.34. Excision of the paracolpos.
The connective tissue between the vaginal mucosa and lower part of the cervix, the paracolpos, is clamped, transected, and suture ligated.

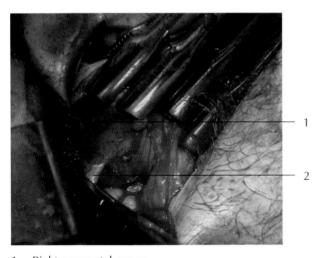

1 – Right pararectal space
2 – Right uterosacral ligament

Figure 10.35. Excision of the right uterosacral ligament.
The pararectal space, which was prepared laparoscopically, is widened by inserting scissors between the uterosacral ligament and the pelvic sidewall. This minimizes the risk to the ureter when transecting the ligament. The contralateral paracolpos and uterosacral ligament are then also transected and suture ligated.

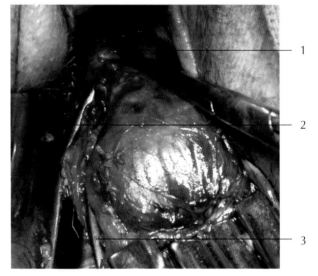

1 – Right ureter
2 – Second clamp
3 – First clamp

Figure 10.36. Resection of the right parametrium.
With the Breisky retractor placed in the paravesical space and a second one placed posteriorly, the ureter can be easily visualized. A curved clamp (Heaney or similar) is placed on the parametrial tissue and adjusted according to the amount of parametrium scheduled for removal. A second clamp (Jean-Louis Faure or similar) is placed in contact with the ureter and lateral to the first clamp. Care must be taken not to injure the ureter when suturing the parametrium. It is important to always be able to visualize the ureter. The parametrium on the other side is grasped, transected, and ligated in a similar fashion.

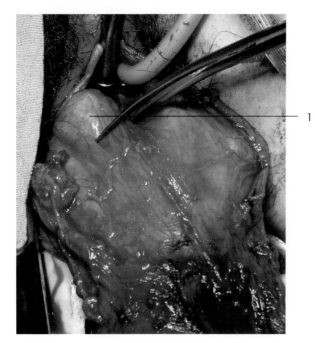

1 – Anterior peritoneum

Figure 10.37. Entering the anterior cul-de-sac.
Once the parametria are excised, the fundus of the
uterus is flipped backwards to delineate the anterior cul-
de-sac. This is opened with the operator's finger serving
as a guide to identify the point of incision. The anterior
cul-de-sac is then incised laterally in both directions.

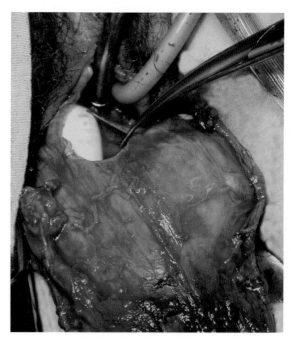

Figure 10.38. Removal of the uterus.
After opening the anterior cul-de-sac, the procedure is
completed by removing the adnexa, as appropriate. If the
adnexa are to be preserved, the utero-ovarian ligaments
are clamped, transected, and suture ligated from below.
If the adnexa were to be removed, the infundibulopelvic
ligaments would have been ligated, cauterized, or stapled
laparoscopically.

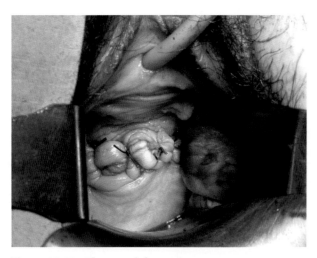

Figure 10.39. Closure of the vagina.
The vaginal vault is closed with interrupted delayed
absorbable (i.e., polyglactin) sutures in a transverse
fashion. The peritoneum is not routinely closed and
drains are not used.

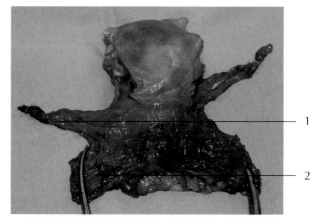

1 – Right uterine artery
2 – Right parametrium

Figure 10.40. Schauta specimen.
The specimen obtained is oncologically satisfactory with
a 3–4 cm parametrium on each side, both uterine arteries
attached to the specimen, and a 1–2 cm vaginal cuff. At
the conclusion of the procedure, a re-evaluation of the
pelvis is conducted laparoscopically to ensure hemostasis
at the surgical sites.

References

1. Schauta F. Die erwierte vaginale Totalexstirpation des Uterus beim Kollumkarzinome. Vienna-Leipzig: *J Safar*, 1908.

2. Wertheim E. *Die erweirte abdominale Operation bei Carcinoma Colli Uteri, auf Grund von 500 Fällen.* (Urban and Schwarzenberg: Berlin, 1911.)

3. Mitra S. Extraperitoneal lymphadenectomy and radical vaginal hysterectomy for cancer of the cervix (Mitra technique). *Am J Obstet Gynecol* 1959; **78**:191–6.

4. Possover M, Krause N, Plaul K et al. Laparoscopic paraaortic and pelvic lymphadenectomy: experience with 150 patients and review of the literature. *Gynecol Oncol* 1998; **71**:19–28.

5. Dargent D, Kouakou F, Adeleine P. L'opération de Schauta 90 ans après. *Lyon Chir* 1991; **87**:323–9.

6. Sardi J, Vidaurreta J, Bermudez A, Di Paola G. Laparoscopically assisted Schauta operation: learning experience at the Gynecologic Oncology Unit, Buenos Aires University Hospital. *Gynecol Oncol* 1999; **75**:361–5.

7. Roy M, Plante M, Renaud MC, Tetu B. Vaginal radical hysterectomy versus abdominal radical hysterectomy in the treatment of early-stage cervical cancer. *Gynecol Oncol* 1996; **62**:336–9.

8. Roy M, Plante M. Pregnancies after radical vaginal trachelectomy for early-stage cervical cancer. *Am J Obstet Gynecol* 1998; **179**:1491–6.

9. Dargent D, Martin X, Mathevet P. Laparoscopic assessment of the sentinel node in early-stage cervical cancer. *Gynecol Oncol* 2000; **79**:411–15.

10. Plante M, Roy M. Radical vaginal trachelectomy. In: (Smith JR, Del Priore G, Curtin J, Monaghan JM, eds) *An Atlas of Gynecologic Oncology, Investigation and Surgery.* (Martin Dunitz: London, 2001.)

11 Vaginal radical trachelectomy

Marie Plante, Marie-Claude Renaud and Michel Roy

There is growing interest in minimally invasive surgical procedures in oncology and a growing emphasis on preserving fertility whenever possible.[1] Vaginal radical surgery (i.e. radical hysterectomy and radical trachelectomy) combined with laparoscopic lymph node dissection is a direct example of both concepts and demonstrates what can be accomplished with minimal scars, bleeding, and morbidity.

The vaginal radical trachelectomy is a new conservative surgical procedure for the treatment of selected cases of early-stage cervical cancer. This procedure has the advantage of preserving the uterine body which, in turn, preserves childbearing potential. Professor Daniel Dargent from Lyon, France,[2] first performed the surgery in 1987. Since then, over 220 cases have been reported worldwide and summarized results are encouraging.[3] The recurrence rate is low (< 5%) and comparable to the results following standard abdominal radical hysterectomy (for similarly sized lesions). Morbidity is also low and childbearing is definitely possible, as is demonstrated by the number of live and healthy babies born to mothers who have undergone the procedure.[3]

In this chapter the surgical technique for radical vaginal trachelectomy will be reviewed step-by-step. First, the procedure requires the surgeon to conduct a complete laparoscopic lymph node dissection, which is fully illustrated in Chapter 6 on laparoscopic radical hysterectomy. Next, the paravesical space is defined laparoscopically, and as much lateral parametrium as possible is removed laparoscopically to reduce the extent of the dissection to be done vaginally (see Chapter 10 on laparoscopic vaginal radical hysterectomy). With regard to the vaginal part of the surgery, the procedure can be divided into six phases: (1) the preparatory phase, which includes vaginal cuff preparation; (2) the anterior phase, which includes opening the vesico-vaginal and paravesical spaces, and mobilization of the ureter; (3) the posterior phase, including opening of the cul-de-sac and pararectal space; (4) the lateral phase, including excision of the parametrium and the descending branch of the uterine artery; (5) the excision of the trachelectomy specimen; and (6) the reconstruction phase, which includes closure of the cul-de-sac, placement of the cerclage and suturing of the vaginal mucosa.

In gynecologic oncology, most radical surgical procedures are performed abdominally. For that reason, gynecologic oncologists, in general, are not comfortable with the vaginal surgical approach for radical procedures. Hopefully, this chapter will help make radical vaginal surgery easier to learn and understand, for the greater benefit of young women affected with cervical cancer who can now envision the preservation of their childbearing potential.

Indications

The indications for this procedure are not definitively established at this point. The eligibility criteria most commonly used are as follows:

- desire to preserve fertility
- no clinical evidence of impaired fertility (relative contraindication)
- lesion size ≤ 2.0 cm
- FIGO Stage IA1 with the presence of lymph–vascular space invasion (LVSI), or FIGO Stages IA2 and IB1
- squamous-cell carcinoma or adenocarcinoma histologic subtypes
- no involvement of the upper endocervical canal as determined by colposcopy or magnetic resonance imaging (MRI)
- no metastases to regional lymph nodes.

As data accumulate, these criteria may change.

Table 11.1. **Recurrence rates following radical trachelectomy.***

Authors/group (ref.)	Recurrences (%)
Dargent et al/Lyon (5)	3/82 (3.7)
Roy and Plante/Quebec (6)	2/44 (4.5)
Covens et al/Toronto (4)	3/58 (5.1)
Shepherd et al/London (7)	0/40 (0)
Total	8/224 (3.6)

*Adapted from Dargent.[3]

Table 11.2. **Risk factors for recurrence following radical trachelectomy.***

Lesion details	Recurrences (%)
Size	
< 2 cm	4/193 (2.1)
≥ 2 cm	4/28 (14.3)
Total	8/221 (3.6)†
Lymph–vascular space invasion	
Absent	2/128 (1.6)
Present	6/56 (10.7)
Total	8/184 (4.3)‡

†Data not available in three cases (Covens et al/Toronto group[4]).
‡Data not available in 40 cases (Shepherd et al/London group[7]).
*Adapted from Dargent.[3]

Oncologic outcome

At the 8th International Gynecologic Cancer Society (IGCS) meeting in Buenos Aires in October 2000, four groups with the largest number of trachelectomy cases presented their data with emphasis on oncologic and obstetrical outcome. Professor Dargent[3] summarized the data of 224 cases. In essence, the rate of recurrence after the trachelectomy procedure is low (< 5%) (Table 11.1). The size of the lesion (≥ 2 cm) and the presence of LVSI seem to be the most important risk factors for recurrence (Table 11.2).

Obstetrical outcome

The collected data on obstetrical outcome is also promising. There have been 92 pregnancies reported from 61 women trying to conceive resulting in 51 live births and 37 pregnancy losses (42%) (Table 11.3). The rate of first trimester miscarriage does not seem to be higher than in the general population, but the rate of second trimester losses is higher. This is most likely secondary to cervical incompetence, resulting in premature cervical dilatation. Additionally, premature labor may occur from subclinical chorioamnionitis due to the shortened cervix or from an inadequate mucus plug. The exact causes remain to be elucidated, but patients should be followed closely during the second and third trimesters. Because a permanent cerclage is placed, women should obviously be delivered by cesarean section. The infertility rate is no higher than in the general population and, in fact, most patients have become pregnant spontaneously without the help of assisted reproductive technology.[1] Covens et al[4]

Table 11.3. **Obstetrical outcome following radical trachelectomy (pregnancies per women attempting conception).***

Authors/group (ref.)	Outcome
Dargent et al/Lyon (5)	47/29
Roy and Plante/Quebec (6)	19/13
Covens et al/Toronto (4)	11/10
Shepherd et al/London (7)	15/9
Total	**92/61**

*Adapted from Dargent.[3]

have estimated the conceptual rate to be 37% at 1 year. Interestingly, some women with a history of infertility have been able to conceive after the trachelectomy procedure, which suggests that a 'history' of infertility should not be considered an absolute contraindication to this procedure.[1]

Based on the collected data available thus far, the radical trachelectomy procedure truly offers a valuable alternative to young women with small early-stage cervical cancer who wish to preserve their fertility potential.

Preparatory phase – vaginal cuff preparation

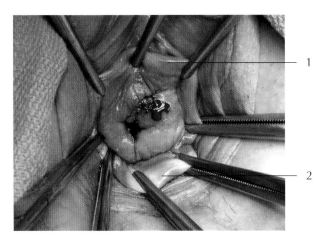

1 – Anterior vaginal mucosa
2 – Posterior vaginal mucosa

Figure 11.1. Defining the vaginal mucosa.
A rim of vaginal mucosa is delineated circumferentially and clockwise using eight straight Kocher clamps placed at regular intervals, about 1 cm distal to the cervix. The bluish coloration is secondary to the subcutaneous injection of Lymphazurin for localization of the sentinel node (see Vaginal radical hysterectomy, Chapter 10). Note that the patient has had a diagnostic conization, so there is no visible residual lesion and the cervix has therefore been shortened.

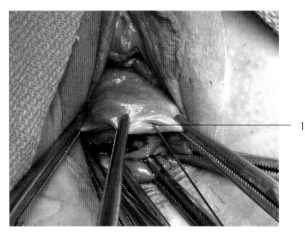

1 – Subcutaneous injection

Figure 11.2. Injection of the vaginal mucosa.
A 10–20 ml solution of 1% Xylocaine mixed with epinephrine 1:100,000 is injected between each Kocher clamp to reduce bleeding and to separate the mucosa from the underlying tissue. Blanching of the overlying anterior vaginal mucosa can be seen.

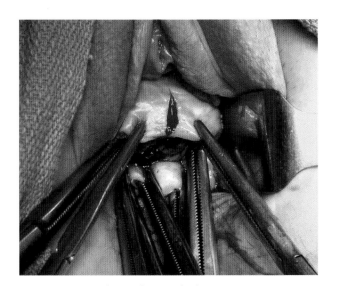

Figure 11.3. Marking of 12 o'clock.
A small vertical incision is made with the scalpel at 12 o'clock as a landmark for future reference. This helps to maintain proper orientation throughout the procedure.

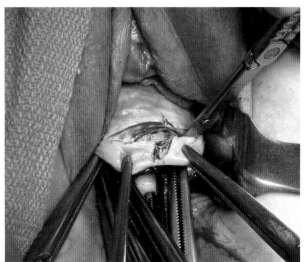

Figure 11.4. Incision of the vaginal mucosa.
A circumferential incision is made with the scalpel just above the Kocher clamps. The mucosa and submucosal layers are incised taking care not to go too deep to avoid tearing the mucosa.

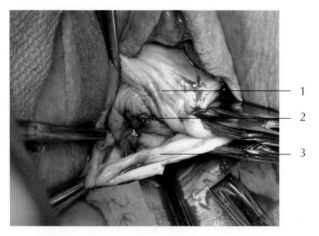

1 – Anterior vaginal mucosa
2 – Cervix
3 – Posterior vaginal mucosa

Figure 11.5. Covering of the cervix.
The anterior and posterior edges of the vaginal mucosa are grasped with Chrobak clamps in order to cover the cervix.

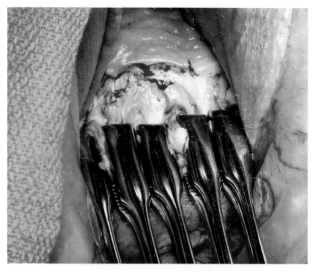

Figure 11.6. Completion of the preparatory phase.
The vaginal cuff preparation is now completed using four to six Chrobak clamps to completely cover the cervix. This allows good traction on the specimen while avoiding potential tumor spillage.

Anterior phase – opening of the spaces, and identification and mobilization of the ureter

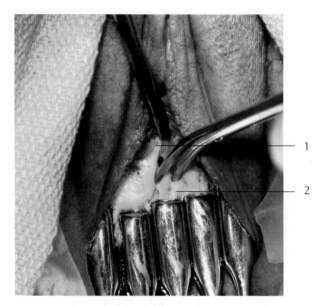

1 – Anterior vaginal mucosa
2 – Cervix

Figure 11.7. Defining the vesicovaginal space.
While maintaining slight downward traction on the specimen, the vesicovaginal space is defined with Metzenbaum scissors held **perpendicular** to the cervix in the midline. A single-tooth forceps is used to hold and retract the anterior vaginal mucosa. Avoid erring laterally because of bleeding from the bladder pillars. Care is taken not to enter the anterior peritoneum as would be done in a simple vaginal hysterectomy.

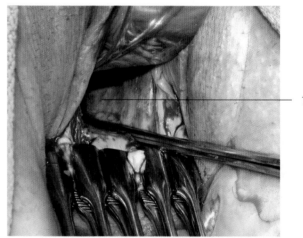

1 – Vesicovaginal space

Figure 11.8. Entering the vesicovaginal space.
If entered correctly, the space should be avascular and allows easy palpation of the anterior surface of the endocervix and uterine isthmus, which has a whitish coloration. The space is stretched upwards with a narrow Deaver retractor.

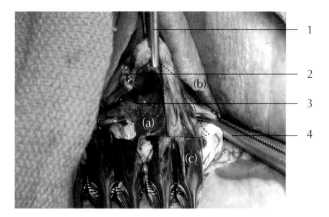

1 – Straight Kocher at 1 o'clock
2 – 12 o'clock mark
3 – Vesicovaginal space
4 – Straight Kocher at 3 o'clock
Triangle – (a) bladder pillars, (b) vaginal mucosa, (c) Chrobak clamps

Figure 11.9. Defining the left paravesical space.
The Chrobak clamps are pulled slightly towards the patient's right side. Straight Kocher clamps are placed onto the vaginal mucosa at 1 and 3 o'clock and stretched out (this is where the 12 o'clock mark made earlier comes useful). This maneuver defines a triangle between the bladder pillars, the vaginal mucosa, and the Chrobak clamps. An areolar opening is seen just medial and slightly anterior to the 3 o'clock clamp indicating where to enter to define the paravesical space.

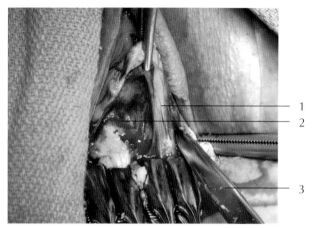

1 – Bladder pillars
2 – Vesicovaginal space
3 – Metzenbaum scissors entering the left paravesical space

Figure 11.10. Entering the left paravesical space.
The left paravesical space is entered blindly by opening and closing the Metzenbaum scissors, with the tips pointing **upwards** and **outwards**. When entering the space, aim laterally with the scissors to avoid bleeding from the lateral aspect of the bladder.

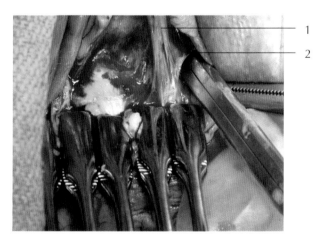

1 – Bladder pillars
2 – Left paravesical space

Figure 11.11. Opening the left paravesical space.
If entered correctly, the space should be avascular and the scissors should slide inside easily. Once entered, the space is widened by rotating the scissors under the pubic bone in a semicircular rotating motion to the patient's contralateral side (not shown).

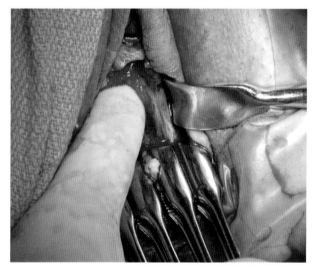

Figure 11.12. Palpation of the left ureter.
Pulling the Chrobak clamps to the right side of the patient, the surgeon's left index finger is placed in the vesicovaginal space while a Breisky retractor (or the back of a forceps) is placed in the left paravesical space. By pulling downward, and pressing the finger and instrument together, the surgeon should feel the characteristic snap of the ureter rolling under the finger. This maneuver orients the surgeon to the location of the ureter in relation to the bladder pillars.

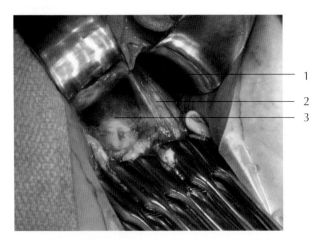

1 – Left paravesical space
2 – Bladder pillars
3 – Vesicovaginal space

Figure 11.13. Identification of the spaces.
A Breisky retractor is placed into the left paravesical space, and a narrow Deaver retractor is placed in the vesicovaginal space; the bladder pillars lie between the two retractors. The knee of the ureter is normally located on the lateral aspect of the bladder pillars and will be identified later in the procedure.

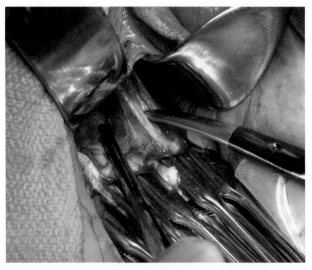

Figure 11.14. Transection of the bladder pillars.
Once the ureter has been located by palpation, the bladder pillars are transected midway between the bladder base and the anterior aspect of the specimen. Bipolar scissors or standard Metzenbaum scissors can be used to minimize bleeding.

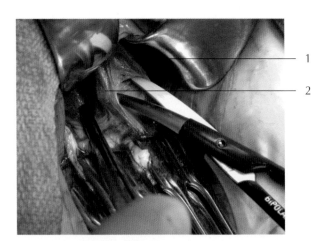

1 – Posterior bladder pillars
2 – Anterior bladder pillars

Figure 11.15. Separating the bladder pillars.
It is recommended that the bladder pillars be stretched open with the scissors before cutting to separate the anterior and posterior pillars. The most distal fibers of the pillars can then be excised.

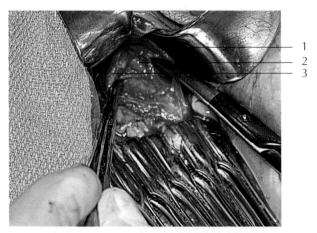

1 – Posterior bladder pillars
2 – Left ureter
3 – Anterior bladder pillars

Figure 11.16. Identification of the left ureter.
The pillars are stretched open again and, usually, the knee of the ureter should appear anteriorly. The anterior and posterior pillars can then be further excised safely. If the ureter is not unequivocally seen, it should be palpated again to relocate its position before cutting the bladder pillars.

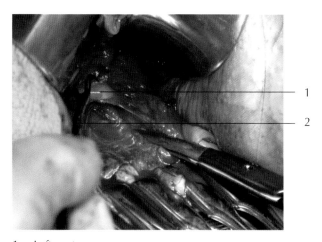

1 – Left ureter
2 – Babcock clamp

Figure 11.17. Completion of the anterior phase.
Once the bladder pillars have been excised, a Babcock clamp is used to elevate the left ureter in order to facilitate transection of the most lateral and posterior fibers (the Babcock clamp is very useful in this step of the procedure). Medial dissection of the ureter should be avoided because of the risk of injury to the bladder base. The anterior phase of the procedure is then performed on the patient's right side.

Posterior phase – opening of the cul-de-sac and pararectal space, and excision of the paracolpos and uterosacral ligaments

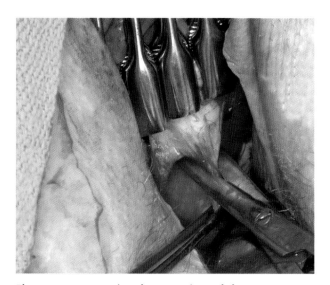

Figure 11.18. Opening the posterior cul-de-sac.
The Chrobak clamps are sharply angulated anteriorly and the posterior cul-de-sac is opened using Metzenbaum scissors.

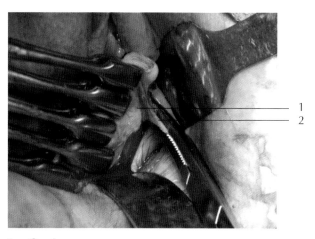

1 – Cervix
2 – Left paracolpos

Figure 11.19. Excision of the left paracolpos.
With the Chrobak clamps rotated to the right, the left paracolpos is clamped using a curved Heaney clamp, excised and suture ligated with 2-0 polyglactin.

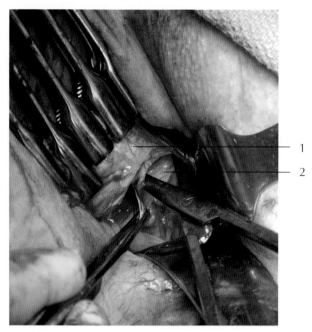

1 – Cervix
2 – Left pararectal space

Figure 11.20. Opening the left pararectal space.
Metzenbaum scissors are used to open the left pararectal space, which is located laterally to the peritoneum and medially to the uterosacral ligament (not yet seen).

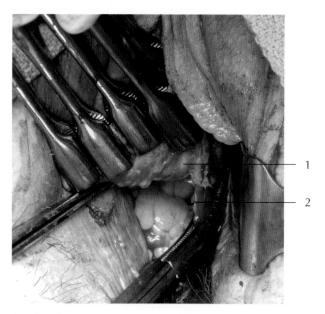

1 – Cervix
2 – Left uterosacral ligament

Figure 11.21. Excision of the left uterosacral ligament.
The proximal part of the left uterosacral ligament is clamped with a curved Heaney clamp, excised, and suture ligated with 2-0 polyglactin. The posterior phase of the procedure is then performed on the patient's right side.

Lateral phase – excision of the parametrium and cervicovaginal artery

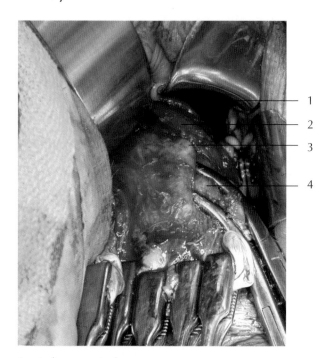

1 – Left paravesical space
2 – Left ureter
3 – Left uterine artery
4 – Left parametrium

Figure 11.22. Excision of the left parametrium
Before clamping the left parametrium, the spaces should be redefined by replacing the Breisky retractor into the paravesical space and the narrow Deaver retractor into the vesicovaginal space. While the Chrobak clamps are pulled and rotated to the patient's right side, a curved Heaney clamp is placed proximally, and then a second clamp is placed higher and more laterally to obtain a wider parametrium. Note the ureter coursing above the parametrium, which can be further dissected if needed, and the bulge of the uterine artery next to the Heaney clamp. The parametrial tissue is excised and suture ligated with 2-0 polyglactin.

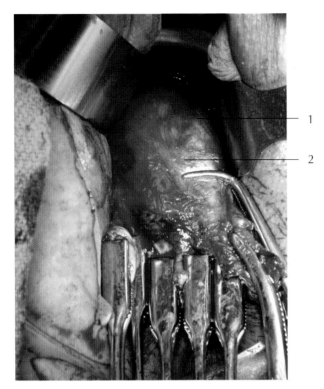

1 – Uterine body
2 – Uterine isthmus

Figure 11.23. Identification of the left cervicovaginal artery.
After precise localization of the isthmus and the cross of the uterine artery, the descending branch of the left uterine artery (the cervicovaginal artery) is clamped with a right angle clamp placed at 90° to the isthmus.

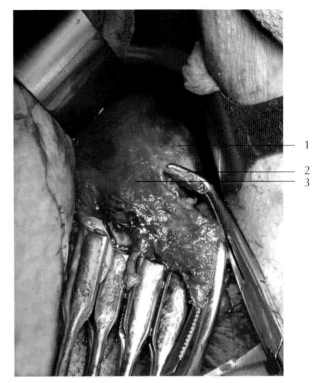

1 – Left uterine artery
2 – Left cervicovaginal artery
3 – Uterine isthmus

Figure 11.24. Excision of the left cervicovaginal artery.
The left cervicovaginal artery is now excised and suture ligated with 2-0 Vicryl. Note the bulge of the cross of the uterine artery above the right angle clamp. Again, an identical procedure is performed on the patient's right side.

Excision of the specimen

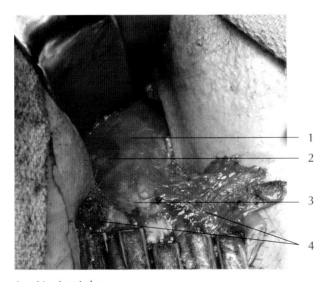

1 – Uterine isthmus
2 – Right uterine artery
3 – Endocervix
4 – Right and left parametrium

Figure 11.25. Identification of the uterine isthmus.
The uterine isthmus and endocervix are precisely located by palpating the uterus both anteriorly and posteriorly. In this case, the narrowing of the uterine isthmus is easily visible. Note again the cross of the uterine artery on the patient's right side.

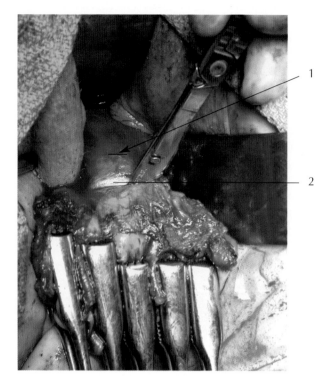

1 – Uterine isthmus
2 – Cervix

Figure 11.26. Transection of the cervix.
The cervix is amputated with a scalpel held perpendicular to the specimen about 1 cm distal to the isthmus.

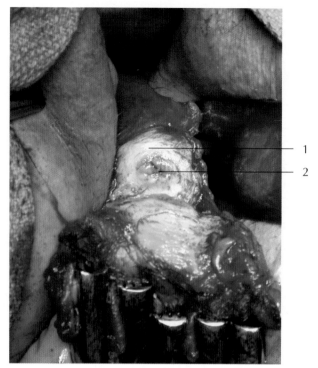

1 – Cervix
2 – Cervical os

Figure 11.27. Excision of the trachelectomy specimen.
As the specimen is excised, the cervical os appears. Care is taken not to angulate the scalpel to avoid removing too much cervix posteriorly.

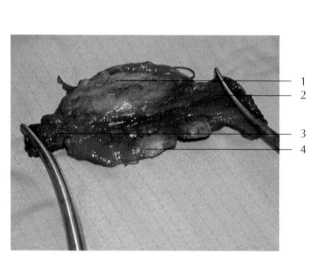

1 – Endocervix
2 – Left parametrium
3 – Right parametrium
4 – Vaginal mucosa

Figure 11.28. Trachelectomy specimen.
Ideally, the specimen should be at least 1–2 cm wide, with 1 cm of vaginal mucosa and 1–2 cm of parametrium. In this case, the specimen is shorter because of the prior conization. The endocervical cut surface appears normal. Since there is no evidence of residual tumor, a frozen section is not performed in this case. The specimen is kept intact for final analysis and will be processed as a cervical cone specimen.

Reconstruction phase – closure of the cul-de-sac, placement of the cerclage and suturing of the vaginal mucosa

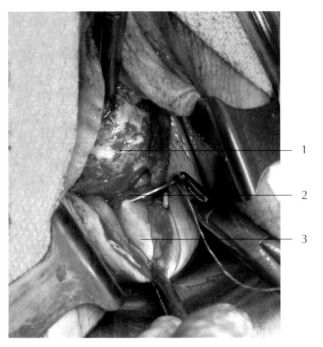

1 – Cervix
2 – Posterior cul-de-sac
3 – Posterior peritoneum

Figure 11.29. Closure of the posterior cul-de-sac.
The posterior cul-de-sac is first closed with a purse-string suture of 2-0 chromic; a straight Kocher clamp is used to lift the cervix anteriorly.

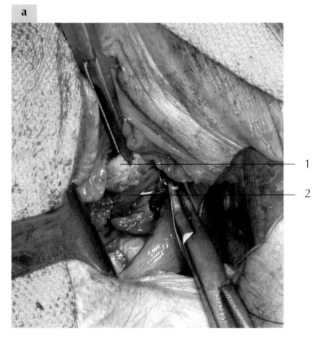

1 – Cervix
2 – Posterior isthmus

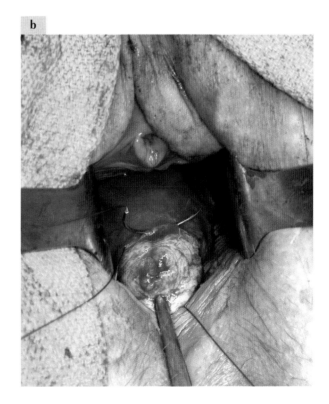

Figure 11.30. Placement of the cervical cerclage.
(a) A permanent cerclage is placed at the level of the isthmus using a non-resorbable 0 polypropylene suture starting posteriorly at 6 o'clock to tie the knot posteriorly; again, a straight Kocher clamp is used to lift the cervix upwards. The cerclage is continued laterally in a counter-clockwise manner. (b) The cerclage is continued anteriorly. Ideally, sutures should be placed at the level of the uterine isthmus and not too deeply within the cervical stroma.

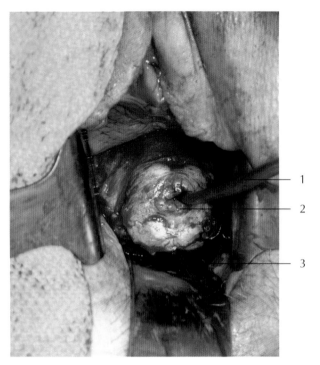

1 – Uterine probe
2 – Cervical os
3 – Cerclage suture

Figure 11.31. Completing the cerclage.
When tying the cerclage knot posteriorly, a uterine probe is in the cervical os to avoid overtightening the knot, as this may cause cervical stenosis.

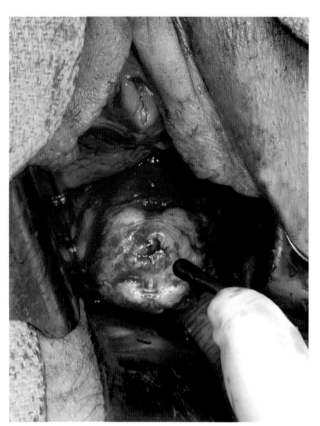

Figure 11.32. Length of the residual endocervix.
The length of the residual endocervix is measured by introducing a uterine probe inside the endocervical canal; ideally, there should be about 1 cm of residual endocervix remaining.

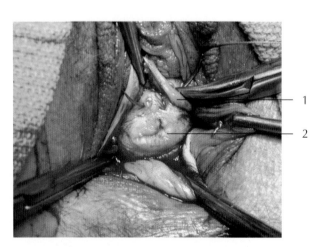

1 – Vaginal mucosa
2 – Cervix

Figure 11.33. Anterior vaginal closure.
Starting anteriorly, the edges of the vaginal mucosa are sutured to the residual exocervical stroma with interrupted figure-of-eight sutures using 2-0 polyglactin. Sutures should not be placed too close to the new cervical os in order to avoid burying the cervix, which may make follow-up examinations more difficult.

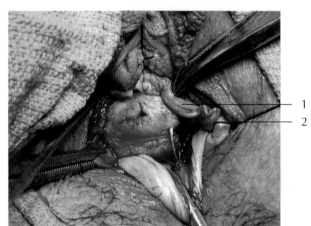

1 – Vaginal mucosa
2 – Lateral vaginal suture

Figure 11.34. Lateral vaginal closure.
Laterally, due to the excess vaginal mucosa, it is preferable to place a separate figure-of-eight suture through the vaginal mucosa only; another suture is then placed to reapproximate the vaginal mucosa to the new exocervix.

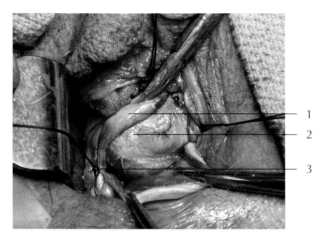

1 – Vaginal mucosa
2 – Cervix
3 – Lateral vaginal suture

Figure 11.35. Contralateral vaginal closure.
An identical procedure is performed on the opposite side. Beginning laterally, the vaginal mucosal sutures are placed. The anterior vaginal mucosa is then sutured to the new exocervix.

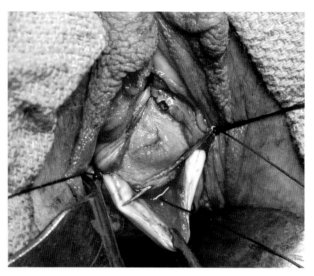

Figure 11.36. Posterior vaginal closure.
The vaginal closure is completed posteriorly in a similar fashion. If needed, additional sutures can be placed in between the previous ones. Sometimes, excess vaginal mucosa may need to be removed with cautery to facilitate the closure (not shown here).

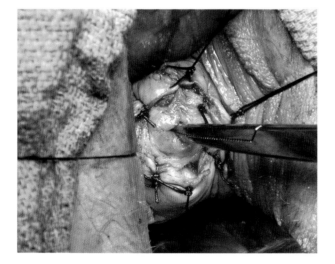

Figure 11.37. Completed vaginal closure.
The cervix is obviously shorter than before the operation, but retains normal anatomical relationships. The new exocervix should remain accessible for monitoring with colposcopic examinations and cytology. At completion of the vaginal trachelectomy, a laparoscopic re-evaluation of the abdomen and pelvis is performed to verify hemostasis and to confirm the integrity of the pelvic structures.

Patient with a macroscopic lesion

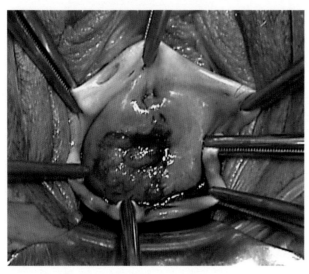

Figure 11.38. Trachelectomy procedure.
The procedure is conducted in a similar fashion for the patient with a macroscopic lesion. Here, it is particularly important to completely cover the cervix during the preparatory phase in order to minimize the risk of tumor spillage.

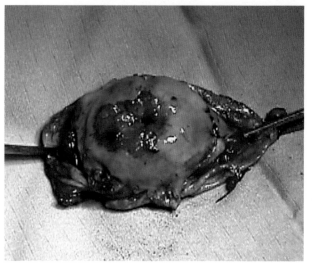

Figure 11.39. Trachelectomy specimen – anterior view.
The anterior/exocervical aspect of the specimen demonstrates the cervix with an exophytic lesion and a rim of vaginal mucosa.

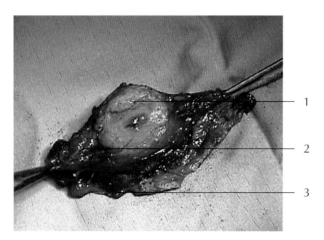

1 – Endocervix
2 – Right parametrium
3 – Vaginal mucosa

Figure 11.40. Trachelectomy specimen – posterior view
The posterior/endocervical aspect of the specimen demonstrates the endocervical resection margin and the proximal parametrium.

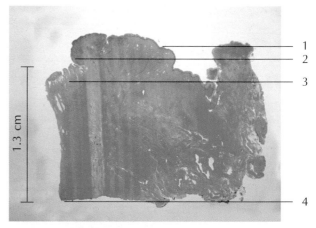

1 – Exocervical squamous epithelium
2 – Cervical cancer
3 – Endocervical glands
4 – Endocervical margin

Figure 11.41. Frozen section.
When residual tumor is seen or suspected, the trachelectomy specimen is sent for immediate intraoperative frozen section to assess the distance from the tumor to the endocervical resection margin. At least 8–10 mm of tumor-free tissue should be present between the tumor and the endocervical resection margin. Otherwise, additional endocervix should be removed, or the trachelectomy should be aborted and a radical vaginal hysterectomy performed instead.

References

1. Plante M. Fertility preservation in the management of gynecologic cancers. *Curr Opin Oncol* 2000; **12**:497–507.

2. Dargent D, Brun JL, Roy M et al. La trachélectomie élargie (T.E.). Une alternative à l'hystérectomie radicale dans le traitement des cancers infiltrants développés sur la face extrerne du col utérin. *J Obstet Gynecol* 1994; **2**:292–5.

3. Dargent D. Fertility preserving management of early stage cancer of the cervix. In: (DiPaola GR, Sardi J, eds) *Gynecologic Oncology Issues. Proceedings of the 8th IGCS Meeting of Buenos Aires.* (Monduzzi Editore, International Proceedings Division: Buenos Aires, 2000) 23–30.

4. Covens A, Shaw P, Murphy J et al. Is radical trachelectomy a safe alternative to radical hysterectomy for stage Ia/Ib carcinoma of the cervix? *Cancer* 1999; **86**:2273–9.

5. Dargent D, Martin X, Sacchetoni A, Mathevet P. Laparoscopic vaginal radical trachelectomy: a treatment to preserve the fertility of cervical carcinoma patients. *Cancer* 2000; **88**:1877–82.

6. Roy M, Plante M. Pregnancies following vaginal radical trachelectomy for early-stage cervical cancer. *Am J Obstet Gynecol* 1998; **179**:1491–6.

7. Shepherd JH, Crawford R, Oram D. Radical trachelectomy: a way to preserve fertility in the treatment of early cervical cancer. *Br J Obstet Gynaecol* 1998; **105**:912–16.

12 Paracentesis

Douglas A Levine

Both gynecologic oncologists and medical oncologists frequently perform paracentesis in the management of patients with ovarian cancer. This simple bedside or office procedure can be employed for diagnostic or therapeutic purposes (Table 12.1). It is usually associated with minimal discomfort and a low rate of complications. Among the many indications for a paracentesis, the most common are to confirm the diagnosis of cancer prior to definitive treatment or to relieve symptoms related to increased intraabdominal pressure. While seeding of the paracentesis tract has been reported in the literature,[1] and is a potential concern, no impact on survival has been shown. This may be due to the high response rate seen with currently available combination chemotherapy. Nonetheless, unnecessary paracentesis should be avoided. In general, if a patient has clinical and radiographic signs of advanced ovarian cancer, a paracentesis for the sole purpose of confirming a cancer diagnosis is not required prior to surgery. A more appropriate indication for paracentesis would be to confirm a cancer diagnosis prior to initiating neoadjuvant chemotherapy in a patient medically unfit to tolerate surgery. In this setting, definitive surgery would be delayed until several courses of cytotoxic chemotherapy had been given.

On the whole, the most common reason to perform a therapeutic paracentesis is to remove symptomatic ascites. This will relieve dyspnea, increase total lung capacity and preload, and diminish nausea, vomiting and abdominal pain. Occasionally, large-volume ascites may interfere with respiratory function to such an extent that preoperative paracentesis is required to allow for the safe induction of general anesthesia. Complications associated with the procedure are relatively uncommon and mainly consist of injury to the bowel or bladder, inadvertent puncture of blood vessels (most seriously the inferior epigastric vessels), or the introduction of infection. If a large volume of ascites is removed, hemodynamic parameters should be closely monitored. Usually, large-volume paracentesis is well tolerated in patients without significant pre-existing cardiac or pulmonary disease. Intravenous fluids should be given throughout the procedure and colloids can be added for symptomatic management as needed. Rarely does hemodynamic instability result, even when > 10 l of ascites are removed.[2]

	Diagnostic	Therapeutic
Advantages	Confirm cancer diagnosis	Relief of symptomatic ascites
	Differentiate from benign ascites	Improve cardiopulmonary function
	Determine general histologic subtype	Reduce intraabdominal pressure
	Provide symptomatic relief prior to surgery	Alleviate gastrointestinal symptoms
Disadvantages	May cause tumor dissemination to abdominal wall	Ascites will recur without further therapy
	Primary site of disease usually not identifiable	Large-volume drainage could lead to hemodynamic instability

Table 12.1. **Indications for paracentesis in gynecologic malignancies.**

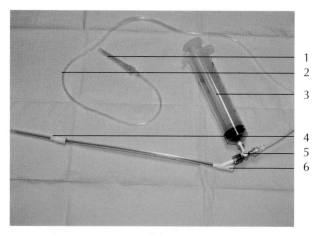

Figure 12.1. Commercial kits.

There are many commercial paracentesis kits available on the market. Most include a tray with all the disposable items needed to perform the procedure, including a local anesthetic, small and large needles, syringes, sterile tubing, and a paracentesis catheter. Usually, sterile gloves, Betadine or another antiseptic solution, and collection bottles must be obtained from hospital supplies. Nowadays, most kits are also prepared latex-free, due to the rising number of patients who report latex allergies. The kit shown here is manufactured by Allegiance Healthcare (McGaw Park, IL). It is also possible to perform the procedure by using readily available hospital supplies, such as a long intravenous angiocatheter, sterile intravenous or other tubing, and an appropriate collection device. While this may offer cost savings, the convenience, completeness, and efficiency of prepackaged kits should be a consideration for a busy gynecologic oncology service. Separate paracentesis needles are also available.

1 – Needle to puncture collection container
2 – Drainage tubing
3 – Aspiration syringe
4 – Paracentesis needle
5 – Three-way stopcock
6 – Paracentesis catheter sheath

Figure 12.2. Assembly.

When properly assembled, the paracentesis catheter attached to sterile tubing provides a sealed system for ascites removal. The tip of the 14-gauge, 5-cm long paracentesis needle is fixed to an 18-cm catheter that has a hub to attach a three-way stopcock, also supplied. An aspiration syringe can be placed onto the stopcock to regulate flow during the procedure and to obtain samples for laboratory analyses. The distal end of the stopcock is connected to a drainage tube with a needle that can be used to puncture sterile collection bottles.

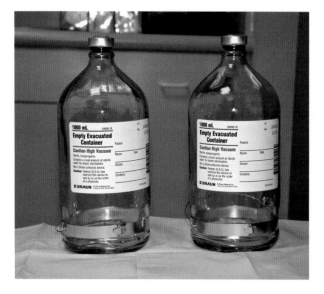

Figure 12.3 Collection bottles.

Ascites can be collected in a number of various collection bags that act by gravity drainage. In this manner the drainage catheter is attached to the collection bag for a period of time (often overnight) and securely affixed to the patient. Shown here are empty glass collection containers with a high-pressure vacuum capable of removing 1 l of fluid in approximately 5 min. In this manner, even large-volume ascites can be removed in a relatively short period of time obviating the need to leave an indwelling catheter in place. The lid of the sterile bottle has a tear-away metal covering through which a large-bore needle can easily be passed. This particular bottle is manufactured by B. Braun Medical, Inc. (Irvine, CA). Bottles come in a variety of volumes.

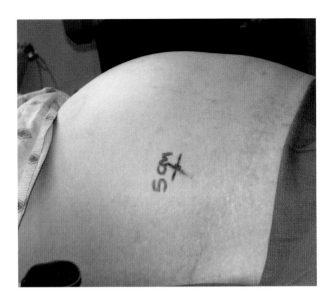

Figure 12.4. Site selection.
In choosing the optimal site to perform the paracentesis, the operator should attempt to minimize the risk of encountering blood vessels, intestines, or tumor. Choosing a site in the lateral quarter of the abdomen should minimize the risk of puncturing the inferior epigastric vessels. Many patients with large tumor burdens will have venous networks in the dermis that can be readily seen and avoided. Typically, when large-volume ascites is present, the bowels will not interfere with site selection in either of the lower quadrants. Tumor location can be assessed by palpating the abdomen or by reviewing a recent computed tomography (CT) scan. Most patients who are candidates for this procedure will usually have undergone a recent imaging study as part of their clinical care that can be used for reference. If site selection based upon physical examination appears difficult and no recent imaging studies are available, a limited abdominal ultrasound can be performed to determine the best location for the procedure. An ultrasound can determine the area of clear passage into the fluid pocket, as well as pocket depth. While many patients have markedly distended abdomens due to ascites, ultrasound can be particularly useful in the morbidly obese patient in whom it may be difficult to distinguish tumor and adipose tissue from fluid. In general, ultrasound marking is not necessary except in the most difficult cases or when an unguided attempt has failed. The patient shown here has been marked by ultrasound, and a depth of 5 cm to the fluid pocket is clearly noted.

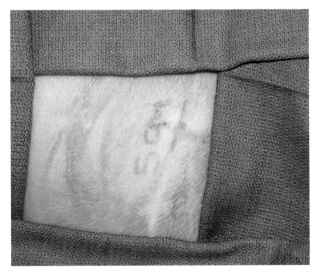

Figure 12.5. Preparation.
After determining the best site for the procedure the abdomen is prepped and draped in the usual sterile fashion. Draping material is often included in commercially available kits, though sterile towels can be readily found in most hospitals. While the risk of infection associated with the procedure is quite low when performed properly, careful attention to aseptic technique is important.

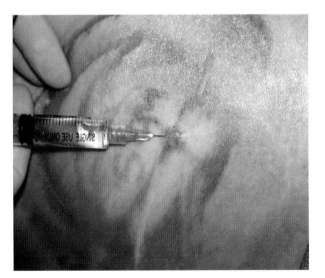

Figure 12.6. Local anesthetic.
One percent local lidocaine without epinephrine is used to anesthetize the skin. This is usually part of the commercially available prepackaged kits. A wheal is created with a short 1.6-cm 25-gauge needle at the site of intended puncture. Several minutes are allowed for the lidocaine to take effect. The tip of the needle is used to ensure that the skin is adequately numb. Usually, only 1–2 ml of local anesthetic is needed to provide sufficient loss of sensation.

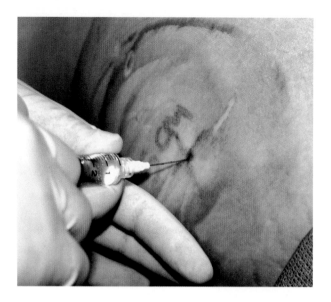

Figure 12.7. Finder needle.

The first needle is then exchanged for a longer 5.1-cm 22-gauge needle to anesthetize the subcutaneous tissue down to and through the peritoneum. This is accomplished by advancing the needle slowly in a direction perpendicular to the abdominal wall while aspirating and injecting 0.5–1 ml of lidocaine every 5–10 mm. If the needle placement is correct, as soon as the peritoneal cavity is entered, ascitic fluid will return into the syringe. This will serve as a mental picture when placing the larger paracentesis needle. Additionally, if blood vessels are encountered, it will be noted by the discoloration of the remaining lidocaine. Pressure can then be applied and a decision made whether or not to attempt the procedure at a different location. The two most sensitive parts of the procedure for the patient are numbing the skin and puncturing the peritoneum. It is a good idea to give a little extra local anesthetic around the time when the peritoneum is likely to be traversed.

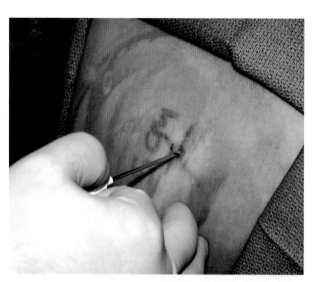

Figure 12.8. Paracentesis needle.

The paracentesis needle is inserted perpendicular to the abdominal wall. The depth of insertion should be slightly more than was required to obtain ascites with the finder needle. It should be placed with slight force, as it is a larger needle (14-gauge) and will meet some resistance when passing through the subcutaneous tissues.

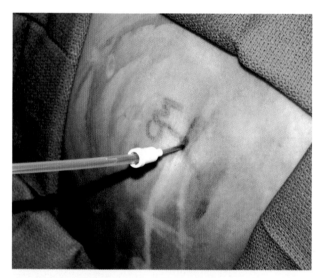

Figure 12.9. Fluid return.

Once the needle is placed at the proper depth, ascites will reflux into the plastic chamber attached to the hub of the needle. This plastic sheath envelopes a catheter that will subsequently be exchanged for the needle. The needle is only 5.1 cm long, and for morbidly obese patients pressure will need to be applied in order to allow the tip to reach into the peritoneum. The paracentesis catheter has previously been attached to a three-way stopcock and sterile tubing. At this point, the needle at the end of the drainage tube (see Fig. 12.2) is inserted into the collection bottle (see Fig. 12.3). A small amount of ascites and the paracentesis catheter can both be seen through the plastic catheter sheath.

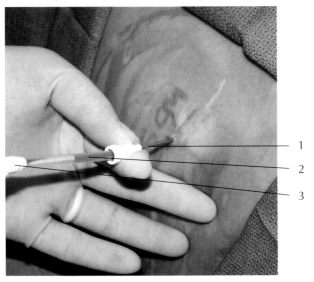

1 – Paracentesis needle
2 – Paracentesis catheter sheath
3 – Hub of paracentesis catheter (see also Fig. 12.2).

Figure 12.10. Catheter exchange.
The catheter is introduced by advancing the plastic sheath while at the same time holding the needle firmly in place. The distal hub of the paracentesis catheter, just proximal to the stopcock, is moved toward the paracentesis needle (see also Fig. 12.2) which will advance the catheter into the peritoneum. During this period, ascites is draining into the collection bottles.

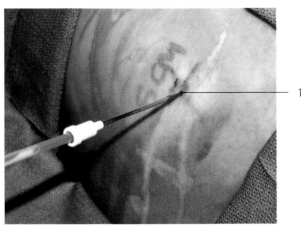

1 – Catheter passing through tip of needle

Figure 12.11. Needle removal.
Once the catheter has been advanced, the needle can be withdrawn until it is no longer in the patient. In this figure, the catheter can be seen coming through the tip of the paracentesis needle. It is very important to never withdraw the catheter through the needle, as this can shear the catheter and result in potential loss within the abdomen. If flow should stop while advancing the catheter, slight readjustment will usually result in continued drainage. The catheter, which is on continuous suction from the high-pressure vacuum within the collection bottle, can get lodged against tissues within the abdomen.

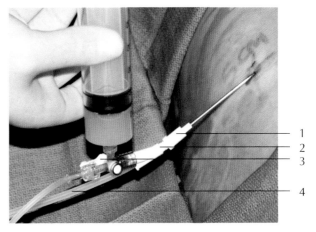

1 – Hub of paracentesis needle
2 – Catheter hub in opposition with needle hub
3 – Valve rotated to stop flow to collection bottles
4 – Catheter sheath now empty

Figure 12.12. Aspiration port.
In this figure the stopcock valve has been turned toward the collection bottles in order to stop the flow and open the channel in the direction of a 60-ml syringe. Ascites is aspirated into the syringe, which can then be sent to the laboratory for cytologic, biochemical, or microbiologic analysis, as indicated. The valve can then be returned to the upright position in order to restore flow to the collection bottle. The aspiration syringe can also be used to regulate flow during catheter repositioning if drainage should cease earlier than expected. Also shown in this figure, the catheter has been completely advanced so that the hub of the catheter (white plastic) is in complete opposition with the hub of the paracentesis needle. The plastic sheath protrudes, but no longer contains the catheter within (contrast with Figs 12.2 and 12.9).

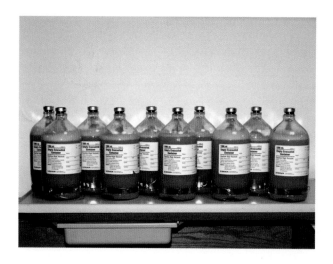

Figure 12.13. Ascites.
This patient had 10.5 l of ascites removed. She was given 1 l of intravenous crystalloid and 500 ml of colloid in order to temporarily compensate for potential fluid shifts. Typically, colloid is not required unless an unusually large amount of ascites has been removed or if the patient has cardiovascular disease that may render her particularly sensitive to fluid shifts. In such a case, the ascites should also be removed over a longer period of time. The patient is also requested to remain at bedrest for up to 2 hours if a large volume of ascites is removed. These collection bottles must be disposed of in accordance with local regulations for biohazardous material. Universal precautions, in addition to sterile technique, should be observed throughout this and other surgical procedures.

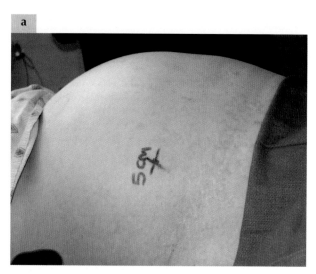
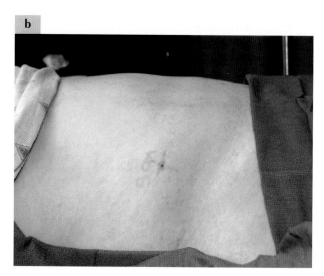

Figure 12.14. Abdominal change.
(a) The patient's abdomen is markedly distended with ascites prior to the procedure. (b) After removing a large volume of ascites, the abdomen is significantly less protuberant and the patient experienced immediate relief of her symptoms. This patient's ascites reaccumulated approximately 3 weeks later, and she underwent a subsequent paracentesis.

References

1. Kruitwagen RF, Swinkels BM, Keyser KG et al. Incidence and effect on survival of abdominal wall metastases at trocar or puncture sites following laparoscopy or paracentesis in women with ovarian cancer. *Gynecol Oncol* 1996; **60**:233–7.

2. Gotlieb WH, Feldman B, Feldman-Moran O et al. Intraperitoneal pressures and clinical parameters of total paracentesis for palliation of symptomatic ascites in ovarian cancer. *Gynecol Oncol* 1998; **71**:381–5.

13 Percutaneous endoscopic gastrostomy tube placement

Mark Schattner and Moshe Shike

In patients with advanced gynecologic malignancies, bowel obstruction is a cause of significant morbidity and mortality. Often, there is complete intestinal obstruction involving multiple segments of bowel, making surgical correction difficult or impossible. Palliation of nausea, vomiting, and abdominal pain in inoperable patients requires gastric decompression. A modification of the percutaneous endoscopic gastrostomy (PEG) tube can safely provide effective drainage of gastrointestinal contents.

The PEG tube was first described as a means to gain access to the gastrointestinal tract for enteral nutrition support. Modification of this technique by using larger (28 French [Fr]) tubes, with a longer intragastric segment and additional drainage ports, allows effective drainage of gastric contents and palliation of obstructive symptoms. Placement of the tube requires 15–30 minutes and can be done under monitored sedation. This chapter describes the 'pull' technique for PEG placement. In this method, a trocar is placed through the skin and into the stomach. A thread is then passed into the stomach and grasped by the endoscopist. This thread is then pulled out of the patient's mouth where it is connected to the PEG tube. The PEG tube can then be pulled into position in the stomach.

A recent review[1] reported success rates of gastrostomy tube placement of 83–100% in patients with inoperable bowel obstruction. Post-procedure survival in this series ranged from 2 to 600 days. After PEG placement, 88% of patients are able to drink and eat soft foods, which are then drained through the PEG.[2] Care of the PEG is easy and requires only flushing of the tube, care of the ostomy site, and emptying of the drainage bag.

PEG placement is a safe procedure with a mortality rate of 1% and a major complication rate of 3%.[3] Major complications include peritonitis due to inadvertent tube removal prior to maturation of the fistulous tract or hemorrhage. Traversing a tumor, the colon, or even the liver by PEG tubes being placed for drainage has not resulted in clinically significant difficulties.[4,5]

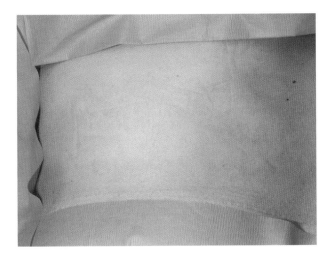

Figure 13.1. Preparing the abdomen.
Ascites is not a contraindication to percutaneous endoscopic gastrostomy placement; however, it may make transillumination from the stomach more difficult and therefore as much ascites as possible should be removed. The abdomen is then cleaned in the usual sterile fashion, after which the Betadine solution is removed with an alcohol wash to facilitate transillumination.

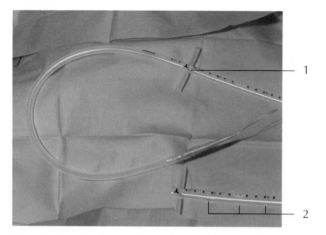

1 – Nonabsorbable suture used to attached crossbar
2 – Side holes cut in intragastric portion of tube

Figure 13.2. Modifying the tube.
To allow for better drainage and less clogging, the standard 28 Fr percutaneous endoscopic gastrostomy tube is modified to create a longer intragastric portion and additional drainage ports. The factory-supplied internal bumper is removed and replaced with a 4-cm crossbar that is positioned to allow 10 cm of the tube to remain within the stomach. The crossbar is attached to the tube using nonabsorbable suture, and three to four side holes are then cut into the intragastric portion of the tube.

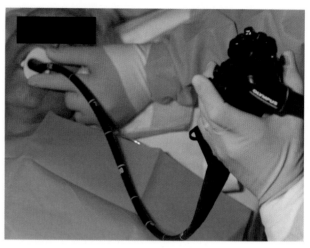

Figure 13.3. Performing the endoscopy.
Endoscopy is performed using a standard upper endoscope. Monitored sedation is typically administered; however, the procedure can also be done with topical anesthesia to the hypopharynx and local anesthesia to the abdominal wall if the patient is unable to tolerate monitored sedation. When the endoscope is in the stomach, the stomach should be fully insufflated with air to help move the liver, spleen, and colon away from the tube site.

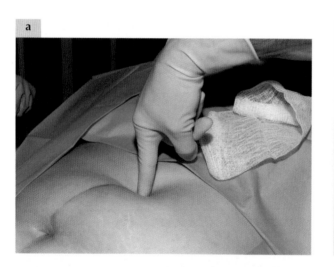

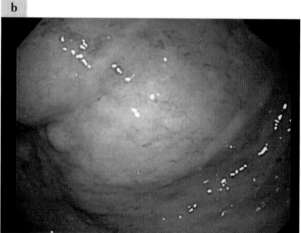

Figure 13.4. Localizing the site for tube placement.
The site for tube placement is determined by finding a discrete point on the skin (**a**) that has been transilluminated by the endoscope while the scope is in the distal body of the stomach (**b**). This area **must** correlate with an area of endoscopically visible indentation when pressure is applied to the site with a finger.

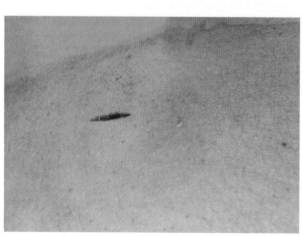

Figure 13.5. Making the incision.
One percent xylocaine is injected at the skin site identified by transillumination and compression above, then a 1-cm incision is made.

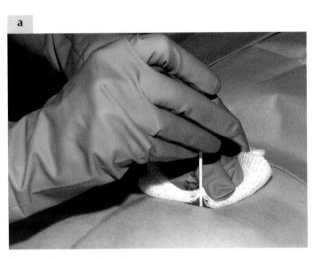

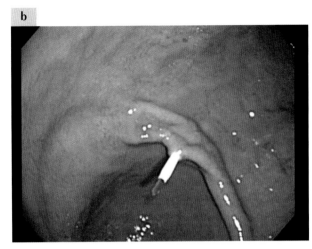

Figure 13.6. Passing the trocar.
(**a**) A 16-gauge trocar is passed through the incision and into the stomach. This must be done with a quick motion in order to pierce all the tissue layers without pushing the stomach out of the way. (**b**) It is important for the endoscopist to ensure that the stomach is fully insufflated as the trocar is passed, and that the endoscope is positioned in such a way that the entry of the trocar into the stomach can be directly visualized.

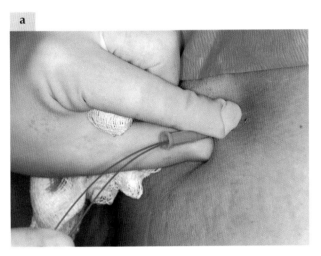

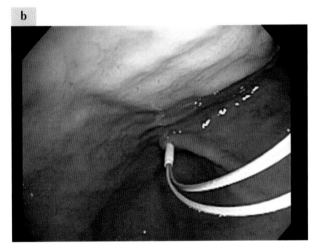

Figure 13.7. Passing the thread.
A thread is passed through the trocar from the skin (**a**) into the stomach (**b**).

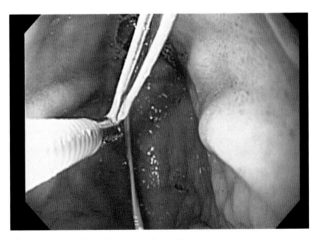

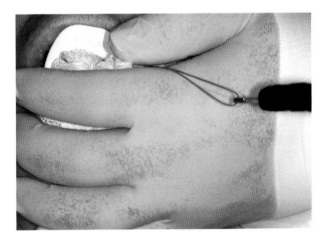

Figure 13.8. Grasping the thread.
The endoscopist grasps the thread in the stomach with standard endoscopic biopsy forceps.

Figure 13.9. Retrieving the thread.
While maintaining a firm grip on the thread, the endoscope is withdrawn out of the patient. As the thread exits the patient's mouth, an assistant grabs it.

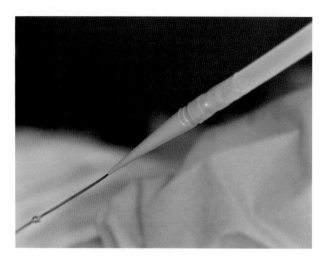

Figure 13.10. Attaching the PEG tube.
The wire loop at the tapered end of the PEG tube is connected to the loop of thread that was pulled out of the patient's mouth.

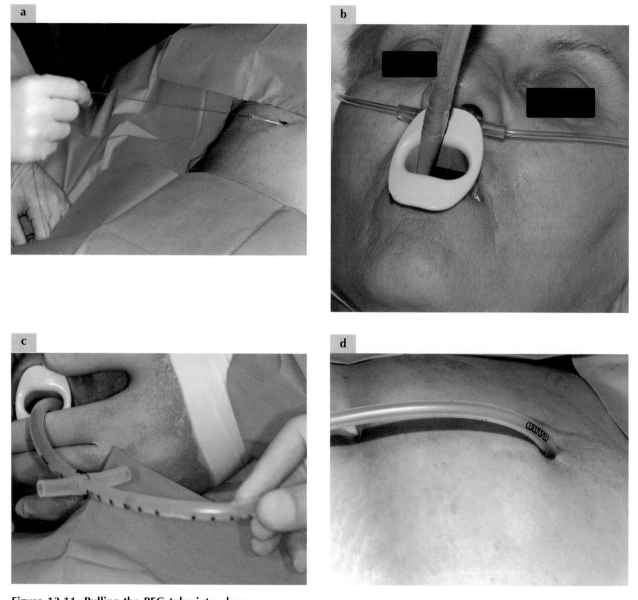

Figure 13.11. Pulling the PEG tube into place.
Using steady, gentle pressure, the free end of the thread is pulled (**a**): this pulls the PEG tube into the patient's mouth (**b**), down the esophagus (**c**), and into place in the stomach (**d**).

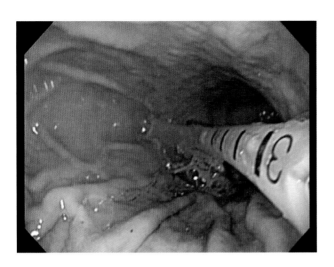

Figure 13.12. Confirming placement.
A repeat endoscopy is performed to confirm the position of the tube and the internal bumper.

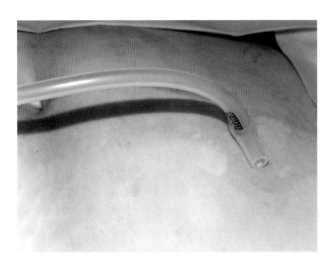

Figure 13.13. Applying the external bumper.
An external bumper is passed over the tapered end of the PEG tube and into position against the skin wall. The bumper should be left 0.5–1.0 cm above the skin to avoid placing excessive pressure on the mucosa under the internal bumper. If the external bumper is pulled tightly against the skin, it will cause the internal bumper to erode through the gastric wall and cause a 'buried-bumper syndrome'. The tapered end of the PEG tube should now be cut off and that end attached to a drainage bag. The patient can now drink and eat soft foods, which will be drained out of the tube.

References

1. Campagnutta E, Cannizzaro R. Percutaneous endoscopic gastrostomy (PEG) in palliative treatment of non-operable intestinal obstruction due to gynecologic cancer: a review. *Eur J Gynaecol Oncol* 2000; **21**:397–402.

2. Herman LL, Hoskins WJ, Shike M. Percutaneous endoscopic gastrostomy for decompression of the stomach and small bowel. *Gastrointest Endosc* 1992; **38**:314–18.

3. Ponsky J, Dunkin B. Percutaneous endoscopic gastrostomy. In: (Yamada T, Alpers DH, Laine L et al, eds) *Textbook of Gastroenterology*, 3rd edn. (Lippincott, Williams & Wilkins: New York, 1999) 2825–33.

4. Stellato TA, Gauderer MW. Percutaneous endoscopic gastrostomy for gastrointestinal decompression. *Ann Surg* 1987; **205**:119–22.

5. Picus D, Marx MV, Weyman PJ. Chronic intestinal obstruction: value of percutaneous gastrostomy tube placement. *AJR Am J Roentgenol* 1988; **150**:295–7.

14 Chest tube placement (tube thoracostomy)

Robert J Korst

Tube thoracostomy refers to placement of a tube, or catheter, into either hemithoracic cavity for drainage purposes. Indications include the drainage of blood (hemothorax), air (pneumothorax), pus (empyema), or fluid (effusion). In the patient with a gynecologic malignancy, tube thoracostomy is usually performed for the drainage of a malignant pleural effusion. Malignant effusions develop as a result of tumor metastases to the parietal and/or visceral pleura, which inhibit the normal reabsorption of pleural fluid, resulting in fluid accumulation. Patients typically present with dyspnea on exertion and pleuritic chest pain, which prompts the performance of a chest radiograph with posteroanterior, as well as upright and lateral decubitus views.

Tube thoracostomy is usually performed at the bedside, using local anesthesia, which may be supplemented with conscious sedation. Care must be taken when administering intravenous sedatives and/or narcotics to patients with compromised respiratory function, mandating the use of telemetry and pulse oximetry for elective cases. It should be emphasized that tube thoracostomy can essentially be performed painlessly with proper technique and placement of the local anesthetic.

The most frequent complications of tube thoracostomy include injury to the underlying lung, resulting in bleeding and air leak, bleeding from intercostal vessels, and malposition. With proper patient selection and technique, these complications should be minimized.

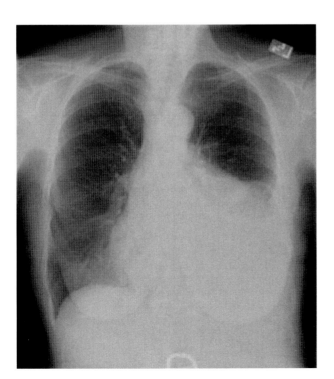

Figure 14.1. Posteroanterior view.
Posteroanterior chest radiograph of a 47-year-old woman with a history of carcinoma of the ovary who presented with the gradual onset of dyspnea on exertion. A left pleural effusion is present, demonstrated by partial opacity of the left hemithorax with a meniscus.

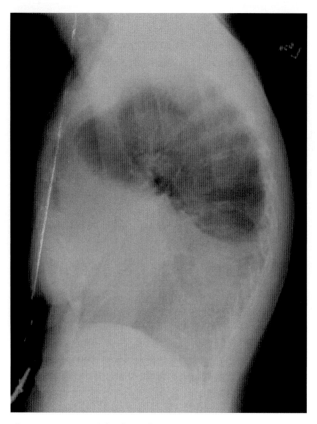

Figure 14.2. Upright lateral view.
Upright lateral chest radiograph clearly demonstrating the partial opacity with a meniscus, implying that pleural fluid is present.

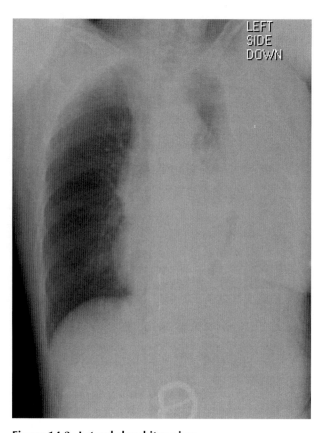

Figure 14.3. Lateral decubitus view.
Lateral decubitus radiograph demonstrating that the pleural fluid is freely mobile and layers out. This view should be performed prior to chest tube placement to differentiate between free pleural fluid and other abnormalities, including atelectatic lung or an intrathoracic mass lesion, both of which are contraindications to tube thoracostomy. If freely mobile fluid is not appreciated on the lateral decubitus radiograph, or the involved hemithorax is completely opacified, computed tomography of the chest with intravenous contrast should be performed to definitively characterize the intrathoracic pathology.

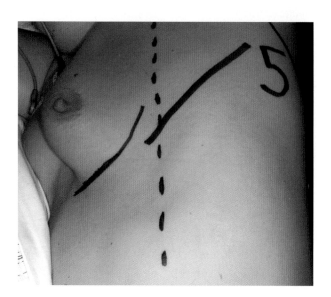

Figure 14.4. Patient position and landmarks.
The patient is placed in the lateral decubitus position with the affected side up. The dashed line indicates the anterior axillary line; the inframammary crease and the fifth intercostal space are marked with solid lines (the fifth intercostal space is usually at the level of the inframammary crease). A common and safe site for tube placement corresponds to the intersection of the anterior axillary line and the fifth intercostal space. Care must be taken not to place the tube posteriorly, as the patient will lie on it, causing discomfort and impaired drainage.

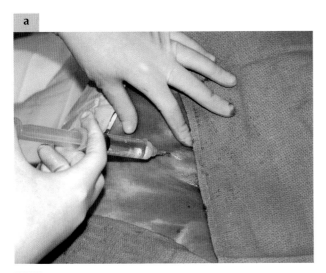

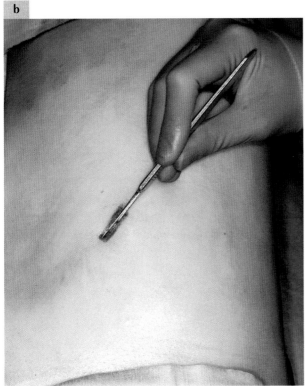

Figure 14.5. Local anesthesia and incision.
Once the incision site is marked, and the patient is prepared and draped in a sterile fashion, 1% lidocaine (without epinephrine) is injected, aimed at anesthetizing three specific sites: (1) the skin; (2) the periosteum of the rib, inferior to the desired intercostal space; and (3) the parietal pleura. In an adult, typically 30 ml of 1% lidocaine is necessary to effectively anesthetize all of these areas. The parietal pleura is anesthetized by inserting the needle (while aspirating) into the chest. When fluid return is obtained, lidocaine is injected while slowly withdrawing the needle (**a**). Local anesthetic will then dissect directly into the extrapleural plane, thereby anesthetizing the pleura. If one is unable to aspirate fluid from the chest, a new site for tube placement should be chosen or the presence of pleural fluid should be questioned. Typically, a #11- or #15-blade scalpel is used to incise the skin (**b**).

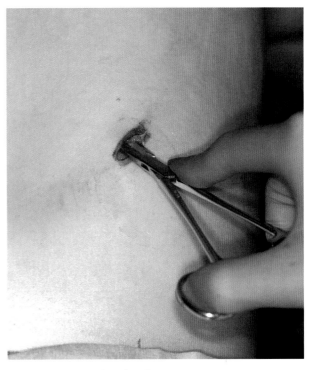

Figure 14.6. Entering the chest.
A blunt-tipped, curved clamp is inserted and used to spread the subcutaneous tissue and muscle down to the periosteum of the rib immediately below the desired intercostal space. Once this rib is delineated, the intercostal muscle immediately **above** the rib is gently spread, and the pleural cavity is entered. Care needs to be taken not to enter the chest immediately **below** the rib, as damage to the intercostal bundle may result in bleeding and/or pain.

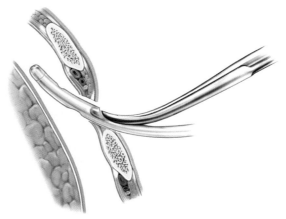

Figure 14.7. Diagrammatic representation of curved clamp being used to insert a chest tube.
Once external air enters the chest, the lung usually collapses slightly, which helps prevent it from being traumatized. Note that the clamp is inserted **above** the rib, avoiding the neurovascular bundle. The tube is then inserted into the desired position as described below. For the sake of simplicity, the extrathoracic musculature is not depicted.

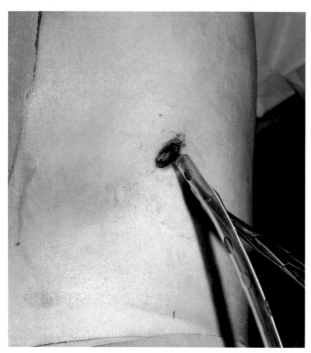

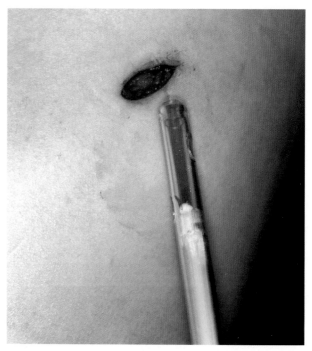

Figure 14.8. Insertion of chest tube – clamp technique.
One technique used for insertion of the tube into the
chest involves directing the tube into the chest using the
blunt-tipped, curved clamp. The tube is grasped with the
clamp at one of the side holes, as shown. Once the tube
is in the thoracic cavity, it is gently placed in the desired
position (posteriorly for fluid, anteriorly for
pneumothorax). All side holes should be well within the
chest – tubes are typically numbered in centimeters from
the last side hole.

Figure 14.9. Insertion of the chest tube – trocar technique.
Another technique that may be used to insert the tube
involves using a tube with a trocar that passes through
the tube. The sharp tip is backed out approximately
1–2 cm from the end of the tube, and is used as a stent
to help guide the tube into the chest. The potential
advantage of this technique is that the tube can be guided
more effectively once inside the thoracic cavity. To
prevent lung laceration, care must be taken to ensure that
the trocar tip does not protrude from the end of the tube.

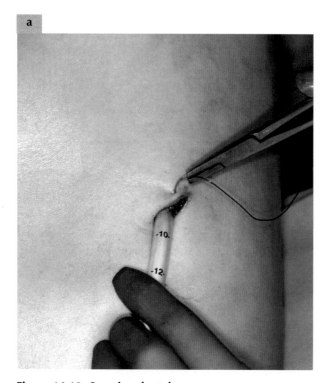

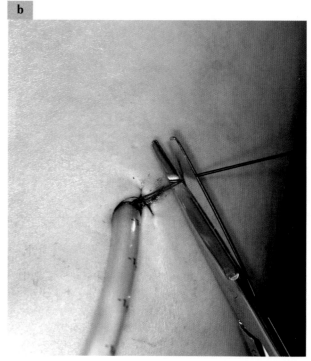

Figure 14.10. Securing the tube.
(**a**) Once the tube has been inserted, a nonabsorbable suture is placed through the skin next to the tube as an
anchoring stitch. (**b**) The suture material is then looped around the tube and tied, securing the tube in place.

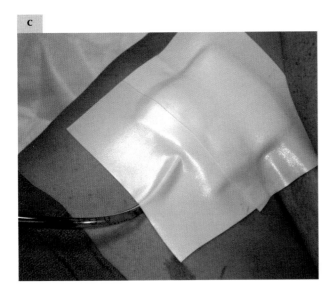

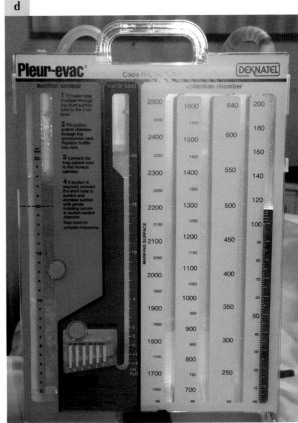

Figure 14.10. Continued.
An occlusive dressing is then applied (**c**) and the tube is attached to a commercially available thoracic underwater drainage unit (**d**).

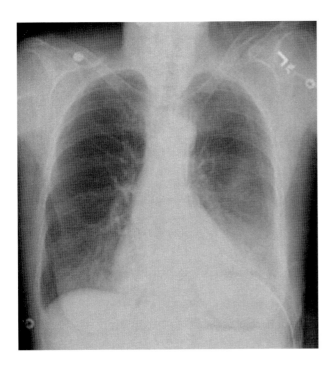

Figure 14.11. Successful drainage.
A post-procedure posteroanterior chest radiograph shows the chest tube in place, having effectively drained from the patient the fluid that was seen in Figures 14.1–14.3. If placed for a malignant pleural effusion, a sclerosing agent, such as talc or doxycycline, may now be instilled to achieve pleurodesis, thereby preventing fluid reaccumulation. If placed for pneumothorax, the tube is removed when the air leak has healed.

15 Central venous catheter placement

Michelle Montemarano and Douglas A Levine

Central venous catheter placement plays an important role in the diagnosis, management, and treatment of the patient with a gynecologic malignancy. Central venous catheter monitoring is frequently employed in the perioperative setting. Indications for central venous catheter placement include pressure monitoring, infusion of large-volume or hypertonic solutions, inaccessible peripheral veins, or hemodialysis. Central venous catheters are placed in the superior vena cava, inferior vena cava or one of their major branches. The subclavian, internal jugular, and external jugular veins are frequently employed when access to the central venous circulation is required, or when peripheral sites are unavailable.

The risks associated with central venous access include pneumothorax, puncture of arteries or lymphatics, air embolus, infection, or thrombus formation. The subclavian and internal jugular veins lie close to the carotid and subclavian arteries, the apical lung, nerves, and other key structures. These structures must be recognized as one is accessing the central venous system. The most commonly recog-

Table 15.1 **Advantages and disadvantages to various central access approaches.**

Approach	Advantage	Disadvantage
Right internal jugular vein	Well-defined landmarks Dome of right lung and pleura lower on the right than on the left Relatively straight line to SVC	Patient discomfort due to fixation of line in mobile portion of neck
Left internal jugular vein	Well-defined landmarks	Patient discomfort Greater potential to injure the left brachiocephalic vein, SVC, or thoracic duct
Right subclavian vein	Patient comfort due to line location outside of mobile areas of body	Higher risk of pleural puncture Sharp vessel curvature at junction of right subclavian vein and brachiocephalic vein, making improper line placement more likely
Left subclavian vein	Patient comfort Lowest risk of infection Lack of sharp vessel curvature; greater likelihood of correct catheter-tip location	Higher risk of pleural puncture

SVC, Superior vena cava.

nized risk, pneumothorax, is apparent when air, instead of blood, is aspirated during location of the vessel. For this reason, all patients undergo a post-procedure chest radiograph to rule out pneumothorax and evaluate line placement. While advantages and disadvantages of the various approaches to central venous access exist, the clinician should choose the technique based on clinical considerations and familiarity with the approach (see Table 15.1). Some patients may have had prior head and neck surgery, or venous thrombi, making certain approaches less desirable. Relative contraindications to central venous catheter placement include marked coagulopathy, patient refusal, and bacteremia. Of note, in coagulopathic states, femoral vein cannulization can result in fewer bleeding complications.

The figures in this chapter illustrate the technique of central venous catheterization via the left internal jugular (IJ) vein. The IJ approach is common because of its well-defined landmarks. The three common approaches for cannulation of the IJ vein are posterior, central, and anterior. Here, the left IJ vein via the central approach (between the two heads of the sternocleidomastoid muscle belly) is depicted, but the figures are applicable to all central venous access approaches. The IJ runs medial to the sternocleidomastoid (SCM) muscle in its upper part, posterior to it in the triangle between the two inferior heads of the SCM in its middle part, and behind the anterior portion of the clavicular head of the muscle in its lower part, terminating above the medial clavicle where it enters the subclavian vein.

The Seldinger technique is frequently used in the placement of central venous catheters. This technique involves puncturing the vein with a small bore needle through which a guidewire is introduced into the vein. The needle is then withdrawn and a catheter is introduced over the guidewire, which is subsequently removed. Most commercially available central venous access trays provide all of the equipment necessary to place a central venous catheter, including needles, guidewires, and dilators (Figure 15.1).

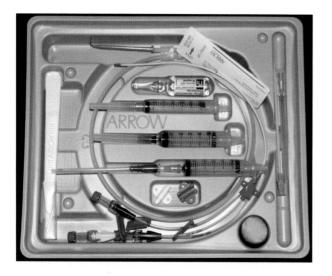

Figure 15.1. Commercially available central venous catheter kit.

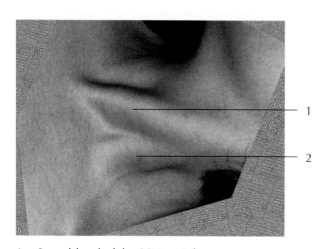

1 – Sternal head of the SCM muscle
2 – Clavicular head of the SCM muscle

Figure 15.2. Positioning the patient.
The patient is supine in the Trendelenburg position, at an angle of at least 15° to reduce the risk of air embolism. The head is rotated to the contralateral side to allow optimal exposure for venipuncture, but not beyond 45°. The sternal head and clavicular head of the sternocleidomastoid (SCM) muscle are demonstrated. Sterile gown, gloves, and mask should be worn.

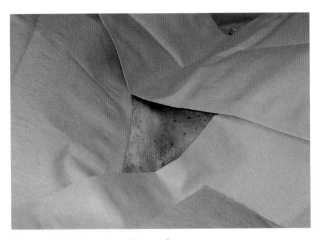

Figure 15.3. Prepping the neck.
The area around the puncture site is prepped and draped in the usual sterile manner. If the patient is awake, the skin should be infiltrated with approximately 5 ml of 1% lidocaine, using a 25-gauge needle.

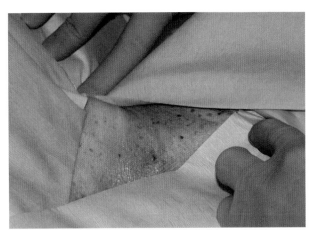

Figure 15.4. Palpation of the suprasternal notch.
The triangle formed by the two heads of the sternocleidomastoid muscle and the clavicle can be found by palpating the suprasternal notch and moving laterally over the sternal head of the muscle. In the conscious patient, it may help to have the patient lift the head up off the bed to visualize the triangle. This can be more difficult in the obese patient.

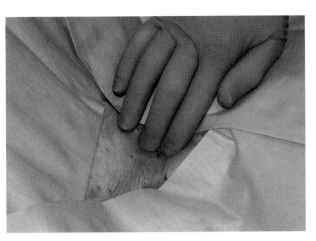

Figure 15.5. Carotid artery.
The carotid pulse can be palpated within the sternocleidomastoid triangle as shown; the internal jugular vein will be found lateral to the artery.

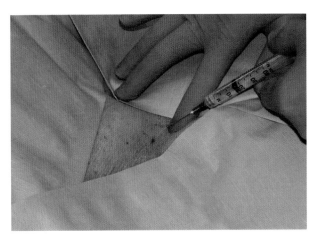

Figure 15.6. Venipuncture.
The needle is directed caudally at an angle of 45° to the frontal plane using negative pressure at all times. The needle is placed laterally and parallel to the carotid artery; it is directed toward the ipsilateral nipple. The vessel is normally entered at a depth of about 2 cm.

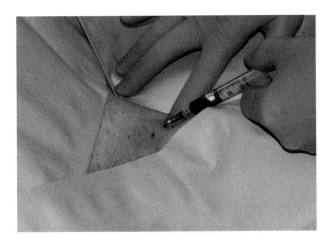

Figure 15.7. Locating the vessel.
Once the lumen of the vessel is penetrated, blood will return; the needle should be advanced a few millimeters to obtain free flow of blood. If bright red blood is noted with rapid and pulsatile filling of the syringe, the carotid artery has most likely been entered. The needle should be removed immediately and pressure applied for at least 10 minutes to ensure hemostasis.

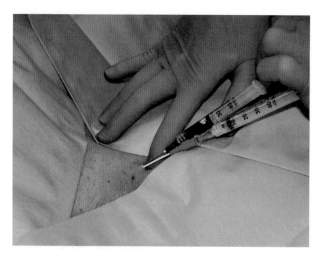

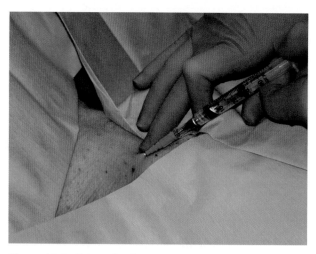

Figure 15.8. Catheter insertion.
Once the vein is located, a 10-ml syringe with an 18-gauge catheter or introducer needle is inserted parallel to the location of the finder needle under negative pressure.

Figure 15.9. Entry of vein.
Once the catheter punctures the vein, return of blood is noted in the syringe. At this point, the syringe and needle are removed from the catheter. The catheter must not be pulled backwards over the needle due to potential shearing of the catheter tip and resultant catheter embolus. The catheter is occluded with a finger to prevent air embolism.

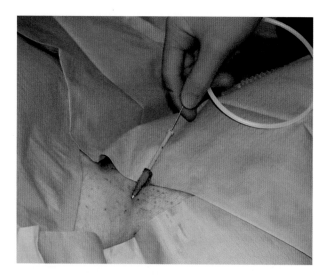

Figure 15.10. Guidewire insertion.
A J-tipped flexible guidewire is advanced through the plastic catheter with the aid of an introducer to straighten the tip. The guidewire should pass freely into the vein; if it does not, the syringe, without the needle, should be reattached to the catheter and blood aspirated to confirm the patency and position of the catheter within the vessel. It is inserted slowly using the introducer to provide stability to the wire as it enters the catheter. The plastic shell provides control of the distal end of the wire. A firm grip on the guidewire must be maintained at all times.

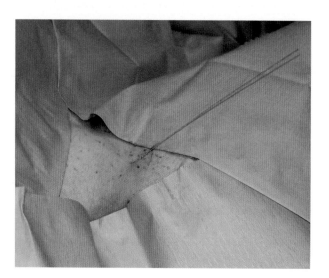

Figure 15.11. Length of guidewire.
The guidewire is usually inserted for most of its length, allowing enough outside of the patient to prevent slippage. If the patient is connected to cardiac monitoring, ventricular ectopy will occur when the right atrium is entered. The catheter is removed from the vessel when the guidewire has been inserted to the appropriate length.

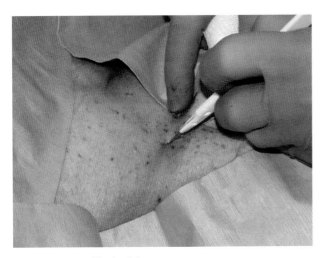

Figure 15.12. Skin incision.
A superficial incision is made in the skin overlying the guidewire with a #11 scalpel blade, to permit access of the catheter through the skin and into the vessel. If the incision is too big, bleeding will occur and the catheter will not be secure.

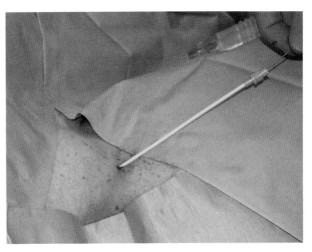

Figure 15.13. Vessel dilator.
A vessel dilator is passed over the wire, through the skin, and into the vessel; this allows the skin and subcutaneous tissues to be dilated for easy passage of the catheter. In addition, the vessel, which can contract around the guidewire, will be dilated to allow unrestricted entry of the catheter. Care is taken not to pull out the guidewire while passing the dilator.

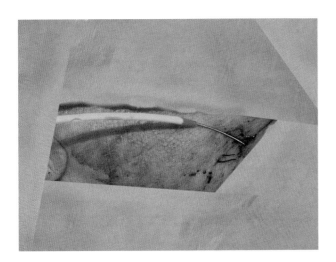

Figure 15.14. Passage of central catheter.
The central venous catheter is passed over the guidewire and advanced into the vein. Large-bore catheters can be passed over the dilator and the wire to provide additional stabilization during catheter placement. The guidewire must be passed through the catheter prior to advancing the catheter into the patient. In this manner, the wire will not be lost in either the patient or the catheter.

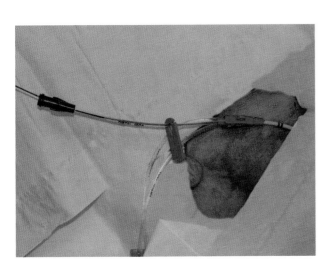

Figure 15.15. Withdrawing the guidewire.
Once the catheter is in place, the guidewire is withdrawn through the largest port; in a standard triple-lumen central venous catheter this is usually the brown port. Blood is aspirated from each port and then each is flushed with approximately 5 ml of normal saline.

246 Central venous catheter placement

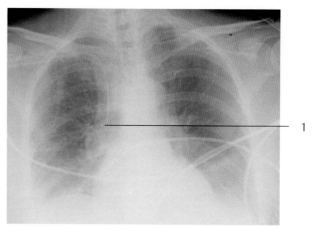

1 – Tip in distal superior vena cava

Figure 15.16. Skin sutures.
The catheter is sutured to the skin with a permanent suture and connected to intravenous tubing (suture material is provided in most standard kits). If the patient is awake, 1% lidocaine is infiltrated into the skin prior to placing the sutures. The puncture site is then covered with a dry sterile dressing.

Figure 15.17. Post-procedure radiograph.
A chest radiograph is obtained to verify placement of the catheter tip and to rule out pneumothorax. Ideally, the catheter tip should lie in the superior vena cava or the right atrium at about the level of the fifth thoracic vertebra. Shown here is a central venous catheter with its tip terminating in the distal superior vena cava.

16 Mediport placement

Anne M Covey and George I Getrajdman

Long-term venous access is important in the treatment and management of patients with gynecologic malignancies. There are several central venous access devices to choose from, which are characterized by catheter size, type (implantable versus external), number of lumens, and longevity ('permanent' versus temporary).

In determining the type of catheter to place in a given patient, several factors should be considered, including the intended use of the catheter, frequency of access, physician preferences, and patient lifestyle.

Implantable ports are ideal for long-term, intermittent central venous access. Compared to external tunneled central venous catheters, implantable ports require less maintenance and have a lower rate of infection. Because implantable ports are completely contained under the skin when not accessed, there is no limitation on range of motion or patient lifestyle. This is an important feature for patients who swim, lift weights, or have small children at home (who may pull on external catheters).

Implantable ports are most often titanium or plastic, both of which are magnetic resonance imaging (MRI) compatible, and connect to valved or open-ended silicone or polyurethane catheters (Figure 16.1). Routine maintenance requires only that the port be flushed with heparinized saline (normal saline for valved catheters) every 4–6 weeks, and after each use.

The role of the interventional radiologist in the placement of central venous access has increased dramatically in the past decade. By using ultrasound, fluoroscopy, intravenous contrast, and specialized catheters with guidewires, interventional radiologists are able to negotiate venous occlusions, deal with vascular anomalies, and provide alternative puncture sites not previously accessible. The lower complication rate and almost 100% success rate may fuel the movement of venous access into the angiography suite.

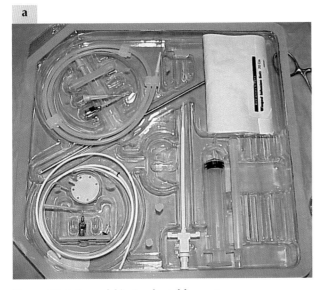
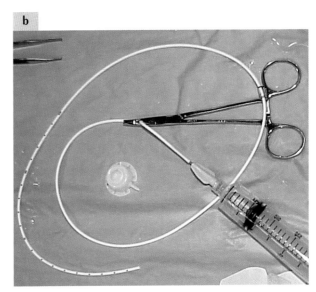

Figure 16.1 (a and b). Implantable port.

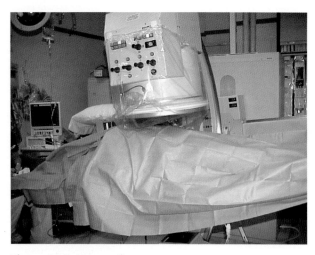

Figure 16.2. Preparation.
Our preferred approach is via the right internal jugular vein, because this eliminates the risk of pneumothorax and subclavian stenosis or thrombosis. The right neck and chest are prepped and draped in usual sterile fashion. A nurse administers conscious sedation that consists of meperidine, fentanyl, and midazolam. The patient is placed in the Trendelenburg position to distend the vein and minimize the risk of air embolism. In this figure, the patient's head is to the left.

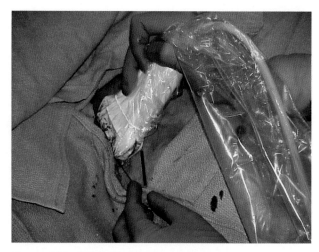

Figure 16.3. Venous puncture.
Using ultrasound for real-time guidance, the internal jugular vein is punctured from a **low posterior** approach. Puncturing just above the clavicle (**low**) and posterior to the posterior belly of the sternocleidomastoid muscle (**posterior**) allows for a transverse needle course parallel to the clavicle, minimizing the risk of pneumothorax and eventually providing for a smooth catheter course. The head of the patient is to the left and the black line represents the approximate location of the clavicle.

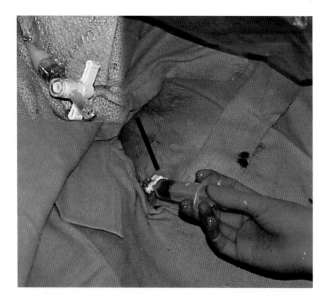

Figure 16.4. Needle exchange.
The needle is then exchanged over a wire for a coaxial dilator. The dilator is flushed and closed with a flow switch (inset) while the port pocket and tunnel are created. The head of the patient is toward the lower left corner of the figure and the black line represents the approximate location of the clavicle.

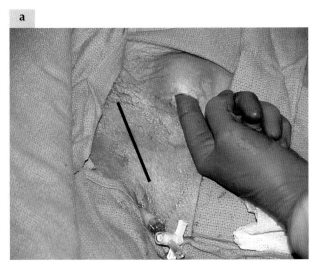
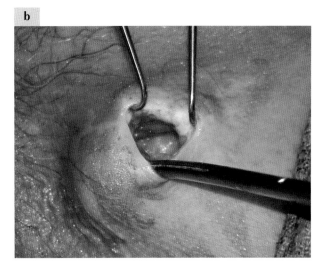

Figure 16.5. Site selection.
Choosing the site of the port pocket is important because it must be both comfortable for the patient and easily accessible. An incision in the subclavicular anterior chest over the ribs is made to fit the port. (**a**) A pocket is created to fit the port using blunt and sharp dissection. (**b**) In thin patients, the pocket may be down to the fascia, whereas in patients with more subcutaneous tissue, the pocket is created to be approximately 5 mm deep so that the port may be easily palpable and accessible in the future. Electrocautery is used occasionally for hemostasis. The head of the patient is toward the lower left corner of the figure and the black line in (**a**) represents the approximate location of the clavicle.

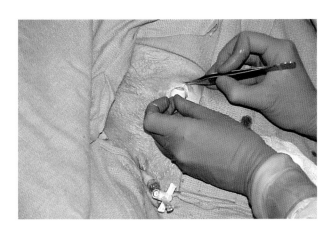

Figure 16.6. Pocket size.
The pocket is flushed with sterile saline and checked to ensure that the selected port fits in the pocket without being directly under the incision. The port is then removed from the pocket and flushed.

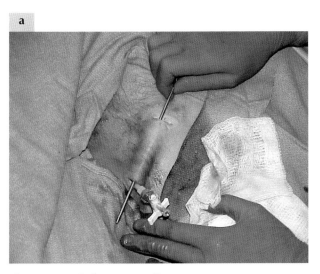
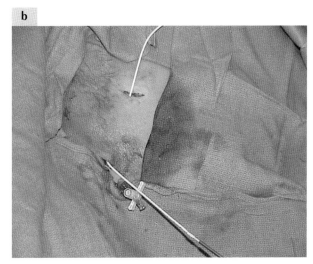

Figure 16.7. Catheter tunneling.
(**a**) The catheter is tunneled from the pocket to the venipuncture site using a metal or plastic tunneler, and the tip of the catheter is cut. (**b**) The back end of the catheter is clamped to prevent air embolism after intravenous placement of the front end.

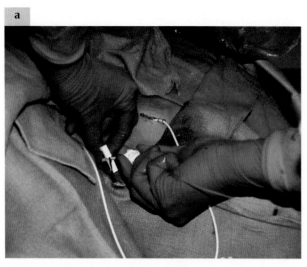
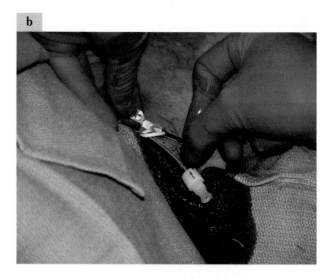

Figure 16.8 (a and b). Dilator exchange.
At the venipuncture site, the coaxial dilator is exchanged over a stiff wire for an appropriately sized peel-away sheath with the patient in the Trendelenburg position. The dilator and wire are removed, and the catheter is advanced through the sheath until the tip is in the right atrium. This is the ideal position, but the position of the catheter may change with a change in position by 1–2 cm, depending on patient body habitus. This may be accounted for in the next step.

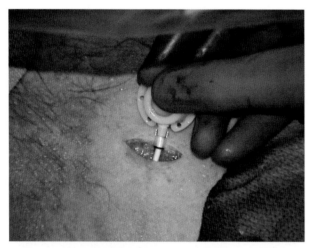

Figure 16.9. Length adjustment.
The back end of the catheter is cut to the desired length, and then affixed and locked to the port stem.

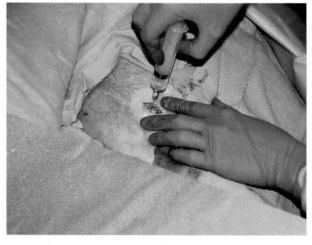

Figure 16.10. Initial flush.
The port is accessed and flushed with sterile saline, to check for function and to look for any leak at the attachment site.

Figure 16.11. Placement into pocket.
The port is placed in the pocket and any slack is pulled from the catheter, providing a gentle course from the port to the right atrium; this is documented fluoroscopically.

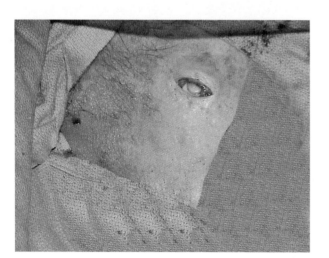

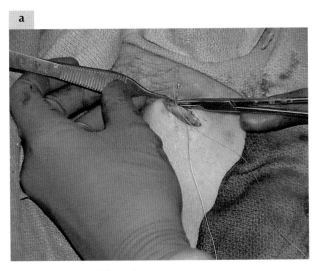 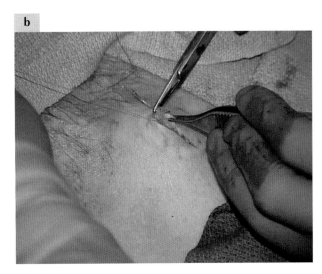

Figure 16.12. Incision closure.
(**a**) The port pocket is closed with interrupted absorbable sutures that serve to limit port mobility and hematoma formation. (**b**) The skin is closed with a running subcuticular monofilament or Dermabond. The venipuncture site is closed with an inverted absorbable stitch, with care not to nick the catheter or Dermabond.

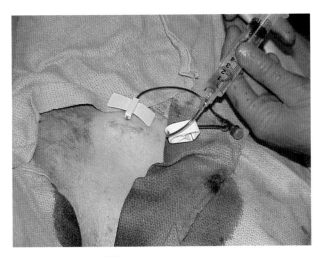

Figure 16.13. Final flush.
At the end of the procedure, the port is accessed with a noncoring needle and flushed with heparinized saline. If the port is to be used the same day, the access may be left in place, otherwise the needle is removed.

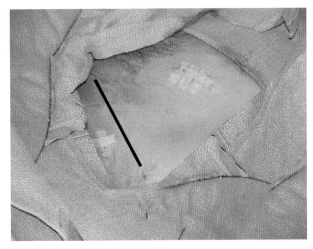

Figure 16.14. Dressing application.
Steri-strips and a sterile dressing are applied. A frontal chest radiograph is obtained. The patient is given a port maintenance booklet and instructed to keep the wound dry for 3 days (1 day for Dermabond) and to call her doctor for pain, erythema, or fever. Each time the port is accessed, the site must be prepped with Betadine or an equivalent. The patient's head is toward the lower left corner of the figure and the black line represents the approximate location of the clavicle.

17 Brachytherapy

Sang E Sim and Kaled M Alektiar

Radiation therapy has a place in the treatment of almost all gynecologic malignancies, although a more limited role in ovarian and fallopian tube carcinomas. Varied modalities are employed in the complete management of an individual patient over time. While external-beam therapy alone is used for certain patients, often, radiation treatment of gynecologic malignancies requires high doses to be delivered for tumor control. Frequently, these doses surpass the safe limits for surrounding normal tissues and so cannot be delivered using conventional external-beam techniques. Therefore, brachytherapy has been utilized to treat gynecologic malignancies with high radiation doses without exceeding critical normal tissue limits.

The most common brachytherapy techniques used to treat cervical, vaginal, endometrial, and recurrent tumors will be discussed in this chapter. In the management of cervical cancer, tandem and ovoids, as well as interstitial implants, are frequently employed. Tandem and ovoids are used in patients with relatively normal vaginal architectures; interstitial implants are reserved for patients with particularly exophytic tumors or vaginal fibrosis/stenosis. Interstitial implants are also used to treat patients with large vaginal tumors from both primary vaginal cancer and, more commonly, recurrent endometrial or cervical cancer after primary surgical therapy.

In the adjuvant treatment of endometrial cancer after initial surgery, intravaginal brachytherapy is used to deliver a prescribed dose to the vaginal mucosa. This has been shown to reduce the likelihood of vaginal recurrences. For recurrent tumors of a number of primary sites, surgical resection is often chosen as the treatment of choice. This may encompass an exenterative procedure, described elsewhere, or local radical resection of an isolated recurrence. In either situation, intraoperative radiation is currently being utilized as a method to reduce the likelihood of recurrence from residual microscopic disease. Applicators are flexible in order to conform to pelvic anatomy and are discussed in detail below.

Tandem and ovoids

Tandem and ovoids are typically used in the treatment of cervical and endometrial cancers. These can be used as sole therapy with small lesions in situations where treatment of draining pelvic lymph nodes is unnecessary (e.g. Stage IA1 cervical tumors). Typically, the tandem and ovoids are used in conjunction with external-beam therapy. Their most common usage is in the treatment of cervical cancer, where either one or two applications can be performed.

There are two common types of tandem and ovoids: the Fletcher–Suit and the Henschke applicator. Differences exist between the two; however, the basic uses and principles of placement and delivery are the same. In this chapter, the Henschke applicator will be discussed. The tandem is placed through the cervical os into the endometrial canal of an intact uterus. The ovoids are placed snugly into the lateral fornices. Both the tandem and the ovoids are loaded with radioactive sources to deliver the dose to the tumor volume.

Cesium-137 (Cs-137) sources are typically utilized for treatment using a low-dose-rate technique. Usually, one source is placed in each ovoid, and an additional three to four sources are placed into the tandem. Cs-137 delivers gamma rays of 662 keV and has a half-life of 30 years. Its energy allows for good local penetration to treat a primary lesion, but still allows limitation of dose to adjacent normal tissue. The standard dwell time ranges from 36 to 60 hours, throughout which time the patient is hospitalized and remains at bedrest. Alternatively, a high-dose-rate technique may be utilized.

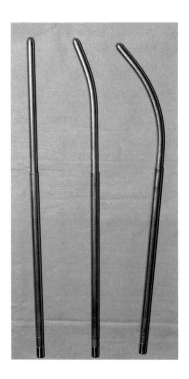

Figure 17.1. Tandems.
Different curvature tandems are available for insertion. The curvature is selected to accommodate the natural flexure of the uterus, as well as to displace the uterus away from either the rectum or the bladder to limit dose to either structure, if necessary.

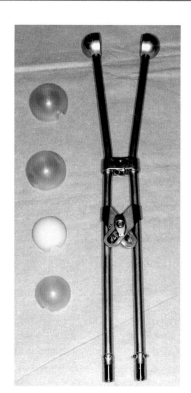

Figure 17.2. Ovoids and caps.
The ovoids are placed into the right and left vaginal fornices. They are 2 cm in diameter, with caps available to increase the diameter of the ovoid to 2.5 or 3.0 cm. The largest diameter ovoids are utilized in order to minimize the dose to the adjacent vaginal surfaces while also contributing dose to point A (see Fig. 17.13).

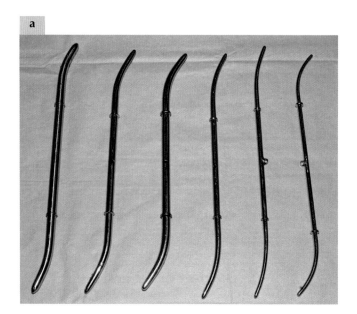

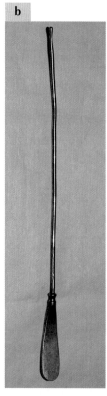

Figure 17.3. Dilators and sound.
(a) The cervix is normally grasped with a single-tooth tenaculum; dilators are sequentially used to dilate the cervical os until a 16-French dilator can be easily accommodated. (b) The sound is gently passed through the cervical os and into the endometrial cavity in order to measure the length of the uterus. This assessment of uterine length is essential so that proper placement of the tandem can be accomplished. If the tandem is placed in too deeply, uterine perforation can occur; if it is too shallow, the dose distribution will be affected.

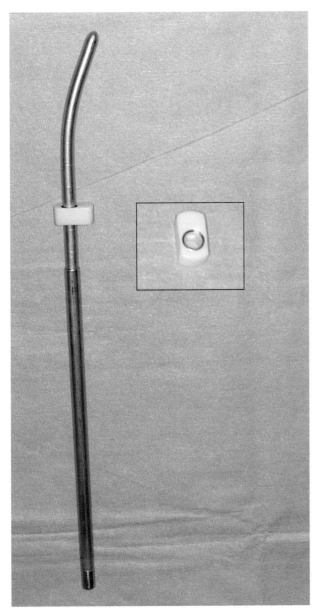

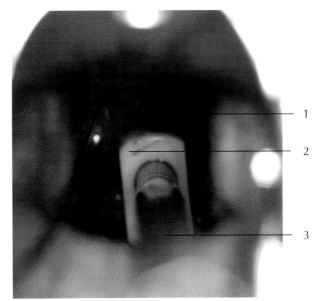

1 – Cervix
2 – Flange
3 – Tandem

Figure 17.5. Tandem in situ.
The tandem is inserted through the cervical os; the flange is seen flush against the external os. The tandem will pass through the ovoids when they are placed, and a stay suture is seen placed into the cervix.

Figure 17.4. Tandem and flange.
The central tandem is inserted through the cervical os after dilatation. A flange, seen in white, is placed on the tandem and secured at a distance from the tip that is equal to the length of the uterine cavity (as measured with the sound).

Therefore, once the tandem is fully inserted through the cervical os and into the uterine canal, the flange should sit flush against the external os. A metal ring is present on one side of the flange (inset) and should lie directly against the os, which allows visualization on radiographs. It is important that the flange is oriented correctly on the tandem so that the metal ring on the radiograph delineates the proper location of the external os. Two inert seeds are inserted into the cervix, one on the anterior right or left side and an additional one on the contralateral side along the posterior aspect (not shown). These seeds should lie only a short distance from the metal ring of the flange on the radiograph, verifying good placement of the tandem.

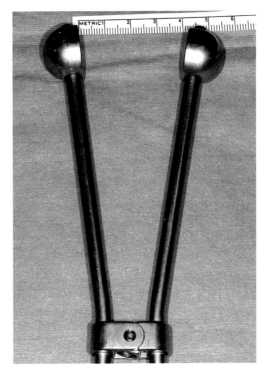

Figure 17.6. Ovoids.
The ovoids are placed into the vaginal canal to lie within the lateral fornices. Typically, the ovoids are separated by approximately 4 cm. Caps can be applied to stretch the vaginal mucosa if it is found to be excessively redundant.

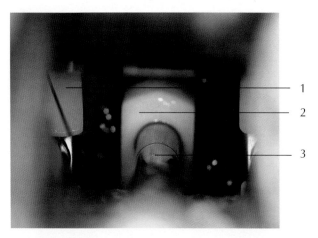

1 – Right ovoid
2 – Flange
3 – Tandem

Figure 17.7. Tandem and ovoids in situ.
The tandem, as described earlier, lies centrally. On either side of the tandem are ovoids that lie in the right and left vaginal fornices. The metal ovoids are covered with a plastic cap to increase the diameter of the ovoids to the maximal diameter that will fit into the fornices. The ovoids are spread apart symmetrically from the tandem, typically 4 cm.

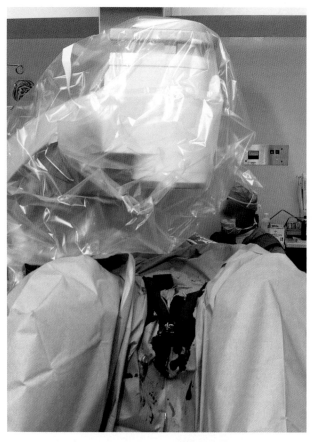

Figure 17.8. Anterior/posterior (AP) fluoroscopy.
Radiopaque gauze is used to pack the tandem and ovoids anteriorly and posteriorly. This secures the tandem and ovoids in place, while displacing the bladder and rectum away from the Henschke apparatus to decrease dose to these structures. Prior to finalizing the packing, fluoroscopy is performed to ensure proper position of the tandem and ovoids. If repositioning is needed, it can be accomplished while the patient is still under anesthesia (see Figs 17.11 and 17.12 for proper positioning). The anterior and posterior packing soaked with Betadine, above and below the intracavitary device, has been preliminarily packed into position.

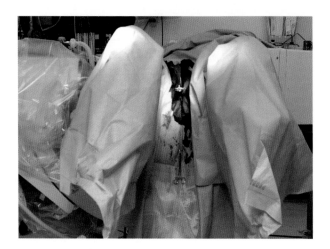

Figure 17.9. Lateral fluoroscopy.
In addition to an AP film, the C-arm of the fluoroscope is rotated 90° to obtain a lateral view; the hips may need to be extended slightly to allow correct positioning of the C-arm. Repositioning of the Henschke apparatus and/or repacking of the gauze may be required if fluoroscopy reveals that the position of the tandem and ovoids is suboptimal.

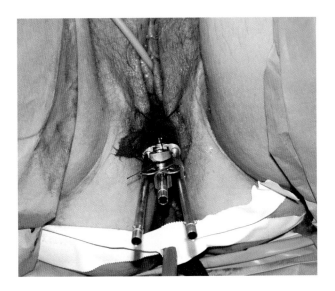

Figure 17.10. Henschke applicator in situ.
When complete, the Henschke applicator is fixed in place with vulvar stay sutures, which will minimize repositioning of the appliance during treatment. Anterior and posterior packing has been placed in position as described in Fig. 17.8. Typically, the applicator will stay in place for 48–72 hours; the patient will remain supine throughout this time. A urinary catheter is placed and the patient is given prophylaxis against the development of deep venous thromboses with low-molecular-weight heparin and intermittent pneumatic compression. Antimotility agents are also given to reduce bowel activity during this period of bed rest. A rectal catheter, seen here, or another rectal marker, is used to facilitate dosimetry. These are removed at the time of afterloading.

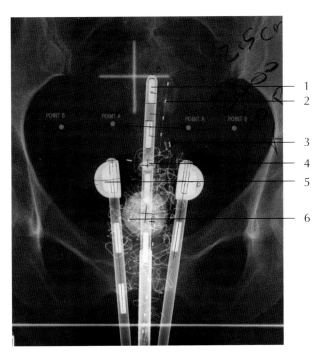

1 – Tandem
2 – Rectal marker
3 – Marker seeds
4 – Flange
5 – Right ovoid
6 – Urinary catheter balloon

Figure 17.11. Anterior/posterior (AP) localization film.
Once the patient has recovered from the procedure, the patient has localization films taken to plan the radiation treatments. The tandem should be in the midline along the vertical axis of the patient and ideally not rotated. The tandem should also be equidistant to each ovoid. The two marker seeds in the cervical os should sit just above the flange, which marks the external os. The Foley balloon, vaginal packing, and rectal marker are also visualized.

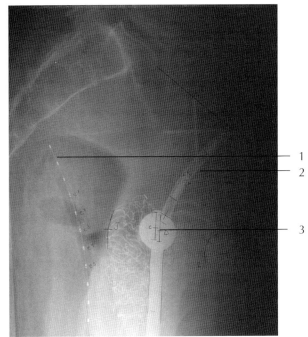

1 – Rectal marker
2 – Tandem
3 – Ovoids

Figure 17.12. Lateral localization film.
The ovoids should overlap each other and bisect the tandem. Again when visualized, the vaginal packing should not extend above the ovoids. The Foley balloon should be visualized in addition to a rectal marker, both being used to define various points for dose measurements.

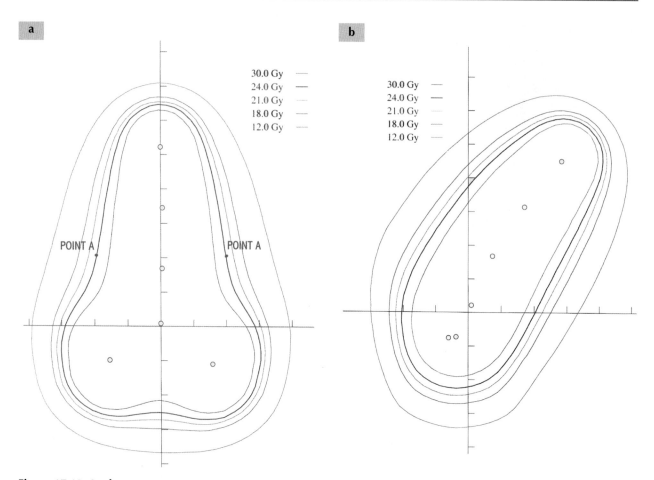

Figure 17.13. Isodose curves.

(**a**) The anterior/posterior view of the isodose line for prescription dose in this patient is noted in green; the isodose is typically described as 'pear-shaped'. (**b**) The lateral view of the isodose line for prescription dose in the same patient is again noted in green. Point A is most often the point of prescription. Two common definitions exist for point A. The classic definition is 2 cm above and 2 cm lateral to a point defined superiorly by the top of the ovoids, and horizontally, at the midpoint of the tandem.[1] A second definition states that point A lies 2 cm above and lateral to the external os marked by the flange.[2] Both definitions define point A in reference to the tandem such that if the flange is tilted, point A moves with its orientation. Point B is defined classically as the location of the obturator nodes, defined as 2 cm above and 5 cm lateral to the points as defined for point A. However, point B is defined in reference to the patient's axis and, therefore, is independent of the tandem orientation.

Interstitial brachytherapy

If the vaginal fornices are replaced by tumor or fibrosed, an interstitial implant may be more appropriate than tandem and ovoids. If significant vaginal extension is apparent, the tandem may still be utilized in conjunction with a vaginal cylinder, or alternatively, for vaginal disease that is deeply penetrant, an interstitial implant may be used.

The timing of placement of the tandem and ovoids varies among practitioners and institutions. It has been the authors' practice to place two insertions when treating cervical cancer definitively. The first applicator is placed after completion of the pelvic portion of the external-beam treatment; the second is placed 1–2 weeks later. If a parametrial boost is utilized, this is delivered between the two applica-tions, in order to minimize the overall treatment time and treatment break.

An interstitial implant may be used in cases of gross disease involving the vagina, where the treatment depth would be too great to allow effective coverage using an intravaginal cylinder, and the geometry would preclude adequate treatment with a tandem and ovoids. Interstitial implants are commonly performed in cases of vaginal cancers and recurrent vaginal tumors of the endometrium and cervix.

Several types of interstitial brachytherapy templates are utilized in the treatment of these tumors. The most common are the Syed–Neblett and the MUPITT templates. While the overall design is different, the treatment principles are the same. The Syed–Neblett template will be described in this section.

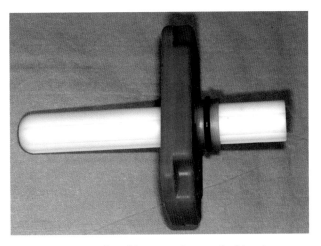

Figure 17.14. Syed–Neblett template and obturator.
The Syed–Neblett template lies against the perineum and a central obturator is inserted into the vagina. After placement of a Foley catheter, its balloon filled with 7 ml of a 30% Renografin solution, the obturator is inserted into the vaginal canal. The template is then attached to the obturator and placed against the perineum.

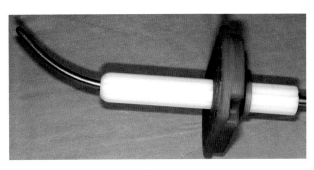

Figure 17.15. Template with tandem.
The obturator has a central opening to accommodate a tandem, which may be utilized for loading Cs-137 sources. This is typically used for patients with an intact uterus. If this is utilized, the cervix should be dilated as described previously for tandem and ovoid insertion. The tandem is locked in position along the obturator at a depth determined by sounding the uterine canal.

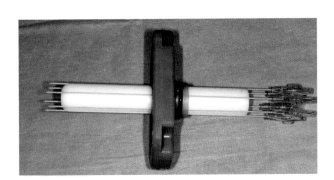

Figure 17.16. Template without tandem.
The obturator also consists of six grooves along the perimeter for placement and loading of needles along the surface of the vaginal mucosa. These are loaded when a central tandem is not used; however, these would be excluded if the tandem were to be loaded.

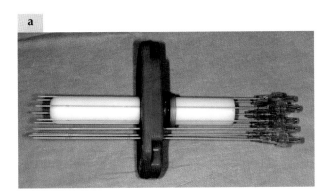

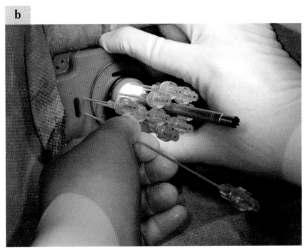

Figure 17.17. Placement of needles.
(a) The Syed–Neblett template consists of circumferential positions for placement of needles to implant into the paravaginal space. The placement of needles into these positions is tailored to the particular volume of tumor to be treated. (b) The Syed–Neblett template is visualized in position. A central obturator with a central tandem is in place. Needles are placed circumferentially around this obturator to treat the paravaginal region. Needle placement is customized for each patient to treat the particular tumor volume.

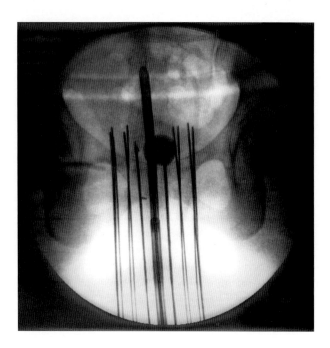

Figure 17.18. Intraoperative fluoroscopy.
Fluoroscopy is performed in the operating room to verify satisfactory placement of the interstitial needles. The needles should cover the tumor volume; they should be relatively parallel in relation to each other and should not deviate towards the rectum or vagina. Shown here is the anterior/posterior fluoroscopy film obtained at the time of needle insertion.

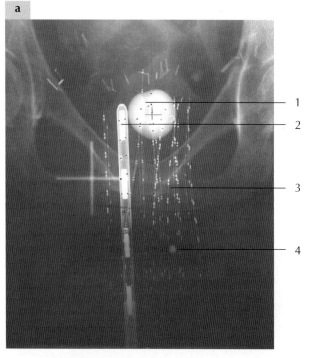

1 – Urinary catheter balloon
2 – Tandem
3 – Interstitial needles
4 – Marker

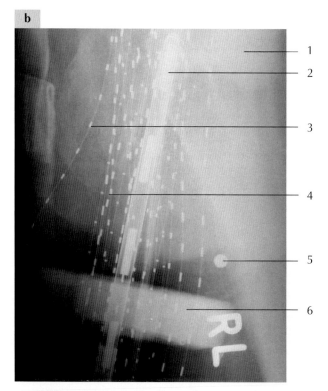

1 – Urinary catheter balloon
2 – Tandem
3 – Rectal marker
4 – Interstitial needles
5 – Marker
6 – Template

Figure 17.19. Localization films.
(a) Anterior/posterior and (b) lateral localization films are obtained for treatment planning. Dose is prescribed to the minimum peripheral dose line of the treatment volume. Dose to the bladder in relation to the urinary catheter balloon, as well as dose to various points along the rectum delineated by a marker wire, are calculated. A metal marker is placed at the vaginal introitus for visualization on a radiograph. Also seen are the central tandem, interstitial needles with dummy iridium wires inserted, and the template.

Intravaginal brachytherapy

The use of IVRT is generally limited to the treatment of the vaginal mucosa when the depth of treatment required is < 5 mm beyond the vaginal surface. Tumors that extend to a greater depth should be treated with alternative methods such as an interstitial implant. This technique is most commonly used in the postoperative treatment of the vaginal cuff for endometrial cancer; however, it may be applicable to other gynecologic malignancies. IVRT can be delivered using either low-dose or high-dose-rate techniques, with the latter becoming more prevalent in current practice in the USA. The total treatment dose is approximately 2100 cGy given in three weekly fractions.

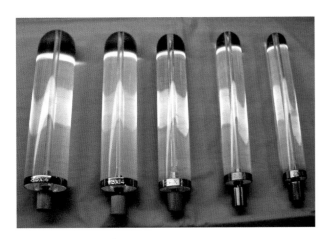

Figure 17.20. Intravaginal cylinders.
These intravaginal cylinders are used for high-dose-rate brachytherapy. Shown are cylinders of 3.5, 3.0, 2.6, 2.3 and 2.0 cm diameters. The patient is placed in the dorsal lithotomy position on the procedure table. Following examination, the length of the vagina is measured. The intravaginal cylinder is placed into the vagina and advanced to the apex. Typically, the largest diameter cylinder that will reasonably fit in the vaginal canal should be utilized. Using a smaller cylinder instead of a larger cylinder will result in a higher relative dose to the vaginal surface than to the prescription point, which is 0.5 cm from the surface.

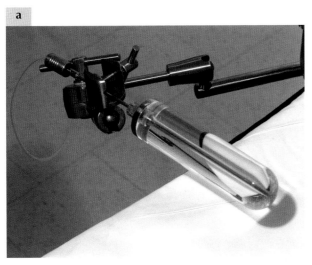
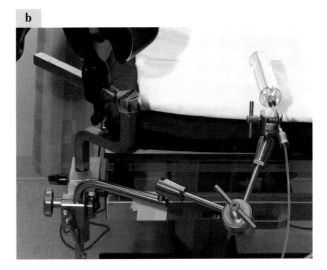

Figure 17.21 (a and b). Intravaginal cylinder positioning.
The intravaginal cylinder is secured in position by connecting it to a bracket that is fixed to the table, which prevents it from moving once satisfactorily placed. Care should be taken to verify that the cylinder is advanced properly to the vaginal apex without deviating to either side of midline. In addition, the cylinder should not be secured in a position that pushes the vaginal mucosa downwards towards the rectum or upwards towards the bladder.

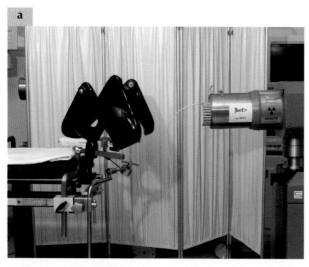 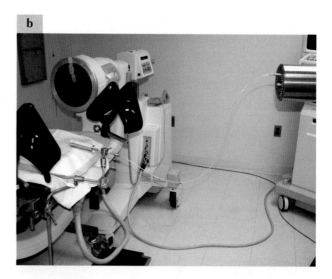

Figure 17.22. Set-up.
(**a**) The procedure table, with leg holders for placement of the patient in the dorsal lithotomy position. The bracket, which is fixed to the procedure table, secures the intravaginal cylinder in the correct location for the duration of the treatment. The cylinder is then connected to the high-dose-rate (HDR) unit with a flexible catheter. Shown at the far right is the Gamma-med 12i unit. (**b**) The C-arm of the fluoroscope is used for obtaining radiographic images to verify correct positioning of the cylinder prior to treatment.

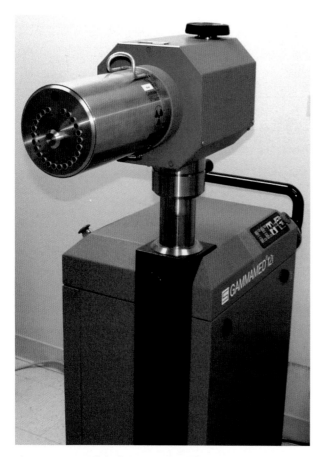

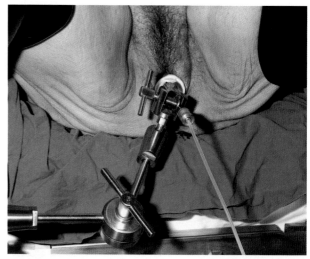

Figure 17.24. Treatment.
The patient is positioned in the dorsal lithotomy position with her legs supported and immobilized with leg holders. After pelvic examination, the vaginal cylinder is inserted and secured in the correct position, as previously discussed.

Figure 17.23. High-dose-rate (HDR) unit.
The Gamma-med 12i unit delivers HDR radiation utilizing a single, high-activity iridium-192 (Ir-192) source. While only one channel is needed for intravaginal radiation therapy, up to 24 channels can be attached to the unit for other purposes.

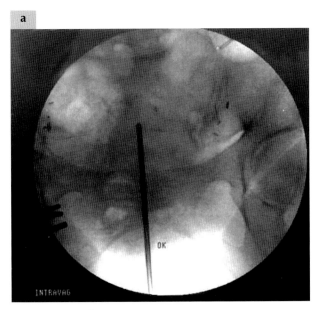 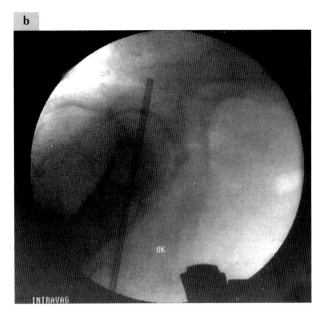

Figure 17.25. Fluoroscopy.
Anterior/posterior (AP) and lateral images are taken prior to the first treatment. This confirms the satisfactory position of the cylinder in reference to the bony anatomy. (**a**) The AP view shows the cylinder correctly positioned in the midline without deviating to either side. (**b**) The lateral view confirms that the cylinder does not deviate posteriorly towards the rectum or anteriorly towards the bladder. Treatment is delivered over an approximately 10-min period using the high-activity Ir-192 source. Following completion of treatment, the cylinder is removed and the patient is discharged. The treatment is usually repeated every 1–2 weeks for a total of three fractions. The total dose delivered is approximately 2100 cGy to a depth of 5 mm below the surface of the vaginal mucosa.

Intraoperative radiation therapy

IORT is utilized for a variety of different sites and malignancies. Typically, IORT is used to deliver focal high doses of radiation to patients who have previously received treatment or to supplement the dose beyond that which would be safely permissible using external-beam therapy alone. The use of IORT allows delivery of high doses of radiation to an operative tumor bed while sparing the adjacent normal tissues. The purpose of IORT is to improve the local control following a surgical resection. In gynecologic malignancies, it is typically used in the recurrent setting. Overall, IORT has had acceptable tolerance with favorable local control rates in patients with recurrent disease following complete surgical resection.

There are two methods for delivering IORT. One provides treatment delivery using electrons produced by a linear accelerator. This method is delivered either with a dedicated linear accelerator in the operating room or by transferring the patient from the operating room to a radiation treatment room. The electron beam is focused on the tumor bed, and the field shape and size is adjusted to encompass the treatment field. The critical normal structures are moved away from the field and the patient is subsequently treated. This technique allows delivery of radiation to a prescribed superficial depth, which can be varied by utilizing different energies of electron beams. Care must be taken when administering radiation using this method. The treatment field must be well exposed with the adjacent structures moved out of the path of the electron beam. This may not be possible with tumors that are deep seated in the pelvis or retroperitoneum, for example. In addition, the electron cone should be set up so that the head of the treatment machine is perpendicular to the surface of the tumor bed. When an electron delivers radiation over a sloped or irregular surface, the dose delivery would be inhomogeneous with varying treatment depths. In addition, larger fields may require that it be split and treated with two separate abutting electron fields, which must be matched carefully.

A second technique of administering IORT is with a high-dose-rate brachytherapy unit, a technique which is becoming more common in the USA. A Harrison–Anderson–Mick (HAM) applicator, composed of flexible silastic material with catheters running parallel through it and spaced 1 cm apart, is used to deliver treatment. This method requires a high-activity Ir-192 source. The distance from each catheter to the treating surface is 0.5 cm. The number of catheters and the length along each catheter that is employed to treat a field can be tailored to the size and dimensions of the tumor bed. The advantage of this form of IORT over that of

electrons is seen when treating deep-seated tumors in the pelvis, or in regions where the normal tissues cannot be moved easily away from the path of an electron beam. With the use of a HAM applicator, small lead blocks can be placed directly against critical adjacent structures to block them from the intraoperative treatment.

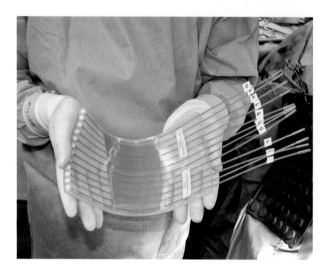

Figure 17.26. Harrison–Anderson–Mick (HAM) applicator.
The HAM applicator is manufactured with a varied number of catheters. Shown here is the 12-channel HAM applicator. Each catheter, colored in green, lies within the silastic material and they are equally spaced 1 cm apart. As demonstrated, the applicator is flexible and, therefore, can conform to the slope/contour of the operative bed. The silastic applicator can also be cut lengthwise to tailor the width to the required number of channels.

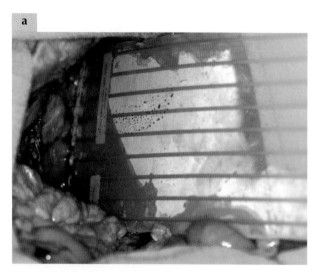
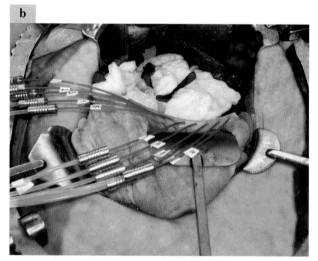

Figure 17.27. HAM applicator positioning.
The HAM applicator is placed directly over the tumor bed. The number of catheters used depends on the treatment area. (a) A nine-channel HAM applicator placed along a pelvic sidewall for treatment. The applicator should lie flat and directly on top of the treatment volume. (b) Positioning for treatment of the anterior surface of the sacrum is demonstrated with a 10-channel applicator.

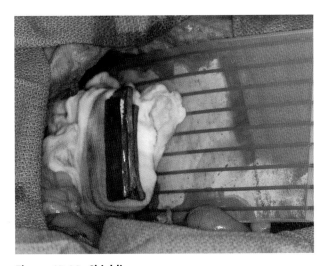

Figure 17.28. Shielding.
The HAM applicator is seen in position along the pelvic sidewall. Lap pads are placed to secure it in position. Lead blocks are also used to shield the adjacent normal structures.

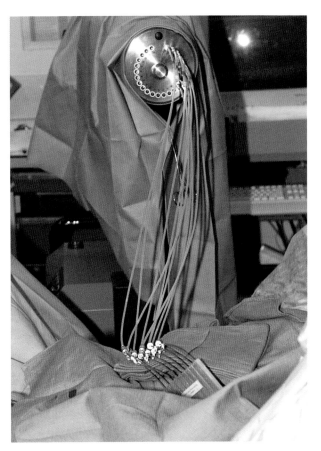

Figure 17.29. High-dose-rate (HDR) unit.
The applicator is then connected to an HDR unit. Shown is the Gamma-med 12i remote afterloading HDR unit.

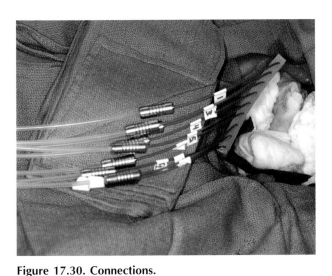

Figure 17.30. Connections.
Sterile transparent catheters are handed off the operative field to a radiation oncology technician who connects them to the high-dose-rate (HDR) unit (see Fig. 17.29). These catheters are then attached to the HAM applicator with a series of interlocking spring-loaded metal components.

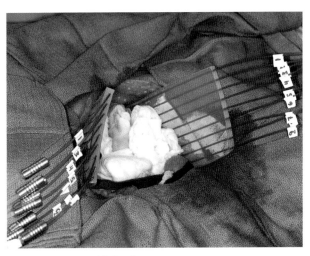

Figure 17.31. Multiple sites.
This system may be used to treat more than one site concurrently. As shown, more than one HAM applicator may be placed and secured in position at a given time. However, the treatments are given sequentially as there is only one source. Treatment times may vary depending on the activity of the source and size of the treatment field. Typical doses of IORT vary depending on the clinical situation; however, they should not exceed 20 Gy in order to avoid excess toxicity to the surrounding previously irradiated tissues.

References

1. Tod M and Meredith W. A dosage system for use in the treatment of cancer of the uterine cervix. *Br J Radiol* 1938; **11**:809–24.

2. Tod M and Meredith W. Treatment of cancer of the cervix uteri – a revised 'Manchester method'. *Br J Radiol* 1953; **26**:252–7.

Appendix: staging systems

FIGO staging classification: vulva

0   Carcinoma in situ; preinvasive carcinoma

I   Tumor confined to vulva or vulva and perineum; 2 cm or less in greatest dimension; nodes are negative

IA   Stromal invasion no greater than 1 mm

IB   Stromal invasion greater than 1 mm

II   Tumor confined to vulva or vulva and perineum; more than 2 cm in greatest dimension; nodes are negative

III   Tumor of any size with adjacent spread to the lower urethra, vagina, or the anus and/or with unilateral regional lymph node metastasis

IVA   Tumor invades upper urethra, bladder mucosa, rectal mucosa, or pelvic bone and/or bilateral regional node metastases

IVB   Distant metastasis

FIGO staging classification: vagina

0   Carcinoma in situ; intraepithelial carcinoma

I   Tumor confined to vaginal wall

II   Tumor involves subvaginal tissues but does not extend to pelvic wall

III   Tumor extends to pelvic wall

IVA   Tumor invades mucosa of bladder or rectum and/or extends beyond the true pelvis

IVB   Distant metastasis

FIGO staging classification: cervix uteri

0   Carcinoma in situ; intraepithelial carcinoma

I   Carcinoma confined to the cervix (extension to corpus should be disregarded)

IA   Invasive carcinoma diagnosed only by microscopy (all macroscopically visible lesions – even with superficial invasion – are Stage IB)

IA1   Stromal invasion no greater than 3 mm in depth and 7 mm or less in horizontal spread

IA2   Stromal invasion more than 3 mm and not more than 5 mm in depth, with a horizontal spread of 7 mm or less

IB   Clinically visible lesion confined to the cervix or microscopic lesion greater than IA2

IB1   Clinically visible lesion 4 cm or less in greatest dimension

IB2   Clinically visible lesion more than 4 cm in greatest dimension

II   Tumor invades beyond cervix but not to pelvic wall or to lower third of vagina

IIA   Without parametrial invasion

IIB   With parametrial invasion

III   Tumor extends to pelvic wall and/or involves the lower third of the vagina and/or causes hydronephrosis or nonfunctioning kidney

IIIA   Tumor involves lower third of vagina; no extension to pelvic wall

IIIB   Tumor extends to pelvic wall and/or causes hydronephrosis or nonfunctioning kidney

IV   Carcinoma has extended beyond the true pelvis or has clinically involved the mucosa of the bladder or rectum

IVA   Tumor invades mucosa of bladder or rectum and/or extends to adjacent organs

IVB   Distant metastasis

FIGO staging classification: corpus uteri

I   Tumor confined to corpus uteri

IA   Tumor limited to endometrium

IB   Tumor invades up to or less than one half of the myometrium

IC   Tumor invades more than one half of the myometrium

II   Tumor invades cervix but does not extend beyond uterus

IIA   Endocervical glandular involvement only

IIB   Cervical stromal invasion

III   Local and/or regional spread

IIIA   Tumor involves serosa and/or adnexa (direct extension or metastasis) and/or cancer cells in ascites or peritoneal washings

IIIB   Vaginal involvement (direct extension or metastasis)

IIIC   Metastasis to pelvic and/or paraaortic lymph nodes

IVA   Tumor invades bladder mucosa and/or bowel mucosa

IVB   Distant metastasis (including intraabdominal and/or inguinal lymph nodes)

FIGO staging classification: fallopian tube

0   Carcinoma in situ

I   Tumor confined to fallopian tube(s)

IA   Tumor limited to one tube, without penetrating the serosal surface

IB   Tumor limited to both tubes, without penetrating the serosal surface

IC   Tumor limited to one or both tube(s) with extension onto or through the tubal serosa, or with malignant cells in ascites or peritoneal washings

II   Tumor involves one or both fallopian tube(s) with pelvic extension

IIA   Extension and/or metastases to uterus and/or ovaries

IIB   Extension to other pelvic structures

IIC   Pelvic extension with malignant cells in ascites or peritoneal washings

III   Tumor involves one or both fallopian tube(s) with peritoneal implants outside the pelvis and/or positive retroperitoneal or inguinal nodes

IIIA   Microscopic peritoneal metastasis outside the pelvis

IIIB   Macroscopic peritoneal metastasis outside the pelvis 2 cm or less in greatest dimension

IIIC   Peritoneal metastasis more than 2 cm in greatest dimension and/or positive retroperitoneal or inguinal lymph nodes

IV   Distant metastasis (excludes peritoneal metastasis) including liver parenchyma or malignant pleural effusion, which must be cytologically positive

FIGO staging classification: ovary

I   Growth limited to the ovaries

IA   Tumor limited to one ovary; capsule intact, no tumor on ovarian surface; no malignant cells in ascites or peritoneal washings

IB   Tumor limited to both ovaries; capsule intact, no tumor on ovarian surface; no malignant cells in ascites or peritoneal washings

IC   Tumor limited to one or both ovaries with any of the following: capsule ruptured, tumor on ovarian surface; malignant cells in ascites or peritoneal washings

II   Tumor involves one or both ovaries with pelvic extension

IIA   Extension and/or implants on uterus and/or tube(s)

IIB   Extension to other pelvic tissues

IIC   Pelvic extension with any of the following: capsule ruptured, tumor on ovarian surface; malignant cells in ascites or peritoneal washings

III   Tumor involves one or both ovaries with peritoneal metastasis outside the pelvis and/or retroperitoneal or inguinal lymph node metastasis

IIIA   Microscopic peritoneal metastasis beyond pelvis

IIIB   Macroscopic peritoneal metastasis beyond pelvis 2 cm or less in greatest dimension

IIIC   Peritoneal metastasis beyond pelvis more than 2 cm in greatest dimension and/or positive retroperitoneal or inguinal lymph nodes

IV   Distant metastasis (excludes peritoneal metastasis) including liver parenchyma or malignant pleural effusion, which must be cytologically positive

FIGO staging classification: gestational trophoblastic disease

I   Disease confined to uterus

II   Disease outside of uterus but is limited to the genital structures – vagina, ovary, broad ligament, and fallopian tube – by metastasis or direct extension

III   Disease extends to the lungs with or without known genital tract involvement

IV   All other metastatic sites

Substages assigned for each stage as follows:

A   No risk factors present

B   One risk factor

C   Both risk factors

Risk factors used to assign substages:

1   Pretherapy serum hCG >100,000 mIU/ml

2   Duration of disease > 6 months

World Health Organization prognostic index score for gestational trophoblastic disease

Prognostic factor	Score 0	1	2	4
Age (years)	≤39	>39	–	–
Antecedent pregnancy	Hydatidiform mole	Abortion	Term	–
Interval from index pregnancy (months)	<4	4–6	7–12	>12
Pretreatment hCG (mIU/ml)	$<10^3$	$10^3–10^4$	$10^4–10^5$	$>10^5$
Largest tumor, including uterine tumor	–	3–5 cm	>5 cm	–
Sites of metastasis	–	Spleen, kidney	Gastrointestinal tract, liver	Brain
Number of metastases identified	–	1–4	5–8	>8
Prior chemotherapy	–	–	Single drug	Two or more

Note: The identification of an individual patient's stage and risk score will be expressed by allotting a Roman numeral to the stage and an Arabic numeral to the risk score, separated by a colon. Total score is interpreted as follows: low risk, 0–4; intermediate risk, 5–7; high risk, ≥8.

Index